# ADOLESCENT MEDICINE: STATE OF THE ART REVIEWS

Infectious Diseases and Immunizations

GUEST EDITORS

Paula K. Braverman, MD
Robert W. Frenck Jr, MD
Cynthia Holland-Hall, MD, MPH

August 2010 • Volume 21 • Number 2

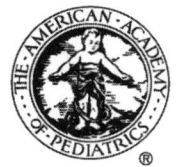

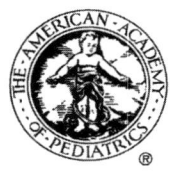

ADOLESCENT MEDICINE CLINICS:
STATE OF THE ART REVIEWS
August 2010
Editor: Diane E. Lundquist
Marketing Manager: Marirose Russo
Production Manager: Shannan Martin

Volume 21, Number 2
ISBN 978-1-58110-365-6
ISSN 1934-4287
MA0524
SUB1006

Copyright © 2010 American Academy of Pediatrics. All rights reserved. No part of this publication may be reproduced or transmitted in any form or by any means, electronic or mechanical, including photocopying, recording, or any information retrieval system, without written permission from the Publisher (fax the permissions editor at 847/434-8780).

*Adolescent Medicine: State of the Art Reviews* is published three times per year by the American Academy of Pediatrics, 141 Northwest Point Blvd, Elk Grove Village, IL 60007-1098. Periodicals postage paid at Arlington Heights, IL.

POSTMASTER: Send address changes to American Academy of Pediatrics, Department of Marketing and Publications, Attn: AM:STARs, 141 Northwest Point Blvd, Elk Grove Village, IL 60007-1098.

Subscriptions: Subscriptions to *Adolescent Medicine: State of the Art Reviews* (AM:STARs) are provided to members of the American Academy of Pediatrics' Section on Adolescent Health as part of annual section membership dues. All others, please contact the AAP Customer Service Center at 866/843-2271 (7:00 am–5:30 pm Central Time, Monday–Friday) for pricing and information.

Supported in part by a grant from Novartis Pharmaceuticals Corporation

# Adolescent Medicine: State of the Art Reviews

Official Journal of the American Academy of Pediatrics
Section on Adolescent Health

## EDITORS-IN-CHIEF

Victor C. Strasburger, MD
Professor of Pediatrics
Chief, Division of Adolescent
Medicine
University of New Mexico
School of Medicine
Albuquerque, New Mexico

Donald E. Greydanus, MD
Professor of Pediatrics
Michigan State University and
Pediatrics Program Director
Kalamazoo Center for Medical
Studies
Kalamazoo, Michigan

## ASSOCIATE EDITORS

Robert T. Brown, MD
Media, Pennsylvania

Cynthia Holland-Hall, MD, MPH
Columbus, Ohio

Martin M. Fisher, MD
Manhasset, New York

Paula K. Braverman, MD
Cincinnati, Ohio

Sheryl Ryan
New Haven, Connecticut

Alain Joffe, MD, MPH
Baltimore, Maryland

## INFECTIOUS DISEASES AND IMMUNIZATIONS

## EDITORS-IN-CHIEF

VICTOR C. STRASBURGER, MD, Professor of Pediatrics, Division of Adolescent Medicine, University of New Mexico, School of Medicine, Albuquerque, New Mexico

DONALD E. GREYDANUS, MD, Professor of Pediatrics, Michigan State University; and Pediatrics Program Director, Kalamazoo Center for Medical Studies, Kalamazoo, Michigan

## GUEST EDITORS

PAULA K. BRAVERMAN, MD, Division of Adolescent Medicine Cincinnati Children's Hospital Medical Center, University of Cincinnati College of Medicine, Cincinnati, Ohio

ROBERT W. FRENCK JR, MD, Division of Infectious Diseases, Cincinnati Children's Hospital Medical Center, Cincinnati, Ohio

CYNTHIA HOLLAND-HALL, MD, MPH, Section of Adolescent Medicine, Nationwide Children's Hospital, Department of Pediatrics, The Ohio State University College of Medicine, Columbus, Ohio

## CONTRIBUTORS

ELISE D. BERLAN, MD, MPH Children's Hospital, Department of Pediatrics, The Ohio State University College of, Section of Adolescent Medicine, Nationwide Medicine, Columbus, Ohio

REBECCA C. BRADY, MD, Division of Pediatric Infectious Diseases, Department of Pediatrics, Cincinnati Children's Hospital Medical Center, Cincinnati, Ohio

TERRILL BRAVENDER, MD, MPH, Section of Adolescent Medicine, Nationwide Children's Hospital, Department of Clinical Pediatrics, The Ohio State University College of Medicine, Columbus, Ohio

LAWRENCE J. D'ANGELO, MD, MPH, Section of Adolescent Medicine, Nationwide Children's Hospital, Department of Pediatrics, The Ohio State University College of Medicine, Columbus, Ohio

SHARON EDWARDS, MD, Department of Pediatrics, Mount Sinai School of Medicine, New York City, New York

**ROBERT W. FRENCK JR, MD,** Division of Infectious Diseases, Cincinnati Children's Hospital Medical Center, Cincinnati, Ohio

**BLANCA E. GONZALEZ, MD,** Division of Pediatric Infectious Diseases and Rheumatology, Rainbow Babies and Children's Hospital, Cleveland, Ohio

**CYNTHIA HOLLAND-HALL, MD, MPH,** Section of Adolescent Medicine, Nationwide Children's Hospital, Department of Pediatrics, The Ohio State University College of Medicine, Columbus, Ohio

**DALE J. HU, MD, MPH,** Division of Viral Hepatitis, National Center for HIV/AIDS, VH, STD, and TB Prevention, Centers for Disease Control and Prevention, Atlanta, Georgia

**W. GARRETT HUNT, MD,** Assistant Professor of Pediatrics, Section of Infectious Diseases, Department of Pediatrics, College of Medicine, The Ohio State University, Nationwide Children's Hospital, Columbus, Ohio

**CORINNE LEHMANN, MD, MEd,** Associate Professor of Pediatrics and Internal Medicine, Section of Adolescent Medicine, Nationwide Children's Hospital, Department of Pediatrics, The Ohio State University College of Medicine, Columbus, Ohio

**JASON M. MEHRTENS, MD,** Division of Adolescent Medicine, Cincinnati Children's Hospital Medical Center, Cincinnati, Ohio

**CHRISANNA MARIE MINK, MD,** Clinical Professor of Pediatrics, Harbor-UCLA Medical Center, Torrance, California

**RODRIGO A. MON, MD,** Pediatric Surgeon, The Children's Hospital of Southwest Florida, Lee Memorial Health Systems, Fort Myers, Florida

**ANNA-BARBARA MOSCICKI, MD,** University of California San Francisco, San Francisco, California

**THAINA ROUSSEAU-PIERRE, DO, MSc,** Adolescent Health Services, Mount Sinai School of Medicine, New York Elmhurst Hospital Center, Elmhurst, New York

**ELIZABETH SCHLAUDECKER, MD,** Division of Infectious Diseases, Cincinnati Children's Hospital Medical Center, Cincinnati, Ohio

**UMID M. SHARAPOV, MD, MSc,** Division of Viral Hepatitis, National Center for HIV/AIDS, VH, STD, and TB Prevention, Centers for Disease Control and Prevention, Atlanta, Georgia

**MICHAEL G. SPIGARELLI, MD, PhD,** Division of Adolescent Medicine, Cincinnati Children's Hospital Medical Center, Cincinnati, Ohio

**SYLVIA HSIN-HUE YEH, MD,** Clinical Associate Professor of Pediatrics, Harbor-UCLA Medical Center, Torrance, California

# INFECTIOUS DISEASES AND IMMUNIZATIONS

## CONTENTS

**Preface**   xii
Paula K. Braverman, Robert W. Frenck Jr, and Cynthia Holland-Hall

**Immunizations in Adolescents—An Update**   173
Sharon M. Edwards and Thaina Rosseau-Pierre

> The past decade has brought a series of new vaccines targeted specifically to adolescents. Recommended vaccinations for adolescents now offer protection against human papillomavirus, *Neisseria meningitidis*, pertussis, and influenza. As the vaccine schedule is ever changing, it is critical that health care providers be up to date and implement current recommendations. In this article, we discuss the major vaccines targeted at adolescents, issues unique to vaccinating adolescents, and strategies for increasing vaccine coverage rates. Forming partnerships with other health professionals, school-based clinics, and most importantly adolescents and their families is a fundamental element of any successful adolescent vaccination effort.

**Acute Sinusitis**   187
Jason M. Mehrtens and Michael G. Spigarelli

> Acute sinusitis is a very common entity that leads to a significant financial medical burden, as well as serious complications when treatment is inadequate. This article investigates the clinical criteria for making the diagnosis of acute sinusitis, the common causative pathogens, and the current treatment and referral guidelines. In addition, the most common complications are outlined, in order for clinicians to develop more familiarity with these conditions and improve recognition when they are present.

**Adolescent Pneumonia**   202
Elizabeth P. Schlaudecker and Robert W. Frenck Jr

> Despite advances in antibiotic treatment and prevention, pneumonia, an acute infection of the pulmonary parenchyma, continues to have a significant impact on adolescent health. Mor-

tality remains low, but pneumonia is associated with significant morbidity at considerable cost to our health care system. The first section of this article focuses on general principles of pneumonia in adolescents, including epidemiology, pathogenesis, etiology, clinical manifestations, radiography, laboratory evaluation, management, complications, and prevention. The final section covers individual pathogens associated with pneumonia in adolescents, including recent updates in diagnosis, management, and prevention of these agents.

## Pertussis in Adolescents and Its Prevention Using Tdap Vaccination 220
ChrisAnna Marie Mink and Sylvia Hsin-Hue Yeh

In industrialized nations, routine use of pertussis vaccines has shifted the burden of pertussis disease from middle childhood to one primarily affecting young infants, adolescents, and adults. Although generally not as severe as observed in infants, pertussis in adolescents and adults can be serious, and these older age groups are often the reservoir of infection for infants. With recognition of the increasing incidence of pertussis in older individuals, reduced-dose acellular pertussis vaccines combined with diphtheria and tetanus toxoids (Tdap) were developed for use in adolescents and adults. The goals of Tdap booster are to protect older vaccinees, reduce circulating disease, and thereby protect young infants.

## Influenza 236
Rebecca C. Brady

Influenza is a disease of global public health significance as evidenced by the 2009 pandemic caused by a novel swine-origin H1N1 virus. Influenza epidemics occur almost every year and are less striking, but nevertheless, account for considerable morbidity and school absences among healthy children and adolescents. Patients with chronic conditions may develop severe illness. This article discusses the epidemiology, clinical manifestations, diagnosis, and management of influenza. Vaccination is the most effective measure available for the control of influenza. Recommendations for use of the inactivated and live attenuated vaccines against seasonal influenza and against the 2009 novel H1N1 influenza viruses are reviewed.

## Epstein-Barr Virus, Cytomegalovirus, and Infectious Mononucleosis
Terrill Bravender

251

Infectious mononucleosis (IM) is a clinical syndrome that is common in adolescents and young adults and is characterized by fever, lymphadenopathy, pharyngitis, and fatigue. IM is most commonly associated with Epstein-Barr virus (EBV) infection in which case laboratory findings include a lymphocytosis with an elevated number of atypical lymphocytes seen on peripheral smear and a heterophile or EBV-specific antibody response. Approximately 10% of those with IM will not be acutely infected with EBV. Many of these individuals will have their symptoms attributed to cytomegalovirus (CMV) infection. This chapter reviews the history, diagnosis, clinical management, and potential complications of both EBV- and CMV-associated IM in adolescents and young adults.

## Viral Hepatitis A, B, and C: Grown-Up Issues
Umid M. Sharapov and Dale J. Hu

265

Viral hepatitis is a major global health problem associated with significant morbidity and mortality. Although there are five major and distinct human hepatitis viruses characterized to date—referred to as hepatitis A, B, C, D, and E, respectively—only hepatitis A, B, and C are epidemiologically and clinically relevant for adolescents in North America. The clinical presentation of acute infection with each of these viruses is similar; thus, diagnosis depends on the use of specific serologic markers and viral nucleic acids. This review provides data on the epidemiology, clinical symptoms, diagnosis, treatment, and prevention of each of these three viral infections, along with points that are important or unique to adolescent patients.

## Meningitis and Encephalitis in Adolescents
W. Garrett Hunt

287

The overall incidence of bacterial meningitis has decreased due to numerous factors, but substantial disease burden remains from both bacterial and nonbacterial meningitis with or without accompanying encephalitis. Recently developed or validated surrogate markers of disease—including polymerase chain reaction, inflammatory markers, and magnetic resonance imaging—enhance diagnostic utility. Current guidelines and studies have modified the use of particular antibiotics and expanded the role of adjunctive steroid therapy in selected patients. This review provides an update to the general diagnostic evaluation, epidemiology, pathophysiology, clinical assessment, antibiotic treatment, adjunctive therapy, prognosis, and prevention of meningitis and encephalitis in the adolescent population.

## *Staphylococcus aureus* Infections in Adolescents  318
Blanca E. Gonzalez and Rodrigo A. Mon

*Staphylococcus* aureus infections are important causes of morbidity and mortality in the pediatric population. Over the past decade, community-associated methicillin-resistant *S. aureus* has emerged as an adolescent pathogen with disease ranging from mild skin and soft tissue infections to severe sepsis syndrome. Various conditions and behaviors common to adolescents render them more susceptible to staphylococcal infections. This review focuses on the problem of *S. aureus* in the adolescent population, including an outline on the approach, treatment, and prevention of these infections.

## Sexually Transmitted Infections in Adolescents: Advances in Epidemiology, Screening, and Diagnosis  332
Elise D. Berlan and Cynthia Holland-Hall

Adolescents are especially vulnerable to acquiring sexually transmitted infections (STIs). Recent national surveillance data and data from population-level studies demonstrate a high prevalence of bacterial and viral STIs in adolescents and striking racial/ethnic disparities. The long-term health consequences of these infections impact heavily on women's reproductive health. Intriguing findings are emerging, suggesting that individual behaviors contribute minimally to risk for STI, and demonstrating the importance of sexual networks for the transmission of STIs. Exciting developments in gonorrhea and chlamydia testing are making routine screening easier for the busy clinician and are acceptable to adolescents. New testing modalities are being used to screen adolescents in nontraditional venues. Recent developments in vaccination against human papillomavirus and new cytological screening recommendations are changing clinical approaches to STI prevention.

## Human Papillomavirus Disease and Vaccines in Adolescents  347
Anna-Barbara Moscicki

Review of the most recent evidence indicates that screening for cervical cancer in females younger than 21 years of age likely leads to more harm than good. In addition, screening during adolescence has not lead to decreased cervical cancers in this age group. The rate of cervical cancer remains extremely low in adolescents. In contrast, abnormal cytology is extremely common, of which most is benign. Hence, referral to colposcopy is unnecessary and costly. New guidelines recommend cervical cancer screening to start at the age of 21 years and to not be based on sexual behavior. The exception is for immunocompromised girls, who should be screened once intercourse is initiated, since they are at increased risk for cervical cancer. Recently, we have also broadened our understanding about human papillomavirus-associated disease in men. In this chapter, we cover the advances in science that have led to new screening recommendation for cervical cancer and the advances in prevention: vaccines for both adolescent women and men.

## Human Immunodeficiency Virus Infection in Adolescents 364
Corinne Lehmann and Lawrence J. D'Angelo

Despite advances in human immunodeficiency virus (HIV) treatment and discovery of effective prevention programs, HIV infection in American youth continues to rise, especially in minority youth. The crisis underscores the lack of access to care and wellness of our adolescent and young adult populations. Primary care practitioners who care for young adults will diagnose and/or encounter HIV-infected patients in their practice. Providers need to become familiar with the basics of HIV prevention and treatment, as well as how adolescence presents unique challenges in HIV care.

**Index** 388

## Preface
# Infectious Diseases and Immunizations

Practitioners caring for adolescents diagnose and treat infectious diseases on a daily basis. New vaccines added to the adolescent platform over the past ten years have the potential to significantly reduce morbidity and mortality from a number of these infectious agents. This issue of *AM:STARs* reviews the clinical presentation, evaluation, and treatment of some of the common infectious diseases seen in the adolescent age group. In cases where a vaccine is available as a preventive strategy, discussion about that vaccine is included in the article. The topics covered include pneumonia, sinusitis, pertussis, influenza, mononucleosis and cytomegalovirus, viral hepatitis (including A, B, and C), meningitis and encephalitis, methicillin resistant *Staphylococcus aureus* (MRSA), and sexually transmitted infections, with separate articles on human papillomavirus and human immunodeficiency virus. Specific discussions are included about Tdap, hepatitis A and B, HPV, and the meningococcal vaccines. In addition, there is an article discussing the updated adolescent immunization platform along with challenges of vaccination in this age group.

The editors hope that this issue will provide a practical, comprehensive update for clinicians caring for adolescents in the primary care setting.

Paula K. Braverman, MD
*Cincinnati Children's Hospital Medical Center*
*University of Cincinnati College of Medicine*
*Cincinnati, Ohio*

Robert W. Frenck Jr, MD
*Cincinnati Children's Hospital Medical Center*
*University of Cincinnati College of Medicine*
*Cincinnati, Ohio*

Cynthia Holland-Hall, MD, MPH
*Nationwide Children's Hospital*
*The Ohio State University College of Medicine*
*Columbus, Ohio*

Copyright © 2010 American Academy of Pediatrics. All rights reserved. ISSN 1934-4287

# Immunizations in Adolescents—An Update

Sharon M. Edwards, MD*[a], Thaina Rousseau-Pierre, DO, MSc[b]

[a]Associate Professor, Mount Sinai School of Medicine, Department of Pediatrics, One Gustave L. Levy Place, Box 1202A, New York, NY 10029
[b]Assistant Professor, Mount Sinai School of Medicine, Attending Physician, Adolescent Health Services, Elmhurst Hospital Center, 79-01 Broadway, Elmhurst, NY 11373

The past decade has brought a series of new vaccines that are targeted specifically to adolescents. Recommended vaccinations for adolescents now offer protection against human papillomavirus (HPV), *Neisseria meningitidis*, pertussis, and influenza. The 2010 recommended childhood and adolescent vaccine schedule[1] developed by the Advisory Committee on Immunization Practices (ACIP) of the Centers for Disease Control and Prevention (CDC) and approved by the American Academy of Pediatrics, and the American Academy of Family Physicians, includes new recommendations regarding immunizing boys 9–18 years of age against HPV. As the vaccine schedule is ever changing, it is critical that health care providers be up to date and implement current recommendations. This article will discuss the major vaccines targeted at adolescents, issues unique to vaccinating adolescents, and strategies for increasing vaccine coverage rates.

One of the objectives of Healthy People 2010 is to achieve a vaccine coverage rate of 90% for adolescents 13–15 years of age. This goal was met for the first time in 2008 for the hepatitis B vaccine and the measles, mumps, and rubella (MMR) vaccine.[2] Adolescent vaccination rates with the quadrivalent vaccine for *N. meningitidis* (MCV4) and the combined tetanus, diphtheria, and pertussis vaccine (Tdap) were 41.8% and 40.8%, respectively.[2] Clearly, there is much work to be done toward reaching the Healthy People 2010 goal for all adolescents and for all vaccines.

In 1996, the ACIP, the American Academy of Pediatrics, the American Academy of Family Physicians, and the American Medical Association issued a consensus statement underscoring the need for a routine adolescent health care visit at age 11–12 years. At this visit, the health care provider should review the vaccination

---

*Corresponding author.
*E-mail address*: sharon.edwards@mountsinai.org (S. M. Edwards).

Copyright © 2010 American Academy of Pediatrics. All rights reserved. ISSN 1934-4287

history and give all recommended vaccines and "catch up" immunizations. This visit is now more critical than ever, since currently many vaccines are targeted specifically at this age group, including the vaccines for pertussis, meningococcal disease, and HPV.

## Human Papillomavirus Vaccines

HPV vaccines are a major advancement in the primary prevention of many HPV diseases. HPV, the most common sexually transmitted viral infection, has >100 different subtypes. Over 30 of these are sexually transmissible. Types 6 and 11 cause >90% of cases of genital warts.[3,4] Furthermore, this virus is responsible for almost all cases of cervical cancers worldwide, with types 16 and 18 implicated in ~70% of these cases.[5] At least half of all sexually active men and women are exposed to HPV in their lifetime.[6]

There are currently two vaccines available, a quadrivalent vaccine and a bivalent vaccine. The quadrivalent vaccine, Gardasil (Merck and Co, Inc.) was approved by the U.S. Food and Drug Administration (FDA) in June 2006.[5] This vaccine was approved for the primary prevention of cervical cancer, cervical precancers, genital warts, and vulvar and vaginal precancers. The quadrivalent vaccine offers protection against HPV types 6, 11, 16 and 18. The bivalent vaccine, Cervarix (GlaxoSmithKline) protects against HPV types 16 and 18 and was approved by the FDA in October 2009.[7] ACIP does not distinguish between the vaccines, recommending the use of either one to reduce the risk of cervical cancer caused by HPV types 16 and 18. The vaccine is ideally given before the initiation of sexual activity; the recommended immunization schedule suggests the administration of the first dose of HPV vaccine at 11–12 years of age. The vaccine is approved for patients as young as 9 years old.[1] On October 16, 2009, the FDA approved the use of the quadrivalent vaccine for males 9–26 years of age for the prevention of genital warts.[8] ACIP gave a permissive recommendation for use in this population. In addition to decreasing their rates of genital warts, it is hoped that use of the vaccine in males may decrease the risk of transmission to their sexual partners. Both intramuscular vaccines are given in a three-dose series given over 6 months. Clinical trials show that both vaccines are safe and highly efficacious. The quadrivalent vaccine has been found to be almost 100% effective in protecting patients against HPV types 6, 11, 16 and 18, when the series is completed before exposure to these types.[9,10] When the quadrivalent vaccine was initially licensed by the FDA, there was some concern that parents would refuse this vaccine for their daughters for fear that it would promote sexual activity. However, recent studies demonstrate most parents support the use of the HPV vaccine.[11,12] The major contraindication to this vaccine is a past history of a hypersensitivity reaction to this vaccine and/or its components.

## Pertussis Vaccine (Tdap)

Because of weakening immunity to pertussis after childhood vaccination, many adolescents are susceptible to this infection.[13] The routine vaccination of adolescents against pertussis was endorsed by the ACIP in 2005.[14] Pertussis is a highly contagious respiratory infection; in adolescents, the presentation is often a protracted cough.[15] Studies estimate a prevalence of pertussis of 12–26% in adolescents and adults with a chronic cough.[13,16] Although complications are not usually severe among teens, infected adolescents remain an important reservoir for infection to neonates and others at high risk of serious illness or pertussis-related death.

There are two formulations of pertussis vaccine currently available to adolescents. Both are available as a single-dose (one-time use) booster vaccine to provide protection against tetanus, diphtheria, and pertussis in adolescents who have completed their primary vaccination series in childhood. Both vaccines contain reduced diphtheria toxoid, tetanus toxoid, and acellular pertussis. Neither contains thimerosal. Boostrix (GlaxoSmith-Kline) is indicated for persons aged 10–18 years, and Adacel (Sanofi Pasteur) is indicated for persons aged 11–64 years.[17] ACIP recommends the routine use of a Tdap vaccine in adolescents aged 11–18 years to replace tetanus and diphtheria toxoid (Td) vaccine.

The recommended age for Tdap vaccination is 11–12 years. Adolescents aged 11–18 years should receive a single dose of Tdap for booster immunization against tetanus, diphtheria, and pertussis if they have completed the recommended childhood DTP/DTaP vaccination series and have not received Tdap in the past. Adolescents who are on the "catch up schedule" should receive Tdap as a single dose; Td should be used for subsequent doses.[1] Adolescents aged 11–18 years who received Td previously are encouraged to receive a single dose of Tdap to provide protection against pertussis. The ACIP recommends an interval of 5 years between Td and Tdap when the vaccine is given as a booster dose; however, studies indicate that a shorter time period can be used if there is an urgent need for protection against pertussis.[1] Absolute contraindications to this vaccine include an anaphylactic reaction to diphtheria, tetanus, and/or pertussis and the vaccine components and a history of encephalopathy within 7 days of receiving the vaccine that was not attributed to another cause.[10] Relative contraindications to receiving Tdap include a history of Guillain-Barré syndrome (GBS) occurring within 6 weeks of the vaccine and an unstable neurologic condition.[10] It is also recommended that people who develop an Arthus reaction after a tetanus vaccine defer vaccination for Tdap for 10 years.

## Meningococcal Vaccine

*N. meningitidis* has become a leading cause of bacterial meningitis in the United States among children aged 2–18 years. Rates of meningococcal disease are highest among infants with a second peak during adolescence.[18] Sequelae of meningococcal disease include neurologic disability, limb loss, hearing loss, renal failure and death.[17] Most invasive disease is attributed to strains A, B, C, Y, and W-135.[19]

There are two vaccines approved against *N. meningitidis* in the United States: the meningococcal polysaccharide vaccine (MPSV4 or Menomune; Sanofi Pasteur) and meningococcal conjugate vaccine (MCV4 or Menactra; Sanofi Pasteur). Both vaccines can prevent infection against four serotypes of meningococcal disease: serogroups A, C, Y, and W-135, but not against serotype B. Research is ongoing to develop an effective vaccine against the B serotype.[20] Clinical trials show that the MCV4 vaccine's immunogenicity is more persistent than that of MPSV4, with a sizeable anamnestic response at reexposure.[21] MCV4 also may be more effective at providing herd immunity. Epidemiologists estimate that ~80% of meningococcal disease in adolescents and young adults is preventable with the conjugate vaccine (MCV4).[19]

In June 2007, ACIP recommended routine vaccination of all people 11–18 years old with MCV4 at the earliest opportunity. In addition, the ACIP continues to recommend that college freshmen living in dormitories, military recruits, and persons who have anatomic or functional asplenia or terminal complement component deficiencies receive vaccination against *N. meningitidis*.[22] Those who remain at increased risk for meningococcal disease and were vaccinated at ages 2–6 years should be revaccinated 3 years after initial vaccination while those who were vaccinated at ages >7 years should be vaccinated 5 years later.[1,23] Adolescents who remain in increased risk groups should continue to be revaccinated at a 5-year interval. This increased risk group includes persons with functional or anatomic asplenia, complement deficiencies, as well as persons traveling to areas with high meningococcal infection rates.[23]

Reports of isolated cases of GBS following vaccination with MCV4 led the FDA to issue an alert about the potential association of GBS with MCV4 in 2005.[24] Since GBS is a rare disorder, it has not been established that there is an increased risk among recipients of MCV4, or that a causal relationship exists. However, the CDC recommends that those with a history of GBS not receive MCV4, although persons with a history of GBS at especially high risk for meningococcal disease might consider vaccination.[24] Otherwise, the current recommendation for vaccination of adolescents remains unchanged. Hypersensitivity to any component of the meningitis vaccine is also a contraindication to receiving this vaccine.

**Influenza and H1N1 Vaccines**

Annual routine vaccination for seasonal flu for children ages 6 months to 18 years has been recommended since February 2008. However, in February 2010 the ACIP issued a statement recommending universal influenza vaccination of all people ages 6 months of age and older who have no contraindications to the vaccine. Immunization is the strongest preventive measure against influenza and its complications. Seasonal influenza causes 36,000 deaths yearly in the United States.[25] Influenza vaccination has always been recommended for adolescents with chronic conditions including asthma, diabetes, human immunodeficiency virus, and sickle cell anemia. Typically, the influenza season occurs in late fall and winter but it can also occur in the spring. Because the circulating influenza virus changes annually, there is a need for annual vaccination against influenza.

There are two vaccines currently available for seasonal influenza: a live attenuated influenza virus vaccine (LAIV) that is administered intranasally, and a trivalent inactivated influenza vaccine (TIV) that is intramuscular. Both are derived from embryonic chicken eggs, so a known severe hypersensitivity to eggs is a contraindication to their use.[26] Fortunately, immediate hypersensitivity reactions to TIV and LAIV are rare.[27]

The TIV is given intramuscularly, usually in the deltoid muscle for adolescents. A large population-based study using data from the Vaccine Safety Data link found no increased medical concerns or visits in children <18 years of age who received the influenza vaccine.[26] For adolescents, the most common side effects are local with some soreness at the injection site. Adolescents with asthma have no increased frequency of wheezing after vaccination.[26] GBS, which is the most common serious adverse event for adults reported to the Vaccine Adverse Event Reporting System (VAERS), is also considered a precaution for receiving the vaccine.[26]

The LAIV contains the same three vaccine antigens as the TIV, but in the live attenuated form. The LAIV is a preservative free vaccine that is administered directly onto the nasal mucosa at a dose of 0.2 mL (0.1 mL to each nostril). The virus in the vaccine replicates in the nasopharyngeal cells; although the precise mechanism of action has not been fully elucidated, it is thought to involve serum and nasal antibodies.[26] The LAIV can be used in healthy, nonpregnant people 2–49 years of age seeking immunization. A major advantage of the LAIV is that it is not an injection and many adolescents may prefer this option. Contraindications and precautions for the use of LAIV include hypersensitivity to LAIV components or eggs, persons <2 years and >50 years of age, certain chronic medical conditions including asthma, immunosuppression, children and adolescents who take salicylates, and pregnancy.[26] The LAIV should not be given to people who are in close contact with immunosuppressed people as there is a small risk of virus transmission from the vaccine.

In July 2009, ACIP recommended vaccination of all persons 6 months to 24 years of age with the monovalent H1N1 vaccine.[28] Like the seasonal influenza vaccine, the H1N1 vaccine is recommended for adolescents and pregnant women, as H1N1 disease may be severe in these populations. The CDC estimates that only

29.4% of children aged 6 months to 18 years of age had been vaccinated as of December 2009.[29] As the vaccine supply has greatly improved, health care providers must continue their vigilant efforts to vaccinate all susceptible persons.

There are also two types of vaccine available for H1N1, an inactivated virus vaccine and a live virus vaccine. The live virus vaccine, like the vaccine for seasonal influenza, is delivered intranasally. The inactivated viral vaccine is given as an intramuscular injection into the deltoid muscle. The side effect and safety profile is similar to that of seasonal influenza vaccine.

It is vital that pregnant adolescents be immunized against seasonal influenza and H1N1. Influenza in pregnancy can have many serious complications; pregnant women's risk of influenza-related hospitalization is more than four times that of nonpregnant women.[30] The American College of Obstetricians and Gynecologists endorses the use of the inactivated seasonal and H1N1 vaccines for pregnant women as this is an essential component of their preventive care.

In many states, the responsibility of immunizing school children for H1N1 was delegated to the school-based health centers along with the Board of Education. Consent packets including the vaccine information statements were sent home and parents were asked to sign the package authorizing the vaccine to be given to their child at school. Many school-based health centers have successfully coordinated this massive effort for vaccination. A major advantage to the school-based model as a method of delivery for this vaccine is that the child does not need to miss school and the parent does not have to miss work.

**Hepatitis B Vaccine**

Although the hepatitis B vaccine was first recommended routinely for infants in 1991, it was not until 1995 that adolescents started to receive catch up immunization at 11–12 years of age.[31] The high coverage rates for adolescents typically seen now are largely attributed to the recommendations for this vaccine in infancy. Hepatitis B vaccines are often given in juvenile justice facilities, sexually transmitted disease clinics, and family planning clinics. Hepatitis B virus (HBV) is transmitted through blood and other body fluids including semen and saliva. Clinical presentation can range from asymptomatic infection to fulminant hepatitis. Once infected with HBV, a person either recovers from the infection and develops lifelong immunity or develops chronic infection. Chronic infection with HBV can lead to hepatocellular carcinoma and vertical transmission to offspring. Strategies to vaccinate neonates, children, and adolescents have had a profound impact on the reduction of HBV infection. In 2004, among U.S. children aged 19–35 months, over 92% had been fully vaccinated with three doses of hepatitis B vaccine.[32]

ACIP recommends that all unvaccinated children and adolescents <19 years of age receive the hepatitis B vaccine series, since HBV causes ~2000–4000 deaths annually in the United States.[33] There are two single-antigen vaccines approved in the United States: Recombivax (Merck & Co, Inc.) and Engerix-B (GlaxoSmith-Kline). Both vaccines are given as a three-dose series using the pediatric/adolescent formulation (given at months 0, 1, and 6) and demonstrate a seroprotection rate that is >95% in adolescents. At 20 years of age and older, an adult dose should be administered. The adult formulation of Recombivax can be given as a two-dose series to adolescents ages 11–15 years at 0 and 4–6 months. Twinrix (GlaxoSmith-Kline), a combined hepatitis A and B vaccine, is indicated for patients age >18 years.[34] As younger adolescents are more likely to have received the full series of vaccine for hepatitis B during infancy as compared with older adolescents, it is essential that health care providers review and clarify this vaccine history at all encounters with adolescents.[35] Adolescents with a history of a severe allergic reaction to the vaccine components including baker's yeast should not receive this vaccine. Pregnant adolescents should receive the hepatitis B vaccine if they are not up to date as soon as possible.

**Hepatitis A Vaccine**

Hepatitis A infection among children is often asymptomatic. Older children and adults are usually symptomatic, with fever, malaise, anorexia, nausea, abdominal discomfort, and jaundice. Hepatitis A vaccines, Havrix (GlaxoSmith-Kline) and Vaqta (Merck & Co, Inc), are currently licensed in the United States as a two-dose series to be given 6 months apart. The combination vaccine Twinrix, which contains both hepatitis A and hepatitis B virus antigens, can be used in adolescents older than 18 years.[34] The ACIP recommends universal vaccination at 12–23 months of age. Hepatitis A vaccine is also recommended for the following populations: persons with chronic liver disease, men who have sex with men, drugs users, recipients of clotting factors, international travelers, persons with occupational risks, children living in areas where infection rates exceed national average, and all individuals who seek immunity to hepatitis A.[34,36] It is appropriate to offer this vaccine to adolescents who have the above risk factors or who wish to reduce their risk of infection with this virus.

**MMR and Varicella Vaccines**

Varicella zoster virus is a member of the Herpesvirus family. Primary infection results in varicella (chicken pox). Symptoms in healthy children and adolescent usually consist of fever and a pruritic maculopapular rash that progresses to vesicles. Complications are rare but more severe among adolescents, adults, and immunocompromised hosts.

Measles is a highly contagious viral illness, characterized by fever, cough, coryza, conjunctivitis, and rash. There was a major measles epidemic in the United States from 1989–1991 that resulted in >11,000 hospitalizations and 120 deaths.[37] The most common symptoms of mumps infections are fever, headache, and enlarged parotid glands. In adults, an infection with mumps is usually more severe and it is more likely to cause orchitis in men as compared with boys.[38] In 2006 and 2009, the United States experienced large-scale outbreaks of mumps, with the highest attack rates among persons aged 18–24 years.[39] Rubella, also known as German measles, is generally a mild disease and causes low-grade fever, lymphadenopathy, and a blotchy rash. However, infection during early pregnancy may cause fetal death or the congenital rubella syndrome that consists of mental retardation, cardiac lesions, neurologic impairment, and eye abnormalities.

There are two varicella vaccines licensed in the United States: Varivax (Merck & Co, Inc), which is a single live attenuated varicella vaccine, and ProQuad (Merck & Co, Inc), which is a combination MMR/varicella vaccine. Varivax is indicated for use among healthy persons 12 months or older, whereas Proquad is licensed for use among healthy children aged 12 months to 12 years.

In June 2006, a second dose of varicella vaccine was recommended because there were reports of cases of varicella in children who had received only one dose of the vaccine.[10] The ACIP continues to recommend two doses of a varicella vaccine, with the first dose to be given at 12 months of age and the second dose at 4–6 years of age.[1] Adolescents 13 years and older who have never been vaccinated should receive two doses of Varivax with a minimum of 28 days between doses. For children younger than 13 years of age, the minimum interval is 3 months.[1] Adolescents who received only one dose in childhood should receive a second dose.

Because the MMR and varicella vaccines are live virus vaccines, they should not be administered to pregnant adolescents. Adolescents who are severely immunocompromised should not be given MMR or varicella vaccines. Vaccination should be delayed after receiving antibody containing blood products (immunoglobulin, whole blood, or packed red blood cells) and interval is based on concentration and quantity of blood product.[40] If tuberculin skin testing is required, it can be administered at the same time as MMR and varicella vaccines; if not, it should be delayed for at least 4 weeks after vaccination. The immune response to live vaccines might be impaired if administered <4 weeks apart. To avoid this, if not administered on the same day, live vaccines should be spaced at least 4 weeks apart.[40] Contraindications to this vaccine also include a severe allergy to the vaccine or any of its components.

**Polio Vaccine**

The eradication of poliomyelitis in the United States and Western hemisphere is a major accomplishment of the polio vaccine. Oral polio vaccine is no longer routinely available in the United States; in January 2000, an all-inactivated polio vaccine schedule was recommended.[41] The ACIP continues to endorse routine childhood vaccination with inactivated polio vaccine. In the United States, routine vaccination 18 years of age and older against polio is not recommended. However, vaccination is recommended for adults traveling to polio-endemic countries and selected laboratory workers.

## Pneumococcal Vaccine

*Streptococcus pneumoniae* is one of the most common causative agents of bacterial pneumonia, meningitis, sinusitis, and otitis media in children and adults. Moreover, it is a frequent cause of secondary bacterial pneumonia among those with influenza. The risk for pneumococcal infection is high among those with chronic renal failure or nephrotic syndrome, functional or anatomic asplenia, diabetes mellitus, and immunosuppression. Adults who have chronic cardiovascular disease, obstructive lung disease, and/or liver disease are also at an increased risk for pneumococcal infection.

There are currently two pneumococcal vaccines available: PPSV23 and PCV7. PPSV23 (Pneumovax; Merck & Co, Inc.) contains polysaccharide antigen from 23 types of pneumococcal bacteria that cause 88% of bacteremic pneumococcal disease.[42] PCV7 (Prevnar; Wyeth-Lederle Vaccines) contains purified capsular polysaccharide of seven serotypes of *S. pneumoniae* that account for 86% of bacteremia, 83% of meningitis, and 65% of acute otitis media among children younger than 6 years of age.[43] PCV7 is part of the routine recommended immunization schedule for infants and young children. PPSV23 is indicated for persons 2 years of age and older with certain underlying medical conditions, including asplenia, HIV, and nephrotic syndrome. A second dose of PPSV23 is recommended 5 years after the first dose of PPSV23 for persons aged >2 years who continue to be at risk for invasive pneumococcal infection.[43,44] Adults age 19–64 years who smoke cigarettes or have asthma should receive a single dose of PPSV23.[40,44]

## Vaccine Safety and Concerns

The VAERS is one of several postmarketing monitoring systems managed by CDC and the FDA to detect adverse reactions to vaccines, particularly rare reactions that were not identified in the premarketing phases of vaccine development. VAERS is a passive surveillance system; that is, reporting is voluntary and data are not collected in a comprehensive, systematic fashion through this system. Causality therefore cannot be established through VAERS alone. CDC and FDA encourage anyone who is aware of an adverse event following administration of a vaccine to report this to VAERS, even if causality is not established. Reporting may be done by vaccine manufacturers, health care providers, parents, or anyone else aware of such an event. The most common side effect for all injectable vaccinations is local tenderness, swelling, and redness at the injection site. Sterile abscesses have also occurred at the injection site. Fortunately, serious adverse events of vaccinations are rare. However, it is prudent that health care professionals report any significant event to VAERS.

Syncope (vasovagal reaction) can occur after vaccination and most commonly occurs in adolescents.[45] From 2005–2006, ACIP recommended the use of three new vaccines in adolescents: MCV4, Tdap, and the quadrivalent HPV vaccine. The CDC and FDA looked at data from VAERS before and after recommendation of these three specific vaccines to investigate trends in adverse events. Their findings show an increase in reports of vasovagal events primarily among females between the ages of 11–18 years.[45] The HPV4 vaccine at the time of this study was recommended only for adolescent females, who may be particularly vulnerable to this phenomenon. The ACIP recommends that health care providers observe patients for 15 minutes after vaccination to avoid possible injuries associated with syncope.[46] It is prudent that health care providers be aware of the potential for syncope after vaccines and take appropriate precautions with their patients. Anecdotal reports and comments from health care providers suggest that inquiring specifically about past vasovagal reactions is useful and some providers prefer to administer vaccines to adolescents in a supine position and have the adolescent use relaxation techniques including slow deep breathing and/or listening to music with headphones.

Thimerosal is a mercury-containing preservative that has been used in vaccines since 1930.[26] It is frequently used in multidose preparations of vaccines to retard bacterial growth. There is no scientific evidence that thimerosal in vaccines is harmful. Furthermore, there is no evidence that thimerosal-containing vaccines given to pregnant women cause any harmful effects to their children.[26] However, the US Public Health Service has recommended the reduction and ultimate elimination of exposures to mercury from all sources including vaccines.[47] Efforts continue to enhance the development of thimerosal-free vaccines.

Reports of patients developing GBS and other neurologic conditions after vaccination with MCV4 led the FDA to issue an alert of a possible association of GBS and MCV4 in 2005.[24] In addition, there are also rare reports of GBS occurring after administration of the quadrivalent HPV vaccine. However, there is no scientific evidence that any vaccine causes GBS or any other neurologic sequelae. VAERS continues to collect and analyze data on vaccine safety and encourages health care providers to use this reporting tool.

**Special Considerations in Adolescent Vaccination Efforts**

In addition to the need for a routine adolescent visit at age 11–12 years, the Society for Adolescent Medicine recommends visits at age 14–15 years and at 17–18 years.[17] These visits were proposed to help with missed vaccinations in addition to promoting preventive care. Moreover, these visits enable immunization of adolescents while they are still covered under the national Vaccines for Children program.[17] Under this program, uninsured or underinsured adolescents may receive recommended vaccinations until their 19th birthday. The high cost of vaccines continues to be a barrier and many insurance companies do not cover vaccines for adolescents >18 years of age. Even for adolescents with private insurance, the rate of reimbursements to health care providers is low. Vaccines may be prohibitively expensive for adolescents and young adults who must pay "out of pocket." For example, as of this writing, an uninsured 20-year-old adolescent may have to pay approximately $375.00 out of pocket to receive the three-dose quadrivalent HPV vaccine.[48]

There are many unique barriers to adolescents receiving appropriate and timely vaccinations. Many adolescents do not regularly seek comprehensive care or even identify a medical home. Some parents and adolescents may have concerns about vaccine safety and the cost of the vaccines. The need for multiple doses (and therefore multiple visits) for vaccine efficacy may be difficult for patients and parents. In addition, providers frequently cite the difficulty in verifying vaccine records for adolescents as a barrier to giving vaccines. Despite the availability of many computer-based vaccine registries, the records are not always complete. Furthermore, most states have laws requiring parental consent for most vaccines, which can also be a barrier to adolescents who seek health care on their own.

Many adolescents do not access health care for preventive services; they are more likely use health care services for crisis and problem-focused visits. However, the Health Plan Employer Data and Information Set 2003 data revealed that the majority of adolescents had seen a health care provider within the past year.[49] It is imperative that adolescent health care providers implement creative solutions to combat low rates of vaccination for this population including reviewing and updating immunizations at problem-focused visits. School-based health centers should not replace the medical home but could complement adolescent health care by increasing vaccination coverage rates at the place where the majority of adolescents spend their time.[50-52] Unfortunately, many school-based health centers have limited funding and resources and are not present in most schools.

Collaborating with school-based clinics, using sick visits and visits other than traditional complete health maintenance encounters is a critical step in improving vaccination coverage rates for adolescents. It is also essential that health care providers continue to educate their adolescent patients about the importance of vaccines using developmentally appropriate language.

## CONCLUSIONS

The past decade has witnessed a tremendous change in the recommended childhood and adolescent immunization schedule. Many new vaccines and new recommendations for the use of existing vaccines have been added in the past 5–10 years. Health care providers need to be facile with the ever changing schedules. It is imperative that providers embrace novel and creative ways to improve immunization coverage in adolescents and continue to advocate for quality adolescent health care. Providing low-cost and free adolescent preventive care must be a national priority if the goals of Healthy People 2010 are to be achieved. Forming partnerships with other health care professionals, school-based clinics, and most importantly our adolescents and their families is a fundamental element of any successful adolescent vaccination effort.

## REFERENCES

1. American Academy of Pediatrics. Recommended childhood and adolescent immunization schedules United States, 2010. *Pediatrics.* 2010;125(1):195–196
2. Centers for Disease Control and Prevention. National, state and local area vaccination coverage among adolescents aged 13–17 years—United States, 2008. *MMWR.* 2009;58(36):997–1001
3. Brown DR, Schroeder JM, Bryan JY, et al. Detection of multiple human papilloma virus types in condyloma acuminate lesions from otherwise healthy and immunosuppressed patients. *J Clinical Microbiology.* 1999;37:3316–3322
4. Garcia F, Saslow D. Prophylactic human papillomavirus vaccination: a breakthrough in primary cervical cancer prevention. *Obstet Gynecol Clin.* 2007;34
5. Moscicki A. HPV vaccines: today and in the future. *J Adolescent Health.* 2008;43:S26–S40
6. Myers ER, McCrory DC, Nanda K, Bastian L, Matchar DB. Mathematical model for the natural history of human papillomavirus infection and cervical carcinogenesis. *Am J Epidemiology.* 2000;151(12):1158–1171
7. FDA approves new vaccine for the prevention of cervical cancer. Available at: http://www.fda.gov/NewsEvents/Newsroom/PressAnnouncements/ucm187048.htm. Accessed January 15, 2010
8. FDA approval letter to expand Gardisil to males. Available at: http://www.fda.gov/BiologicsBloodVaccines/Vaccines/ApprovedProducts/ucm186991.htm. Accessed January 12, 2010
9. Diaz M. Human papilloma virus–prevention and treatment. *Obstet Gynecol Clin North Am.* 2008;35:199–217
10. Ackerman L. Update on immunizations in children and adolescents. *Am Family Physician.* 2008;77:1561–1568
11. Rodewald L, Orenstein W. Vaccinating adolescents—new evidence of challenges and opportunities. *J Adolescent Health.* 2009;45:427–429
12. Bernat D, Harpin S, Eisenberg M, Bearinger L, Resnick M. Parental support for the human papillomavirus vaccine. 2009;45:525–527
13. Wright S, Edwards K, Decker M, Zeldin M. Pertussis infection in adults with persistent cough. *JAMA.* 1995;273:1044–1046
14. Pichiero M, Blatter M, Kennedy W, Hedrick J, Descamps D, Friedland L. Acellular pertussis vaccine booster combined with diptheria and tetanus toxoids for adolescents. *Pediatrics.* 2006;117:1084–1093
15. Craig A, Wright S, Edwards K, Greene J, et al. Outbreak of pertussis on a college campus. *Am J Med.* 2007;120:364–368
16. Nennig M, Shinefield H, Edwards K, et al. Prevalence and incidence of adult pertussis in an urban population. *JAMA.* 1996;275:1672–1674
17. Middleman A, Rosenthal S, Rickert V, Neinstein L, Fishbein D, D'Angelo L. Adolescent immunizations: A position paper of the Society for Adolescent Medicine. *J Adolescent Health.* 2006;38:321–327
18. Centers for Disease Control and Prevention. Prevention and control of meningococcal disease: Recommendations of the Advisory Committee on Immunization Practices. *MMWR.* 2005;54(RR-07):1–21
19. Harrison L, Pass M, Mendelsohn A, et al. Invasive meningococcal disease in adolescents and young adults. *JAMA.* 2001;286:694

20. Beernink P, Welsch J, Harrison L, et al. Prevalence of factor H- binding protein variants and NadA among meningococcal group B isolates from the United States: Implications for the development of a multicomponent group B vaccine. *J Infectious Dis.* 2007;195:1472
21. Keyserling H, Papa T, Koranhyi K, et al. Safety, immunogenicity, and immune memory of a novel meningococcal (groups A,C,Y and W-135) polysaccharide diptheroid toxoid conjugate vaccine (MCV-4) in healthy adolescents. *Arch Pediatr Adolesc Med.* 2005;159:907
22. Centers for Disease Control and Prevention. Revised recommendations of the advisory board on immunization practices to vaccinate all persons aged 11–18 years with meningococcal conjugate vaccine. *MMWR.* 2007;56(31):794–795
23. Centers for Disease Control and Prevention. Updated recommendation from the Advisory Committee on Immunization Practices for revaccination of persons at prolonged increased risk for meningococcal disease. *MMWR.* 2009;58(37):1042–1043
24. Centers for Disease Control and Prevention. Update: Guillain-Barré syndrome among recipients of menactra meningococcal conjugate vaccine—United States, June 2005–September 2006. *MMWR.* 2006;55(41):1120–1124
25. Thompson W, Shay D, Weintraub, et al. Mortality associated with influenza and respiratory syncytial virus in the United States. *JAMA.* 2003;289:179–186
26. Hannoun C. Immunogenicity and protective efficacy of influenza vaccination. *Virus Res.* 2004; 103:133–138
27. Fiore A, Shay D, Broder K, et al. Prevention and control of seasonal influenza with vaccines. *MMWR.* 2009;58:1–52
28. Recommendations of the Advisory Committee on Immunization Practices (ACIP), 2009: Use of the influenza A (H1N1) 2009 monovalent vaccine. *MMWR.* 2009;58:1–8
29. Singleton J, Santibanez T, Lu P, et al. Interim results: Influenza A (H1N1) 2009 monovalent vaccination coverage—United States. *MMWR.* 2009;59:44–48
30. Center for Disease Control and Prevention. Epidemiology and prevention of vaccine-preventable diseases. 11th edition. Washington, DC: Public Health Foundation, 2009
31. Centers for Disease Control. Notice to readers update: recommendations to prevent hepatitis B virus transmission—United States. *MMWR.* 1995;44:574–575
32. Mast E, Margolis H, Fiore A, et al. A comprehensive strategy to eliminate transmission of hepatitis B virus infection in the United States: recommendations of the ACIP. *MMWR.* 2005; 54(RR-16):1–33
33. Centers for Disease Control and Prevention. Surveillance for acute viral hepatitis—United States, 2006. *MMWR.* 2008;198:299–304
34. Centers for Disease Control and Prevention. Prevention of hepatitis a through active or passive immunization: recommendations of the ACIP. *MMWR.* 2006;55(RR07):1–23
35. Jain N, Hennessey K. Hepatitis B vaccination coverage among US adolescents, National Immunization Survey—Teen, 2006. *J Adolescent Health.* 2009;44:561–567
36. Committee on Infectious Diseases. Hepatitis A Recommendations. *Pediatrics.* 2007;120:189–199
37. National Immunization Program, Centers for Disease Control and Prevention. *Needle Tips and the Hepatitis B Coalition News.* 1999;9:13–15
38. Weisberg S. Mumps. *MMWR.* 2007;53:484–487
39. Centers for Disease Control and Prevention. Mumps Outbreak–New York, New Jersey, Quebec, 2009. *MMWR.* 2009;58:1270–1274
40. Centers for Disease Control and Prevention. Epidemiology and prevention of vaccine-preventable diseases. 11th ed. Washington, DC: Public Health Foundation, 2009
41. Centers for Disease Control and Prevention. Poliomyelitis prevention in the United States: updated recommendations of the Advisory Committee on Immunization Practices. *MMWR.* 2000;49:RR-05
42. Centers for Disease Control and Prevention. Prevention of pneumococcal disease recommendations of the Advisory Committee on Immunization Practices (ACIP). *MMRW.* 1997;46:RR-8

43. Centers for Disease Control and Prevention. Bacterial Co-infections in lung tissue specimens from fatal cases of 2009 pandemic influenza A (H1N1)—United States, May–August 2009. *MMRW*. 2009;58:1–4
44. Centers for Disease Control and Prevention. ACIP Provisional Recommendations for Use of Pneumococcal Vaccines. Available at: http://www.cdc.gov/vaccines/recs/provisional/downloads/pneumo-oct-2008-508.pdf. Accessed January 14, 2010
45. Centers for Disease Control and Prevention. Syncope after vaccination—United States, January 2005–July 2007. *MMWR*. 2008;57:457–460
46. Centers for Disease Control and Prevention. General recommendations on immunization: recommendations of the ACIP. *MMWR*. 2006;55:RR-15
47. McCormick M, Bayer R, Berg A, et al. Report of the Institute of Medicine. Immunization safety review: vaccine and autism. Washington, DC: Institute of Medicine; 2004
48. Gardasil pricing information. Available at: www.cdc.gov/std/hpv/STDFact-HPV-vaccine-young-women.htm#hpv. Accessed January 18, 2010
49. Central for Disease Control and Prevention. Health United States 2005. Available at: http://www.cdc.gov/nchs/data/hus/hus0.5.pdf. Accessed July 1, 2009
50. Lindley M, Boyer-Chu L, Fishbein D, Kolasa M, et al. The role schools in strengthening delivery of new adolescent vaccinations. *Pediatrics*. 2008;121:S46–S54
51. Schaffer S, Fontanesi J, Rickert D, et al. How effectively can health care settings beyond the traditional medical home provide vaccines to adolescents? *Pediatrics*. 2008;121:S35–S45
52. Middleman A. Adolescent immunizations: policies to provide a shot in the arm for adolescents. *J Adolescent Health*. 2007;41:109–118

# Acute Sinusitis

Jason M. Mehrtens, MD[a], Michael G. Spigarelli, MD[a], PhD*

[a]Division of Adolescent Medicine, Cincinnati Children's Hospital Medical Center, 3333 Burnet Avenue, Cincinnati, OH 45229-3039

Sinusitis, also referred to as rhinosinusitis, can be defined as inflammation of the paranasal sinuses. In the United States, ~31 million cases of acute sinusitis are diagnosed yearly,[1] making it one of the most common primary care issues. Nearly 16% of the adult population is affected by this condition,[2] resulting in $5.8 billion of annual health care costs in 1996, the last year data for sinusitis specifically were extensively analyzed.[3]

Based on the length of symptoms, sinusitis is divided into three broad categories: *acute* (symptoms lasting <4 weeks), *subacute* (symptoms lasting 4–8 weeks), and *chronic* (symptoms present over 8 weeks). Sinusitis can be further classified as *recurrent*, defined as 4 or more discrete episodes in the course of a year. Chronic sinusitis accounts for over 18 million office visits per year; however, this is most commonly a disease of people 20–59 years of age.[1] Thus, this article focuses primarily on acute sinusitis and its complications because this is the clinical entity that most commonly affects adolescents.

## Anatomy

Four symmetrical air-filled cavities comprise the paranasal sinuses: maxillary, frontal, ethmoid, and sphenoid. These sinuses are lined with ciliated pseudostratified columnar epithelium. Small tubular openings, called sinus ostia, connect the sinuses and drain into the nasal cavity. The sphenoid and posterior ethmoid sinuses open into the superior meatus, and the anterior ethmoid, frontal, and maxillary sinuses open into the middle meatus. These structures form the osteomeatal complex, which is the common drainage area of the ethmoid, frontal, and maxillary sinuses. Ciliary action moves mucus and other material from the sinuses into the osteomeatal complex; when this is blocked or inflamed and ciliary clearance is impaired, bacterial infection can occur. The floor of the frontal sinus is also the roof of the orbit, and the anterior wall of the cranial fossa comprises the posterior wall of the frontal sinus. This anatomic location explains

---

*Corresponding author.
*E-mail address:* michael.spigarelli@cchmc.org (M. G. Spigarelli).

why infections of the frontal sinus can spread to the central nervous system and/or the orbit. Additionally, the sphenoid sinuses can be a focus for the spread of infection to the central nervous system since they are surrounded by the cavernous sinuses, the internal carotid arteries, and the optic nerve and are located directly anterior to the pituitary fossa.[4]

Although the nasal cavities are colonized with multiple bacteria that comprise the normal flora, the sinuses are typically sterile. When the bacteria colonizing the nasal cavities reach the sinuses, they are the organisms most commonly associated with sinusitis. If the defenses of mucociliary clearance and immune responses (nasal secretions contain immunoglobulin A, E, G, and M and lysozymes)[5] fail, infection of the sinuses can ensue.

**Predisposing Factors**

Although the anatomy of the sinus region plays a major role in the development of sinusitis, that alone cannot explain why some individuals are more likely to develop sinusitis than others. At least three other categories of predisposing factors also contribute to the onset of sinusitis: systemic, local insult, and mechanical obstruction. Systemic factors include viral upper respiratory infections (URI), tobacco smoke, allergic inflammation, cystic fibrosis, and immune disorders.[4] It is thought that viral infections impair ciliary motility, resulting in impaired mucociliary clearance and occlusion of the sinus ostium. Cystic fibrosis, a well-known cause of immotile cilia, also has impaired mucociliary clearance and may be a reason why this population is at increased risk of sinusitis as well.[6] Lastly, children who attend day care have twice the rate of sinusitis as age-matched children who do not attend day care, thought to be due in part to the significant increase in viral upper respiratory tract infections children in day care contract. The risk of sinusitis among family members of children attending day care is also increased compared with the general population. This is likely due to the children becoming colonized with respiratory bacterial pathogens associated with sinusitis such as *Streptococcus pneumoniae* and *Staphylococcus aureus* and then transmitting the organisms to family members.[4]

Local insult factors include facial trauma, overuse of nasal decongestants, swimming/diving, and nasal intubation.[4] These insults can create pathways for normal nasal flora to be introduced into the sinuses, whether directly through facial trauma and nasal intubation, through pressure changes as seen with diving and swimming, or through induced obstruction from overuse of decongestants.

Mechanical obstruction factors include choanal atresia, deviated septum, nasal polyps, foreign body, tumor, and ethmoid bullae.[4] These factors physically block the flow of normally functioning mucociliary clearance.

## Specific Microbiology

As the nasal cavity is directly connected with the sinuses, it is common practice to culture the nose and use the results as a surrogate of findings from the sinus. Unfortunately, isolation of bacteria from the nasal cavity has a low predictive value for the organisms infecting the sinus and can lead to an incorrect diagnosis and inappropriate prescription of antibiotics. An accurate microbiologic diagnosis thus requires direct culture of the sinuses, but the procedure is very invasive and involves puncture of the maxillary antrum for aspiration analysis.[2]

When maxillary aspiration is undertaken, the bacterial pathogens most commonly isolated from the sinuses are *S. pneumoniae* (20–43% of cases); *Haemophilus influenzae*, predominantly nontypable (22–35%); and *Moraxella catarrhalis* (2–10%).[1] Studies including younger children often find a higher proportion of sinus disease due to *Moraxella catarrhalis,* whereas in adults the organism is rarely isolated. Anaerobes and *S. aureus* have been isolated from the sinuses as well, particularly in cases of subacute and chronic sinusitis. In ~33% of cases, the etiology of acute sinusitis is polymicrobial.[7]

In ~30–40% of aspirate samples obtained from patients with acute sinusitis, no bacteria are isolated, which leads to the presumption that the illness is of viral etiology, although viruses are rarely cultured from the sinuses. Possibly, viruses are not commonly isolated from the sinuses because culturing often does not occur until the patient has been ill for 7–10 days, at which time the preceding viral infection is clearing.[4] When viruses have been isolated from the sinuses, rhinovirus is the most common organism, found in ~10% of the cases.[8] The ease of transmission of rhinovirus, with 95% of exposed individuals becoming infected and 75% developing symptomatic disease, makes it understandable why this virus has been the one most commonly associated with sinus disease.[9]

Fungal sources have also been implicated in sinus infections, although these tend to be more common in an immunocompromised host.[7] Given its relative rarity, fungal sinusitis and in particular the devastating invasive fungal sinusitis will not be further discussed in this article. The astute clinician, however, should consider fungal sources when treatment regimens for bacterial sinusitis are failing, particularly in patients with underlying conditions that can suppress the immune response, such as diabetes, conditions causing or resulting from neutropenia, HIV infection, or in patients in critical care units.

Nosocomial infections should also be considered in the differential diagnosis of sinusitis. These infections primarily occur in patients in the critical care setting, and causative agents include *Pseudomonas* species, *Escherichia coli, Proteus mirabilis, S. aureus, Candida* species, and *Streptococcus viridans*.[10] Presence of a nasogastric tube is a major risk factor for the development of nosocomial sinusitis. In one study, presence of a nasogastric tube was associated with a

9.8-fold increase in the likelihood of sinusitis translating to 15.7 cases per 1000 patient days with a nasogastric tube, compared with 1.6 cases per 1000 patient days in patients without history of a nasogastric tube.[10] Nasotracheal intubation is another risk factor for the development of nosocomial sinusitis, with ~25% of the patients intubated for more than 5 days contracting a sinus infection.[7] In adolescent populations, nasoenteric tubes could be of particular importance when treating patients with eating disorders or other conditions requiring nasogastric delivery of their nutrition over a prolonged period of time.

**Diagnosis**

Acute sinusitis is diagnosed almost exclusively on a clinical basis. One of the most important factors for diagnosis is duration of symptoms. Symptoms of acute sinusitis can mimic viral URI. However, while a viral URI tends to last 5–7 days, with significant improvement by day 10, bacterial sinusitis, in the absence of treatment, often persists. Another scheme for the diagnosis of acute sinusitis relies on the use of major and minor criteria (Box 1).[7]

In a study of suspected sinusitis, clinical findings most commonly associated with the disease included maxillary toothache, little or no response to decongestants, history of discolored nasal discharge, purulent rhinorrhea on examination and abnormal transillumination of the frontal or maxillary sinuses. When all five

Box 1
Major and minor clinical criteria suggestive of bacterial sinusitis

---

A strongly suggestive history requires the presence of two major criteria or one major and two or more minor criteria. A suggestive history requires the presence of one major criterion or two or more minor criteria

*Major criteria*
  Facial pain or pressure (requires a second major criterion to constitute a suggestive history)
  Facial congestion or fullness
  Nasal congestion or obstruction
  Nasal discharge, purulence or discolored postnasal drainage
  Hyposmia or anosmia
  Fever (for acute sinusitis; requires a second major criterion to constitute a strong history)
  Purulence on intranasal examination

*Minor criteria*
  Headache
  Fever (for subacute and chronic sinusitis)
  Halitosis
  Fatigue
  Dental pain
  Cough
  Ear pain, pressure, or fullness

---

Adapted from: Brook I. Acute and chronic bacterial sinusitis. *Infect Dis Clin N Am.* 2007;21:427–448.

findings were present, the clinical diagnosis of sinusitis was correctly predicted in 92% of the cases. The presence of maxillary tooth pain had a 93% specificity for the diagnosis of sinusitis but its relatively rarity (18% of cases) detracted from the clinical utility of the finding. Alternatively, abnormal transillumination had a 73% sensitivity but a specificity of only 54%.[11] One limitation of this study was the reliance on plain radiographs as the gold standard because many experts do not recommend this test for diagnosis.

A clinical practice guideline for adult sinusitis was compiled in 2007 by a panel of experts. The three cardinal symptoms of acute sinusitis include purulent nasal drainage, nasal obstruction, and facial pain/pressure/fullness. Additionally, this panel recommended the current guidelines due to the higher sensitivity and specificity as compared with diagnosis based on minor and major criteria discussed above.[1] This guideline also states that "clinicians should not obtain radiographic imaging for patients who meet diagnostic criteria for acute rhinosinusitis, unless a complication or alternative diagnosis is suspected."[1] Based on a meta-analysis, radiography of the sinuses has a sensitivity of 76% and a specificity of 79%, as compared with the standard of maxillary aspirate to confirm bacterial infection. Sinus involvement is common with a viral URI, and thus distinguishing viral infection from bacterial sinusitis is not possible by using imaging alone. However, imaging is useful in cases of failed treatment or when there is a concern for a complication from sinusitis. CT is usually the best available imaging modality, but even CT imaging cannot determine a difference between viral and bacterial sinusitis.[8]

No parameter for diagnosing sinusitis is perfect, as none are both sensitive and specific. The true gold standard of documenting bacterial presence in the sinuses, maxillary aspirate, is invasive and highly impractical in the primary care clinical setting. Therefore, a combination of key symptoms, as well as the duration and severity of these symptoms, is used to determine suspicion for bacterial infection.

**Treatment**

Antibiotics are commonly used when sinusitis is diagnosed in the primary care setting. However, according to the adult sinusitis guidelines, watchful waiting is acceptable even in cases of suspected bacterial infection in patients with "uncomplicated acute bacterial rhinosinusitis who have mild illness (mild pain and temperature <38.3°C or 101°F) and assurance of follow-up."[1] This statement is based largely on the high level of spontaneous resolution of sinusitis in placebo arms of randomized controlled studies, as well as only a modest benefit in the antibiotic treatment arms. According to the Centers for Disease Control and Prevention, clinical improvement is noted in 81% of patients treated with antibiotics, as compared with 66% of controls, providing an absolute benefit of only 15% attributable to antibiotic therapy.[12] Watchful waiting without use of antibiotic therapy is acceptable in mild, uncomplicated cases for up to 7 days after diagnosis, with recommendation to start antibiotics if there is no improvement after 7 days, or if there are worsening symptoms at any time.[1]

When the decision to prescribe antibiotics has been made, amoxicillin is often recommended as the first-line choice for acute uncomplicated sinusitis. In studies comparing different antibiotic agents, no significant differences in clinical outcome have ever been observed.[1] Therefore, the favorable safety profile, cheap cost, clinical efficacy, and relatively narrow antimicrobial spectrum of amoxicillin make it an excellent choice for treating sinusitis. In cases of children who attend day care, adults who have children attending day care, or those who have been on antibiotics in the past 4–6 weeks, high-dose amoxicillin regimens (up to 90 mg/kg) may be needed due to emerging resistance to penicillin, with up to 50% of *S. pneumoniae* demonstrating moderate or high resistance (>2 μg/mL) to penicillin.[2] Although resistance to *S. pneumoniae* is due to an alteration of the penicillin-binding protein, resistance to *H. influenzae* (50% of strains) and *M. catarrhalis* (90% of strains) is a result of the organism producing a β-lactamase, which deactivates penicillin and amoxicillin. To overcome this type of resistance, amoxicillin combined with a potassium clavulanate salt (Augmentin) should be used.

First-generation cephalosporins such as cefadroxil and cephalexin should not be used, as they have poor coverage against *H. influenzae*. Second- and third-generation cephalosporins have variable efficacy, with cefuroxime and cefprozil (second generation) and cefpodoxime and cefdinir (third generation) having the best activity against the common causative agents.[2] For those with penicillin allergies, trimethoprim-sulfamethoxazole is an acceptable alternative, as are macrolide antibiotics,[1] although there is increasing resistance of *S. pneumoniae* to these agents as well.[2]

The duration of antibiotic treatment required to eradicate the infection is not well defined. A 10- to 14-day course is usually chosen, although some clinicians recommend treatment for 7 days beyond resolution of symptoms.[2] Treatment failure is defined as worsening signs or symptoms or failing to improve within 7 days after the initial diagnosis is made.[1] Patients who experience treatment failure should then be reevaluated to ensure accurate diagnosis and/or exclude other potential causes of the illness or symptoms, and to monitor for complications.

Analysis of the use of adjunctive therapies, such as intranasal corticosteroids and antihistamines, has shown no significant added benefit in acute sinusitis. However, steroids may be beneficial in those patients with allergic rhinitis as an underlying cause for their sinusitis. The use of nasal saline may provide some symptom improvement, with large-volume irrigation tending to be more effective than simple nasal sprays. This modality has been noted to be more effective in patients with chronic sinusitis.[4]

**Referral Indications**

Although the vast majority of sinusitis and its related conditions are managed in the primary care setting, there are some presenting symptoms that merit consideration for referral to a subspecialist. According to the Joint Task Force on Practice Parameters for Sinusitis,[2] subspecialist referral is indicated in the following cases:

- When the condition or its treatment is interfering with a patient's performance or causing significant loss of school or work on a chronic or recurrent basis or when the patient's quality of life is significantly affected.
- When there are complications of sinusitis, such as otitis, asthma, bronchiectasis, nasal polyps, or bronchitis.
- When there is consideration for an allergic or immunologic basis for the sinusitis or when immunocompetence needs to be assessed.
- When the condition becomes chronic, persists for several months, or recurs 2–3 times per year, despite treatment by the primary care physician.
- When there is the need for complex pharmacology to treat recalcitrant infections caused by underlying allergies, allergic fungal sinusitis, resistant pathogens, or aspirin desensitization.

**Complications**

With the advancement of antibiotic treatment, complications of sinusitis are fortunately relatively rare, occurring at a rate of 1 per 10 000 cases.[13] When treatment failure occurs, however, complications should always be considered. Symptoms and physical examination findings that suggest a developing complication include severe headache, mental status changes, changes in vision, proptosis, abnormal extraocular movements, and erythema or edema of the periorbital region.[1] Sinusitis complications can be divided into three major categories based on location of the complication: local, orbital, and intracranial. The major anatomy of the sinuses and their proximity to the regions where the most common sinusitis complications occur are demonstrated in Fig. 2.

*Local*

The two most common local complications are mucoceles and Pott's puffy tumors.

*Mucoceles* Mucoceles are slowly expanding cystic lesions that can take over a decade to become evident. Primary mucoceles (mucus retention cysts) form due to blockage of a minor salivary gland duct, located within the lining of the paranasal sinus, usually in the maxillary sinus. Secondary mucoceles, most

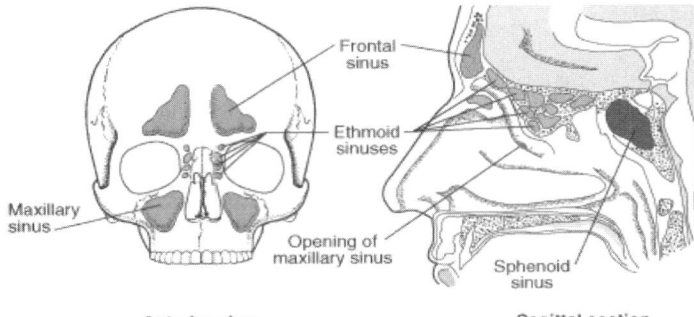

Fig 1. Sinus locations. (From The Merck Manuals Online Medical Library. *Approach to the patient with nasal and pharyngeal symptoms.* Available at: http://www.merck.com/mmpe/sec08/ch089/ch089a.html. Accessed February 9, 2010).

frequently occurring in the frontal and ethmoid sinuses, develop following sinus ostium blockage, a result of chronic sinusitis, trauma, nasal polyps, or tumors. Frontal sinus mucoceles tend to present with frontal headaches and proptosis and outward and downward displacement of the globe, sometimes accompanied with periorbital or deep nasal pain. When the mucocele is located in the sphenoid

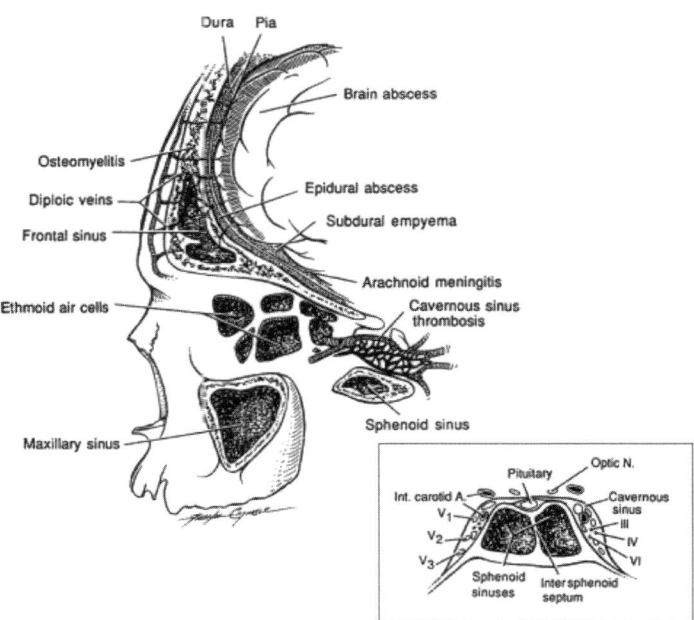

Fig 2. Complications associated with sinusitis. (From Chow AW. Infections of the sinuses and parameningeal structures. In: Gorbach SL, Bartlett JG, Blacklow NR, eds. *Infectious Diseases*. 3rd Ed. Philadelphia, PA: Lippincott Williams & Wilkins, 2004:431).

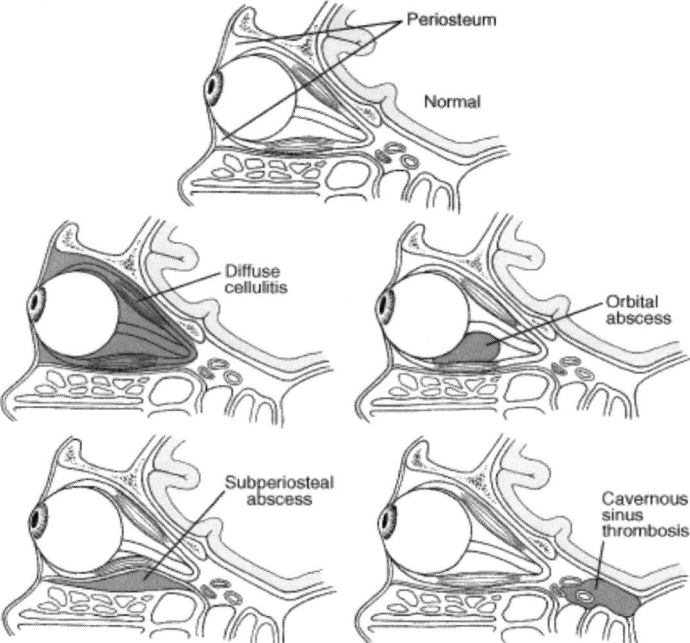

Fig 3. Orbital complications. (From The Merck Manual Online Medical Library. *Preseptal and orbital cellulitis.* Available at: http://www.merck.com/media/mmpe/figures/Fig.1sec9ch108_eps.gif. Accessed February 9, 2010).

sinus, worsening vision and headaches are most often the presenting symptoms.[14] Computed tomography (CT) and magnetic resonance imaging (MRI) both are useful diagnostic tools and gadolinium-enhanced MRI can help differentiate mucoceles from tumors.[15] Surgical intervention is the treatment of choice.

*Pott's Puffy Tumor* Pott's puffy tumor is a subperiosteal abscess of the frontal bone that was first identified by Sir Percivall Pott in 1760. It is usually accompanied by frontal osteomyelitis and clinically appears as swelling over the forehead. This entity was classically described as being secondary to trauma, although it is more frequently associated with sinusitis. Pott himself stated that symptoms "appear some few days after the head has suffered injury from external mischief."[16] Other risk factors include dental sepsis, chronic cocaine use, and neurosurgical complications.[17]

Overall, Pott's puffy tumor has become relatively infrequent most likely due to current antibiotic treatment regimens for sinusitis. It can be a complication of either acute or chronic sinusitis, and is more common in adolescents and young adults. The age predilection is perhaps due to frontal sinus growth and peak vasularlity of the diploic system, a set of thin-walled valveless veins that drain the frontal sinuses, seen in adolescence.[17] Sinus infection can travel hematogenously through these veins to the frontal bone, or occasionally to intracranial or orbital regions.[18]

The most common pathogens associated with Pott's puffy tumor are *S. aureus*, *Streptococcus* species, and oral anaerobes. Symptoms typically are mild, including headache with or without fever. The characteristic "puffy" lesion arises when the infection pushes through the outer frontal bone and develops an abscess between the bone and the periosteum, resulting in a tender and erythematous swelling at the middle forehead region.[17] CT is the best choice for imaging, although MRI is indicated if concerns for concomitant intracranial complications are present. Surgical intervention (drainage and debridement) is necessary, and since this condition is osteomyelitis, at least 6 weeks of IV antibiotics should be administered.

*Orbital*

Infection most commonly spreads from the sinus to the orbit. Orbital infection secondary to sinusitis is the leading cause of childhood unilateral proptosis.[19] The organisms most frequently associated with orbital complications include *Streptococcus* species, *Staphylococcus* species, anaerobes and Gram-negative bacilli.

*Periorbital Cellulitis* Periorbital cellulitis, which is also referred to as preseptal cellulitis or inflammatory edema, is the most common orbital complication, making up 70% of these complications.[20] The development of periorbital cellulitis is the end result of the obstructed sinus blocking venous and lymphatic drainage. Physical examination reveals eyelid erythema, edema, and tenderness to palpation. There are no visual/ophthalmic findings; the individual has normal visual acuity, normal intraocular pressure, no pupil abnormalities, fully functional extraocular motions, and no proptosis. If intracranial complications are suspected based on the clinical presentation or if any abnormal ophthalmic findings occur in 24–48 hours after therapy has been initiated, a CT scan is imperative for further evaluation.[21] Treatment is most often initiated on an outpatient basis with oral antibiotics, warm packs, and head elevation. Close follow-up must occur to ensure that no further complications are developing and the infection is responding to treatment.[22]

*Orbital Cellulitis* Orbital cellulitis is defined as an infection within the orbit, and behind the orbital septum. Orbital swelling follows increased venous pressure in the sinus, which then places pressure on the orbital blood vessels. Findings include eyelid swelling, chemosis, and mild proptosis. Orbital pain is present in 85% of the patients.[23] Visual changes are usually absent. Ophthalmologic consultation should be obtained for complete evaluation when this condition is suspected. Contrast-enhanced CT is the most common imaging modality used for diagnostic purposes. Patients with this complication are admitted for administration of intravenous antibiotics and for serial ophthalmic evaluations, monitoring for changes in visual acuity, pupil activity, color vision, and extraocular movements.[24] Surgical intervention is indicated in cases of visual acuity of 20/60 or worse on initial presentation (when visual acuity was better than this at baseline), presence of an abscess on CT, severe orbital findings (such as pupil abnormalities or blindness) on initial presentation, a worsening clinical picture, or lack of improvement within 48 hours despite antibiotic treatment.[21]

*Subperiosteal Abscess* Subperiosteal abscess is most often associated with infection of the ethmoid sinus, when the infection expands through the ethmoid foramina. Fluid builds up in the subperiosteal space and can cause blindness as it expands by elevating intraorbital pressure, compressing the optic nerve directly, or stretching the optic nerve with proptosis.[24] High suspicion for subperiosteal abscess should arise when someone with orbital cellulitis has worsening proptosis or decreased extraocular mobility. Increased intraorbital pressure can lead to color-blindness before loss of visual acuity, so color vision testing may be a better marker of progression.[19] CT is the diagnostic test of choice, and ophthalmology consultation is crucial, since the decision about whether to pursue medical versus surgical approaches is at times controversial.[24]

*Orbital Abscess* When sinusitis is present, progression to orbital abscess is most often associated with a delay in diagnosis and/or treatment, or is seen in a patient with a compromised immune system. Patients present with significant proptosis, ophthalmoplegia, chemosis, and visual changes. Purulent discharge may even be visualized from the eyelid. CT scans will show marked proptosis and sometimes even gas formation. Surgical drainage is the most important treatment, although the condition may progress to irreversible blindness before intervention occurs.[24]

*Intracranial*

Complications affecting the intracranial region are rare but can be particularly dangerous. Mortality associated with intracranial complications of sinusitis has declined to an estimated 4%, but morbidity ranges from 13–35%, and includes impaired cognition, epilepsy, cranial nerve palsy, hydrocephalus, visual/hearing loss, and other long-term neurologic deficits.[24] Major intracranial complications, due to direct extension of the infection, include meningitis, cavernous sinus thrombosis, epidural abscess, intracerebral abscess, superior sagittal sinus thrombosis and subdural abscess, with the latter the most commonly reported intracranial complication.[25]

Although the intracranial complications of sinusitis in children and adolescents typically occur in the setting of acute sinusitis, in adults such complications are more commonly found with chronic sinusitis. Intracranial complications also can occur together with extracranial complications, particularly orbital infections.[24]

Extension from the orbit is a common factor leading to intracranial complications, particularly in children over 7 years of age, CT scan findings of frontal sinus opacification, delayed response to therapy, male sex, African-American race, and surgical drainage of an orbital abscess.[26]

*Subdural Abscess* Subdural abscess usually follows an infection of the ethmoid or frontal sinus.[24] It is a particularly devastating complication, with mortality as high as 25%, and with additional morbidity of 30% among those who survive.[27] Symptoms include headache, neck stiffness, and fever, mimicking symptoms of meningitis. This is important to consider because lumbar puncture is contraindicated in patients with subdural abscesses due to increased intracranial pressure.[28] Subdural abscess can progress quickly to more profound neurologic findings such as altered consciousness or focal deficits.[24] Seizures are more common with this condition than any other intracranial complication.[27] An MRI with gadolinium contrast is the diagnostic tool of choice.[29] Treatment involves surgical drainage and broad-spectrum antibiotics. Since seizures are commonly associated with this condition, prophylactic use of anticonvulsants is also sometimes recommended.[24]

*Epidural Abscess* Although epidural abscess is almost exclusively seen following infections of the frontal sinus, it is among the more common intracranial complications and is associated with less morbidity. Presenting symptoms are often mild, including headache, fever, and scalp pain and may take weeks to develop. The diagnosis is usually made with contrast CT, although imaging is often delayed due to the paucity of symptoms. While the condition does require surgical drainage and broad-spectrum intravenous antibiotics, the long-term prognosis is good.[24] *S. aureus* and *Streptococci* are the most common pathogens.[27]

*Intracerebral Abscess* Intracerebral abscess most often follows frontal sinusitis, but the complication may also occur in association with sphenoid or ethmoid sinusitis.[27] A nonspecific headache followed by an asymptomatic period is a common prodrome. As the abscess enlarges, the headache recurs and other neurologic findings, such as seizures and focal deficits, may appear.[30] Imaging provides the definitive diagnosis and MRI is the best imaging modality. As in the case of subdural abscess, lumbar puncture can be life-threatening, with the risks far outweighing any diagnostic value.[24] Treatment involves surgical drainage and broad-spectrum antibiotics. Mortality of the condition ranges from 20–30% with neurologic and developmental morbidity of up to 60% among survivors.[27]

## Meningitis

Meningitis most commonly occurs after infection of the ethmoid or sphenoid sinuses, and *S. pneumoniae* is the organism most frequently associated with this complication.[31] Although a detailed discussion of meningitis is included in another section of this publication, it is important to note that when meningitis is a complication of sinusitis, the classic findings of meningitis are seen in addition to those of sinusitis—the latter of which actually may have been the original reason the patient sought medical care.

*Venous Sinus Thrombosis* Venous sinus thrombosis is most commonly seen following sphenoid, ethmoid, and frontal sinuses involvement since these sinuses are in close proximity to the cavernous sinus or the superior sagittal sinus. Cavernous sinus thrombosis is quite devastating and can progress rapidly to meningitis, vision loss, and even death, despite the correct diagnosis and treatment.[24] Symptoms include bilateral orbital involvement, often within 24 hours of the initial presentation, due to posterior extension of phlebitis into the cavernous sinus. Other findings include high fever, chemosis/ophthalmoplegia, and retinal engorgement with resultant papilledema and/or retinal hemorrhages noted on examination.[32] Contrast CT can show irregular filling in the cavernous sinus, but MRI and magnetic resonance venograms are more sensitive diagnostic modalities.[24] Although *S. aureus* is the most commonly identified causative agent, broad-spectrum intravenous antibiotic coverage is needed to treat both anaerobes and aerobes, as well as methicillin-resistant *S. aureus*. Surgical drainage is also indicated in most cases.[24] Since this is a thrombotic condition, the use of anticoagulation has been considered, although its efficacy is still unproven.[32]

## Prevention

A 2007 task force for adult sinusitis suggest that simple measures including handwashing, especially when in contact with ill individuals, and elimination of smoking can significantly decrease the risk of developing sinusitis.[1] In patients with sinus disease that has required surgical intervention, postsurgical use of nasal saline irrigation has been found to decrease the risk of recurrence of sinus disease. The benefits of irrigation seem to be decreased edema in the nasal mucosa, enhanced mucociliary function, and rinsing of allergens and infectious debris.[33]

In patients who present with multiple episodes of sinusitis or in cases of sinusitis that respond poorly to treatment, investigation for potential presence of previously discussed underlying conditions should be instigated. To date, no vaccine has been associated with a decrease in sinus infections. However, routine vaccinations should be administered to all adolescents, including annual influenza immunizations as the decrease in influenza may have a secondary drop in sinusitis by preventing the ciliary dysfunction and local tissue damage associated with acute influenza.[4]

## CONCLUSIONS

Acute sinusitis is a very commonly encountered condition in the primary care setting, particularly among adolescent populations. The astute clinician will be able to recognize the clinical signs and symptoms suggestive of the diagnosis, understand the treatment options, and be cognizant of the potential complications that may arise. In addition, clinicians should understand when specialist referral is indicated, especially when complications are present. In the vast majority of cases, acute sinusitis can be readily handled in primary care offices. However, complications can be devastating when present, so providers should consider these complications when treatment options fail.

# REFERENCES

1. Rosenfeld RM, Andes D, Bhattacharyya N, et al. Clinical practice guideline: Adult sinusitis. *Otolaryngol Head Neck Surg*. 2007;137:S1–S31
2. Slavin RG, Spector SL, Bernstein IL. The diagnosis and management of sinusitis: A practice parameter update. *J Allergy Clin Immunol*. 2005;116:S13–S47
3. Ray NF, Baraniuk JN, Thamer M, et al. Healthcare expenditures for sinusitis in 1996: Contributions of asthma, rhinitis, and other airway disorders. *J Allergy Clin Immunol*. 1999;103:408–414
4. DeMuri GP, Wald ER. Sinusitis. In: *Mandell, Douglas, and Bennett's Principles and Practice of Infectious Diseases, 7th Ed.* Philadelphia, PA: Churchill Livingston; 2009
5. Jones N. The nose and paranasal sinuses physiology and anatomy. *Adv Drug Deliv Rev*. 2001;51:5–19
6. Alho OP. Nasal airflow, mucociliary clearance, and sinus functioning during viral colds: Effects of allergic rhinitis and susceptibility to recurrent sinusitis. *Am J Rhinol*. 2004;18:349–355
7. Brook I. Acute and chronic bacterial sinusitis. *Infect Dis Clin N Am*. 2007;21:427–448
8. Leung RS, Katial R. The diagnosis and management of acute and chronic sinusitis. *Prim Care Clin Office Pract*. 2008;35:11–24
9. Gwaltney JM Jr, Hayden FG. Psychological stress and the common cold. *N Engl J Med*. 1992;326:644–646
10. George DL, Falk PS, Umberto Meduri G, et al. Nosocomial sinusitis in patients in the medical intensive care unit: A prospective epidemiological study. *Clin Infect Dis*. 1998;27:463–470
11. Williams JW Jr, Simel DL, Roerts L, et al. Clinical evaluation for sinusitis. Making the diagnosis by history and physical examination. *Ann Intern Med*. 1992;117(9):705–710
12. Centers for Disease Control and Prevention. Acute Bacterial Rhinosinusitis information sheet. Available at: http://www.cdc.gov/getsmart/campaign-materials/info-sheets/adult-acute-bact-rhino.pdf. Accessed February 9, 2010
13. Piccirillo JF. Acute bacterial sinusitis. *N Engl J Med*. 2004;351:902–910
14. Haloi AK, Ditchfield M, Maixner W. Mucocele of the sphenoid sinus. *Pediatr Radiol*. 2006;36(9);987–990
15. Eggesbo HB. Radiological imaging of inflammatory lesions in the nasal cavity and paranasal-sinuses. *Eur Radiol*. 2006;16(4);872–888
16. Pott P. *Observations on the nature of consequences of wounds and contusions of the head, fractures of the skull, concussions of the brain*. London, UK: Hitch & Lowes, 1760:38–58
17. Forgie SE, Marrie TJ. Pott's puffy tumor. *Am J Med*. 2008;121(12);1041–1042
18. Lang EE, Curran AJ, Pati N, et al. Intracranial complications of acute frontal sinusitis. *Clin Otolaryngol*. 2001;26:452–457
19. Osguthorpe JD, Hochman M. Inflammatory sinus diseases affecting the orbit. *Otolaryngol Clin North Am*. 1993;26(4):657–671
20. Goldberg AN, Oroszlan G, Anderson TD. Complications of frontal sinusitis and their management. *Otolaryngol Clin North Am*. 2001;34(1):211–225
21. Younis RT, Lazar RH, Bustillo A, et al. Orbital infection as a complication of sinusitis: Are diagnostic and treatment trends changing? *Ear Nose Throat J*. 2002;81(11):771–775

22. Donahue SP, Schwartz G. Preseptal and orbital cellulitis in childhood: A changing microbiologic spectrum. *Ophthalmology*. 1998;105(10):1902–1905
23. Jackson K, Baker SR. Clinical implications of orbital cellulitis. *Laryngoscope*. 1986;96(5):568–574
24. Epstein VA, Kern RC. Invasive fungal sinusitis and complications of rhinosinusitis. *Otolaryngol Clin N Am*. 2008;41:497–524
25. Singh B, Van Dellen J, Ramjettan S, Maharaj TJ. Sinogenic intracranial complications. *J Laryngol Otol*. 1995;109:945–950
26. Herrmann BW, Forsen JW Jr Simultaneous intracranial and orbital complications of acute rhinosinusitis in children. *Int J Pediatr Otorhinolaryngol*. 2004;68(5):619–625
27. Younis RT, Lazar RH, Anand VK. Intracranial complications of sinusitis: A 15-year review of 39 cases. *Ear Nose Throat J*. 2002;81:636–638
28. Jones NS, Walker JL, Bassi S, et al. The intracranial complications of rhinosinusitis: Can they be prevented? *Laryngoscope*. 2002;112:59–63
29. Osborn MK, Steinberg JP. Subdural empyema and other suppurative complications of paranasal sinusitis. *Lancet Infect Dis*. 2007;7(1):62–67
30. Clayman GL, Adams GL, Paugh DR, et al. Intracranial complications of paranasal sinusitis: A combined institutional review. *Laryngoscope*. 1991;101(3):234–239
31. Younis RT, Anand VK, Childress C. Sinusitis complicated by meningitis: Current management. *Laryngoscope*. 2001;111(8):1338–1342
32. Cannon ML, Antonio BL, McCloskey JJ, et al. Cavernous sinus thrombosis complicating sinusitis. *Pediatr Crit Care Med*. 2004;5(1):86–88
33. Friedman M, Vidyasagar R, Joseph N. A randomized, prospective, double-blinded study on the efficacy of dead sea salt nasal irrigations. *Laryngoscope*. 2006;116:878–882

# Adolescent Pneumonia

Elizabeth P. Schlaudecker, MD[*,a], Robert W. Frenck Jr, MD[a]

[a]*Division of Infectious Diseases, Cincinnati Children's Hospital Medical Center, Cincinnati, OH 45229*

Despite advances in antibiotic treatment and prevention, pneumonia, an acute infection of the pulmonary parenchyma, continues to have a significant impact on adolescent health. Mortality remains low, but pneumonia is associated with significant morbidity at considerable cost to our health care system.

The first section of this article focuses on general principles of pneumonia in adolescents, including epidemiology, pathogenesis, etiology, clinical manifestations, radiography, laboratory evaluation, management, complications, and prevention. The final section covers individual pathogens associated with pneumonia in adolescents, including recent updates in diagnosis, management, and prevention of these agents.

## General Principles

*Epidemiology*

On an annual basis in the United States, pneumonia is estimated to occur in up to 2.6% of children <17 years of age and in ~7 per 1000 adolescents 12–15 years of age.[1,2] Despite this high incidence, pneumonia mortality in the developed world is <1 child per 1000 annually.[3] In contrast, pneumonia remains the leading cause of childhood deaths in the developing world, with an estimated 2 million deaths annually.

In temperate climates, the incidence of pneumonia is markedly increased in the winter months, attributed to enhanced person-to-person respiratory droplet spread in addition to impaired mucociliary clearance in dry indoor air. The increased number of viral infections in the winter months leads to primary viral pneumonias, as well as secondary bacterial pneumonias.

Risk factors for the development of pneumonia include tobacco use and alcohol consumption, presumably by impairing mucociliary clearance and causing aspi-

---

*Corresponding author.
*E-mail address*: michele.dritz@cchmc.org, elizabeth.schlaudecker@cchmc.org (E. P. Schlaudecker).

Copyright © 2010 American Academy of Pediatrics. All rights reserved. ISSN 1934-4287

ration, respectively.[4] Despite educational campaigns, it is estimated that ~100 000 young people daily start smoking worldwide.[5] Other risk factors associated with an increased risk of pneumonia and its complications include sickle cell disease, asthma, cystic fibrosis, and immunodeficiency syndromes. Seizure disorders and neuromuscular disorders are associated with an increased pneumonia risk secondary to aspiration.

*Pathogenesis*

Upper respiratory infections are usually the precursor to lower respiratory tract infections. Organisms are typically spread by close contact, person-to-person respiratory droplets, or contaminated fomites. Organisms may colonize the nasopharynx and be inhaled, or an initial bacteremia may lead to a pulmonary focus of infection.

The pulmonary defense system consists of multiple mechanical barriers, including nasal hair, mucociliary clearance, saliva, the epiglottis, and the cough reflex. Immunoglobulins play a role in microbial killing, whereas cell-mediated immunity attacks certain pathogens. Adaptive and innate immune responses both play important roles in the defense against pneumonia.

## Etiology

Etiologic agents associated with pneumonia (Table 1) are often categorized by the age of the child (ie, infant, toddler, or school-age), with adolescents commonly included as part of the school-age group. The wide age range associated with "school age" makes it difficult to discern the frequency of various pathogens occurring

Table 1
Common causes of pneumonia in adolescents

| Pathogen | Unique Features |
| --- | --- |
| Parainfluenza, influenza, human metapneumovirus, adenovirus, rhinovirus | More common in toddlers |
| *Streptococcus pneumoniae* | Complications, including empyema, are common |
| *Mycoplasma pneumoniae* | Major cause in adolescents Radiographic findings vary |
| *Chlamydophila (Chlamydia) pneumoniae* | Common in school-aged children as well as adolescents |
| *Staphylococcus aureus* | Formally uncommon, but methicillin-resistant *Staphylococcus aureus* is rising in prevalence |
| *Mycobacterium tuberculosis* | Major concern in areas with high prevalence of tuberculosis or human immunodeficiency virus |

among adolescents. Etiologic studies are also influenced by regional and seasonal variation of pathogens associated with pneumonia. Lastly, the microbiologic diagnosis of pneumonia is typically based on indirect methods such as nasopharyngeal culture, blood culture, polymerase chain reaction (PCR), and serology, as direct diagnosis requires obtaining lung tissue through invasive techniques. With these caveats, when aggressively pursued, a specific etiology for the pneumonia has been reported in 79% to 85% of patients tested.[6,7] A brief review of the major organisms associated with pneumonia in adolescents will be described later in this review.

**Clinical Manifestations**

In all age groups, fever and cough are the hallmark symptoms of pneumonia.[3] Tachypnea and other signs of respiratory distress may be absent or mild unless there is significant disease or pleural effusions. The World Health Organization (WHO) uses tachypnea and retractions to effectively diagnose pneumonia in children under the age of 5 years,[8] but tachypnea becomes much less sensitive and specific as age increases.[9] A recent study demonstrated a lack of predictive value of tachypnea in the diagnosis of children under the age of 5 years.[10] However, children with tachypnea as defined by the WHO's respiratory rate thresholds were more likely to have pneumonia than children without tachypnea.

Both viral and bacterial pneumonias are often preceded by a few days of low-grade fever and upper respiratory tract illness symptoms. However, the onset of bacterial pneumonia may be abrupt and severe. Cough often occurs later in the course of disease when debris from the infected lung is swept into the upper airway.

Auscultation is also limited by low sensitivity and specificity. Crackles and bronchial breathing are reported to have a sensitivity of 75% but a specificity of only 57%.[11] Wheezing is also a poor predictor of clinical pneumonia, although it may be present in young children with bronchiolitis. A recent study conducted in a pediatric emergency department demonstrated a very low rate of pneumonia (2.2%) among afebrile children 21 years of age or younger presenting with wheezing.[12] This article discouraged the use of chest radiography in the diagnosis of children with wheezing but no fever.

Various clinical prediction models have been developed to assist in the diagnosis of pneumonia.[13,14] However, these models have focused on younger age groups and do not specifically address the diagnosis of pneumonia in adolescents. In general, a full history should include duration of illness, respiratory symptoms, and history of fever, headache, abdominal pain, sore throat, myalgias, and lethargy. It is also important to focus on the patient's past medical history, including any recent illnesses or antibiotics, vaccination history, chronic illnesses, ill contacts, or other unusual exposures. A physical examination should include vital signs (temperature, pulse, respiratory rate, and oxygen saturation), in addition to a close observation of the adolescent's general appearance.

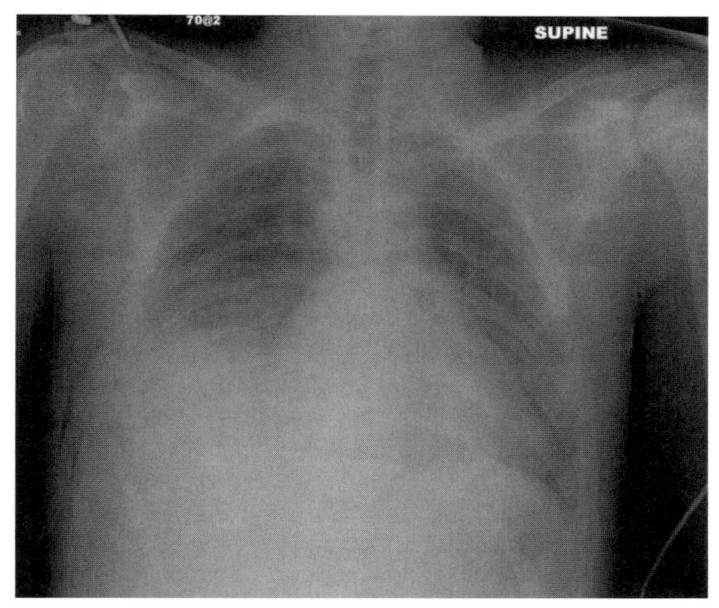

Fig 1. Supine chest radiograph demonstrating lobar pneumonia.

## Radiography

Chest radiography does not change the clinical outcome for most pediatric or adolescent patients when they are being treated in an outpatient setting.[3] A recent systematic review evaluated two trials, one with 522 outpatient children and one with 1502 adults presenting to an emergency department.[15] This review concluded that there is no evidence that chest radiography improves outcome in outpatients with acute lower respiratory infection. However, chest radiography is important in patients who have chronic or recurrent disease, or if complications such as significant pleural effusion are suspected on physical examination. A chest radiograph may also assist with diagnosis in febrile adolescents who have no discernible source of infection (Figure 1).

## Laboratory Evaluation

Elevated white blood cell or neutrophil counts, erythrocyte sedimentation rate (ESR), and C-reactive protein (CRP) are associated with more invasive infections, such as complicated bacterial pneumonia (Table 2). Complete blood count with differential, ESR, and CRP therefore are not recommended in the routine outpatient setting.[16] Influenza and other viruses may also have a heightened inflammatory response, so acute-phase reactants cannot be used to predict bacterial versus viral disease.[17]

Table 2
Diagnosis of pneumonia in adolescents

| Laboratory Test | Unique Features |
| --- | --- |
| Complete blood count with differential, erythrocyte sedimentation rate and C-reactive protein | Important for following response to therapy; cannot predict bacterial versus viral |
| Blood culture | Very specific but not sensitive |
| Diagnostic thoracentesis, lung biopsy, or other sampling technique | May be beneficial in seriously ill patients or patients with complications |
| Nasopharyngeal samples | Excellent for viral polymerase chain reaction |
| Mycoplasma serology | Good sensitivity but varying specificity |
| Chlamydophila (Chlamydia) pneumoniae culture, serology, polymerase chain reaction | Not readily available |
| Purified protein derivative | Used in high-risk situations |

*Diagnosis of Bacterial Pneumonia*

Because the finding of organism in the nasopharynx or sputum does not correlate well with the etiology of bacterial pneumonia, cultures from the sites can be problematic, resulting in the use of blood cultures to try to determine the bacterial etiology. Although blood cultures are insensitive, when they are positive, they provide a specific diagnosis and can guide therapy. A prospective, observational, cohort study of 414 adults presenting to an emergency department analyzed patients with radiographic evidence of pneumonia, clinical evidence of pneumonia, and blood cultures.[18] Blood cultures were positive in only 29 of 414 (7.0%) cases, resulting in altered therapy for only 15 patients (3.6%), of which 4 (1.0%) had their therapy broadened due to antibiotic resistance to empiric therapy.

A diagnostic thoracocentesis should be considered in patients with pleural effusions.[16] Additionally, lung biopsy, bronchoalveolar lavage, and other surgical procedures may be necessary to confirm the diagnosis in seriously ill patients who are not responding to empiric therapy.

*Diagnosis of Other Pathogens*

If the patient's diagnosis is unclear and the treatment response is poor, other etiologies of pneumonia should be considered. These agents include *Histoplasma capsulatum, Coccidioides immitis, Blastomyces dermatitidis, Legionella pneumophila, Francisella tularensis, Pseudomonas pseudomallei, Brucella abortus, Leptospira, Chlamydophila psittaci, Coxiella burnetii*, and Hantavirus.[19]

## Management

Choice of antibiotic in the treatment of pneumonia in adolescents is largely based on severity of disease. Because the etiologic agent is usually difficult to deter-

Table 3
Outpatient and inpatient treatment of adolescent pneumonia

| Antibiotic | Comments |
| --- | --- |
| First-line therapy for outpatients | |
| Azithromycin | Covers *Mycoplasma pneumoniae, Chlamydophila (Chlamydia) pneumoniae*, and most *Streptococcus pneumoniae* |
| Second-line therapy for outpatients | |
| Doxycycline | Covers atypical organisms |
| Levofloxacin | Not yet approved for younger adolescents, but highly effective against *M. pneumoniae, C. pneumoniae, S. pneumoniae, Legionella* |
| First-line therapy for inpatients | |
| Ampicillin | Less commonly used now |
| Cephalosporins | Usually able to overcome resistance to *S. pneumoniae* |
| PLUS | |
| Azithromycin | Covers atypical organisms |
| Second-line therapy for inpatients | |
| Vancomycin | Covers methicillin-resistant *Staphylococcus aureus* (MRSA) |
| Clindamycin | Provides additional anaerobic coverage and also covers MRSA |
| Linezolid | Broad-spectrum coverage, including MRSA |

mine, therapy is usually empiric and based on likely etiologies in the adolescent population (Table 3). For patients over the age of 5 years, a macrolide is the treatment of choice for community-acquired pneumonia.[16] Both macrolides and doxycycline are highly effective in treating atypical organisms, such as *Mycoplasma* or *Chlamydophila pneumoniae*. A macrolide may also treat *Streptococcus pneumoniae*, thereby providing therapy for the majority of etiologic agents in adolescent pneumonia. Recommended treatment duration is 7–10 days, although a 5-day course of azithromycin may be used.[20,21]

If pyogenic bacterial pneumonia is suspected, initial treatment with intravenous ampicillin is appropriate.[19] However, decreasing penicillin susceptibility in *S. pneumoniae* isolates has led more and more experts to recommend cefuroxime, ceftriaxone, cefotaxime, or ampicillin-sulbactam for empiric therapy.[3,16,22] However, penicillins and cephalosporins administered at appropriate doses are usually sufficient to overcome resistance and will treat penicillin-nonsusceptible *S. pneumoniae* organisms. In general, a $\beta$-lactam agent and a macrolide will provide broad coverage for adolescents with more severe pneumonia.

If pneumonia secondary to methicillin-resistant *Staphylococcus aureus* (MRSA) is suspected, or if the adolescent fails to respond to initial empiric therapy, the addition of vancomycin, clindamycin, or linezolid is recommended.[23] These antibiotics are also helpful in the setting of $\beta$-lactam allergy.

Fluoroquinolones, such as levofloxacin and moxifloxacin, may be used to treat pneumonia in older adolescents. These agents are highly effective against *S. pneumoniae, M. pneumoniae,* and *C. pneumoniae.* Fluoroquinolones are also very effective against *Legionella pneumophila,* a rare but potentially serious cause of pneumonia in this age group. While increasing data suggest quinolones are safe in children and adolescents, this class of drugs is not approved by the U.S. Food and Drug Administration (FDA) for routine use in patients under 18 years of age.[24]

## Hospitalization

Hypoxemia with oxygen saturation <92% is the most important indication for hospitalization, as these patients are at greatest risk of death. Other indications for hospitalization (Figure 2) include dehydration, respiratory distress, toxic appearance, poor oral intake, recurrent pneumonia, underlying medical condition, or less than optimal home situation.[3,16,19]

Adolescents admitted to the hospital should undergo chest imaging and laboratory tests, including complete blood count, blood culture, ESR, CRP, and renal panel. Adolescents are also usually capable of expectorating sputum, so sputum cultures may be beneficial in this setting. Hospitalization usually includes intravenous antibiotics with the support of oxygen therapy, fluid therapy, and fever management. Critically ill adolescents may require ventilatory support and supplementary nutrition.

## Complications

Effusions and empyemas are potential complications of pneumonia. A pleural effusion is the presence of fluid between the visceral and parietal pleurae. Parapneumonic effusions are inflammatory fluid collections adjacent to a pneumonic process, while an empyema is a parapneumonic fluid collection that has become purulent or seropurulent. Empyemas are associated with 3% of all pediatric hospitalizations[25] and up to one third of admissions for pneumococcal pneumonia.[26,27]

## Pleural Effusions

### Etiology of Pleural Effusions

*S. pneumoniae* is the most common causative organism for pleural effusions, though MRSA is emerging as a frequent cause of complicated parapneumonic effusions.[27,28] *S. pneumoniae* replaced methicillin-sensitive *Staphylococcus aureus* as the most common etiologic agent in the 1990s,[28] although *S. aureus* remains the most common cause of empyema in South Asia.[29] Recent data from the Kids' Inpatient Database, a national pediatric hospital discharge database for 2000, 2003, and 2006, demonstrated an increase in annual empyema-associated hospitalization rates in children, despite decreased rates of bacterial pneumonia

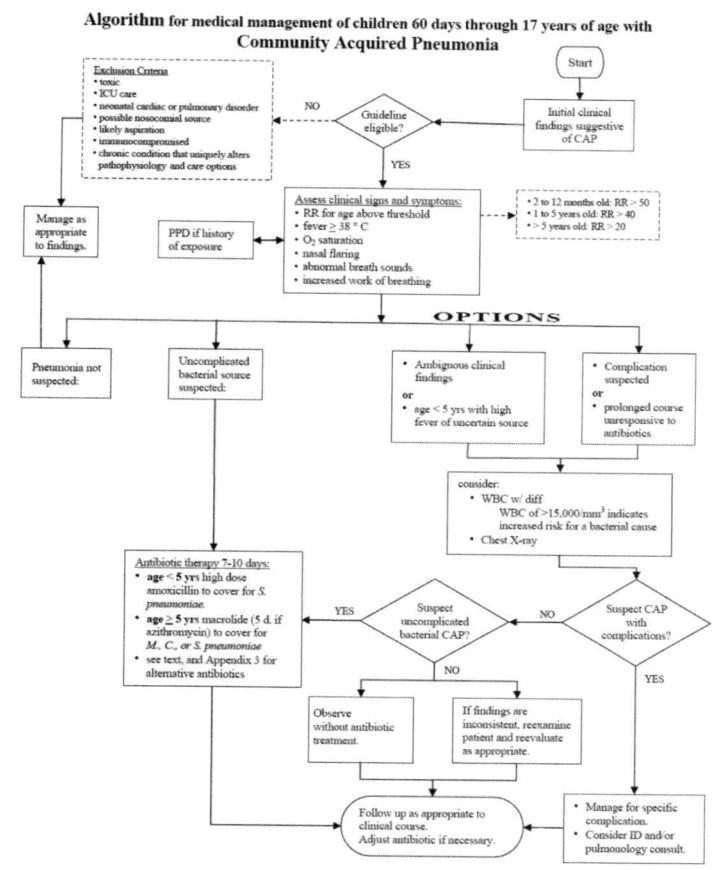

Fig 2. Algorithm for medical management of community acquired pneumonia. Adapted from **Community Acquired Pneumonia Guideline Team, Cincinnati Children's Hospital Medical Center:** Evidence-based care guideline for medical management of Community Acquired Pneumonia in children 60 days to 17 years of age, http://www.cincinnatichildrens.org/svc/alpha/h/health-policy/ev-based/pneumonia.htm, Guideline 14, pages 1–16, December 22, 2005.

and invasive pneumococcal disease.[30] However, the increased incidence of empyema did not extend to the adolescent population. Increasing age and white race are other risk factors associated with the development of empyema.[26,27]

*Radiography of Pleural Effusions*

The diagnosis and management of pleural effusions and empyemas are guided by imaging. Blunting of the costophrenic angle, thickening of the pleural shadow, and a subpulmonic density on chest radiograph all suggest pleural effusion.[19] Chest radiographs are very sensitive for the detection of pleural effusions, while chest ultrasounds are usually used in the management of pleural effusions. The

British Thoracic Society guidelines for the management of pediatric empyema recommend the use of chest ultrasound for guiding chest tube placement.[31] Chest computed tomography (CT) is not routinely necessary for identifying or managing pleural effusions. Chest ultrasound and chest CT are similar in their ability to detect loculated effusions and lung abscesses in the pediatric and adolescent population.[32] However, chest CT can be useful for diagnosing parenchymal disease not readily visible on chest radiographs or ultrasounds.

*Laboratory Evaluation of Pleural Effusions*

Pleural fluid should be analyzed with biochemical methods (pH, glucose, and lactate dehydrogenase), hematologic methods (white blood cell count and differential), special pathologic staining techniques, and culture. Effusions that require aggressive management can be identified by gross appearance of pus, or low pH ($<7.1$), a glucose level $<40$ mg/dL, and a lactate dehydrogenase concentration $>1000$ IU/mL.[19]

*Management of Pleural Effusions*

The best management of pleural effusions and empyemas in the pediatric and adolescent population remains controversial. Most studies have been conducted in the adult population; there has thus far been only one prospective, randomized trial comparing medical and operative management in the pediatric and adolescent populations.[33]

The traditional approach to management of pleural effusions and empyemas is to obtain a pleural fluid sample by needle aspiration, initiate antimicrobial medication, and observe the patient's clinical course. If the patient has persistent symptoms, toxicity, or respiratory compromise, a chest tube for drainage is recommended. Using the traditional approach, surgical intervention is only recommended in severe cases.

*Video-Assisted Thoracoscopic Surgery*

With the advent of the less invasive video-assisted thoracoscopic surgery (VATS), opinion is shifting to support surgical management. A prospective, randomized trial comparing VATS to thoracostomy tube drainage in children demonstrated a decrease in hospital length of stay, number of chest tube days, narcotic use, number of radiographic procedures, and interventional procedures in the patients who underwent primary VATS.[33] However, this study was limited by the small number of subjects[18] and the high prevalence of loculations on computed tomography scan of the chest (89%).

Two recent retrospective cohort studies and a meta-analysis support early VATS or thoracotomy in the treatment of empyema and complicated pneumonia. The first study used data from the Kids' Inpatient Database on 1173 patients aged 18 or younger. The use of early VATS or thoracotomy decreased length of stay, hospital charges, and likelihood of transfer to another short-term hospital, compared with nonoperative management.[34] The other study obtained data from the Pediatric Health Information System on all patients between 12 months and 18 years of age with complicated pneumonia.[35] Out of 2862 complicated pneumonia patients, 961 underwent early pleural fluid drainage, including chest tube placement, VATS, and thoracotomy. Compared with primary chest tube placement, primary VATS was associated with shorter length of stay and fewer procedural interventions. Similar findings were demonstrated in the systematic review comparing operative and nonoperative management, including a lower in-hospital mortality rate, a lower reintervention rate, decreased length of stay, decreased time with tube thoracostomy, and decreased time of antibiotic therapy in patients undergoing operative management.[36]

*Antimicrobial Therapy for Pleural Effusions*

Empiric therapy of complicated pneumonia in adolescents should treat *S. pneumoniae*, MRSA, and group A streptococcus. Coverage with doxycycline for atypical organisms, such as *Mycoplasma*, should be considered. Complicated pneumonia is usually treated for a minimum of 3–4 weeks, following inflammatory markers for response to treatment.

## Specific Agents of Pneumonia in Adolescents

*Bacterial Causes*

*Streptococcus pneumoniae* remains an important cause of pneumonia in adolescents. Invasive pneumococcal disease, including pneumonia, meningitis, and sepsis, result in almost 1 million childhood deaths annually, although largely in younger children.[37] The introduction of the 7-valent pneumococcal vaccine (PCV7) in late 2000 has dramatically decreased the number of pneumonia cases caused by pneumococcus. Initial vaccine uptake was slow but it is estimated that 93% of children born in 2006 had received 3 or more doses of PCV7 by 24 months of age.[38] Over the 10 years since the vaccine was introduced, invasive pneumococcal disease, including pneumonia, has dropped significantly in children in the United States.[39] As there have not been an aggressive catch-up vaccine campaign for pneumococcal immunization among adolescents, rates of disease elimination have not been as dramatic in this group. However, as the birth cohort ages, it is likely that significant drops in pneumococcal pneumonia will be noted among adolescents.

*S. pneumoniae* typically causes pyogenic pneumonia, and complications such as pleural effusion and empyema are common. Diagnosis is made by isolating the organism from blood or pleural fluid culture. Adolescents are often able to expectorate sputum for Gram-stain and culture. Rapid antigen tests, latex agglutination, and PCR assays are in development for the diagnosis of pneumococcal pneumonia. Rapid antigen tests have been used effectively in the diagnosis of pneumococcal meningitis,[40] but it is difficult to obtain pleural fluid for diagnosis of pneumonia. A rapid immunochromatographic test for the detection of the C polysaccharide antigen in pleural fluid has recently been shown to effectively diagnose pneumococcal pneumonia in children.[41]

Initial treatment with an oral macrolide is appropriate in the outpatient setting, offering additional coverage for *M. pneumoniae* and *C. pneumoniae*. For hospitalized patients, penicillins and cephalosporins administered at appropriate doses are usually sufficient to overcome resistance and treat $\beta$-lactam-nonsusceptible *S. pneumoniae* organisms.

There have been several significant trends in pneumococcal pneumonia over the past decade. First, the incidence of pneumococcal pneumonia has decreased dramatically. Invasive disease caused by all types of *S. pneumoniae* decreased by 43% from 1998–1999 to 2007.[38] Secondly, the incidence of invasive disease caused by serotype 19A increased significantly (212%), whereas other nonvaccine serotypes remained fairly stable in the 5- to 17-year-old age group.[38] The 19A serotype is now the most common serotype among all age groups.

On February 24, 2010, a 13-valent pneumococcal conjugate vaccine was licensed by the FDA for prevention of invasive pneumococcal disease caused by the 13 pneumococcal serotypes covered by the vaccine, including the 19A serotype.[42] This vaccine is recommended for children aged 6 weeks to 71 months and is expected to further decrease the incidence of invasive pneumococcal disease. With this new vaccine, the spectrum of serotypes may continue to change, although it is unclear if evolution of pneumococcal serotypes is secondary to vaccination or natural variation.

Once children reach school age, *Mycoplasma pneumoniae* and *Chlamydophila (Chlamydia) pneumoniae* become important pathogens. Both were thought to cause pneumonia primarily in adolescents and young adults, but new evidence suggests that *Mycoplasma* may be a significant cause of lower respiratory tract disease in young children as well.[43] However, the relative importance of *M. pneumoniae* as a causative agent increases with increasing age.

*C. pneumoniae* is also becoming increasingly prevalent in younger children.[44] One prospective, population-based study in Seattle demonstrated high incidences of acute infection in school-aged and adolescent individuals. The highest incidence was in 5- to 9-year-olds (9.2 per 100 person-years), followed by 10- to 14-year-olds (6.2 per 100 person-years) and 15- to 19-year-olds (2.2 per 100 person-years).[45] Additional studies to confirm these findings are needed.

*M. pneumoniae* can be detected most effectively via PCR; however, this test is not readily available. Cultures can take up to 3 weeks to become positive. Cold agglutinins (immunoglobulin M antibodies that agglutinate human red cells) are used to diagnose acute *M. pneumoniae* illness, but this test is not highly reliable. A positive result may occur due to infections such as adenovirus, influenza, Epstein-Barr virus, and cytomegalovirus. A cold agglutinin titer of 1:64 or greater has a high predictive value of infection, but low values do not eliminate *Mycoplasma* as a cause. An early study demonstrated that only 30–75% of individuals with *M. pneumoniae* pneumonia had detectable cold agglutinins during the acute phase of the illness.[46]

The most sensitive test that is readily available for the diagnosis of *M. pneumoniae* is serology for IgM and IgA antibodies, with sensitivities up to 92% reported in the literature.[47] However, specificity and reproducibility vary. The recent introduction of PCR opens the possibility for improved diagnosis of *M. pneumoniae*; however, this test continues to have limited availability in most clinical settings.[48]

*C. pneumoniae* can be diagnosed with serology, tissue culture, or PCR, although none of these tests may be readily available. The diagnosis is therefore largely based on clinical findings. New technologies, including different nucleic acid amplification techniques, are under investigation at this time.[49]

Although both macrolides and doxycycline are highly effective in treating these atypical organisms, a macrolide, due to ease of administration and safety profile, is typically the treatment of choice for both *M. pneumoniae* and *C. pneumoniae*.

Infections caused by methicillin-resistant *Staphylococcus aureus* (MRSA) have been increasingly reported worldwide. Several studies suggest that MRSA is replacing methicillin-susceptible *Staphylococcus aureus* (MSSA) as the leading cause of invasive infections.[50,51] In a recent study from Illinois, all children 18 years of age or younger with community-acquired *Staphylococcus aureus* infections were identified from a computer-assisted laboratory-based surveillance and medical record review.[52] Of 199 patients, 67 (34%) had invasive infections, and pneumonia with empyema was more likely to be caused by MRSA than by MSSA. A retrospective study conducted at a pediatric hospital in Texas identified all patients with complicated parapneumonic effusions discharged between January 1, 1994, and March 31, 2004.[28] No cases of MRSA were detected among the 36 cases of parapneumonic effusion that occurred between 1994 and 2001. However, between 2002 and 2004, 4 of 18 cases were caused by MRSA. This is in contrast from the late 1980s through the 1990s, when *S. pneumoniae* was found to be the most common cause of parapneumonic effusions.[27]

MRSA has demonstrated the ability to be resistant to all classes of antimicrobials. *S. aureus* acquired β-lactamase genes in the 1940s, and hospital-associated MRSA (HA-MRSA) has been spreading within hospital settings ever since. Community-associated MRSA (CA-MRSA) isolates are distinguished from HA-

MRSA by their lack of common risk factors for acquiring *S. aureus*. Additionally, due to different antibiotic resistance carried on the smaller staphylococcal chromosomal cassette (SCC) as compared with the SCC of HA-MRSA, most CA-MRSA isolates are susceptible to clindamycin, trimethoprim-sulfamethoxazole, and doxycycline (see MRSA chapter for more details). While hospitalized patients are at risk for HA-MRSA infections, higher rates of CA-MRSA colonization can be found in patients with dermatologic conditions, frequent needle use, indwelling intravascular devices, and health care employment.

MRSA is also a significant cause of necrotizing pneumonia following influenza infection. A recent study examined all pediatric patients admitted to Atlanta pediatric hospitals from October 2006 to April 2007 with laboratory-confirmed influenza or *S. aureus* cultured from a respiratory or sterile site.[53] Coinfected children were more frequently admitted to the intensive care unit (71%) than other patients with influenza (28%) or *S. aureus* (36%) alone. Coinfected children also had a significantly higher case fatality (29% coinfected, 0% influenza, 5% *S. aureus*).

*Mycobacterium tuberculosis* is the second leading cause of death from infectious diseases in the world.[54] From 1990 through 2003, the incidence of tuberculosis increased steadily around the world, predominantly in resource-poor countries.[55] This trend has clearly affected the incidence of tuberculosis in developed countries, as global migration has increased concurrently. A recent study analyzed tuberculosis screening and follow-up data among U.S.-bound immigrants and refugees from the Centers for Disease Control and Prevention (CDC). This study identified active cases of tuberculosis in immigrants and refugees between 1999 and 2005 who were diagnosed with smear-negative tuberculosis or inactive tuberculosis in their countries of origin.[56] Active pulmonary tuberculosis was diagnosed in 7.0% of immigrants and refugees with an overseas diagnosis of smear-negative tuberculosis and in 1.6% of those with an overseas diagnosis of inactive tuberculosis. Foreign-born persons, including adolescents, are clearly at high risk of having tuberculosis, despite overseas screening. Other populations at risk for tuberculosis include HIV-infected individuals and individuals in contact with infected adults. Additionally, adolescents are at higher risk of tuberculosis during puberty and in pregnancy.[3]

Multidrug resistant (MDR) tuberculosis is becoming a worldwide problem. A recent epidemiologic study identified drug susceptibility data on 90 726 patients in 83 countries and territories between 2002 and 2007.[57] The median prevalence of resistance to any drug in new cases of tuberculosis was 11.1%. China and the former countries of the Soviet Union had the highest prevalence of MDR tuberculosis, whereas data on drug resistance are largely unavailable in most African countries.

Placement of a purified protein derivative skin test with or without a control is recommended in adolescents with history of exposure to tuberculosis, including personal or family travel in areas with high tuberculosis prevalence.[58] On May 2, 2005, a new test, QuantiFERON-TB, received final approval from the FDA as an aid in diagnosing *M. tuberculosis* infection. This enzyme-linked immunosorbent assay test detects the release of interferon-γ in fresh blood from sensitized persons when it is incubated with mixtures of synthetic peptides simulating two proteins present in *M. tuberculosis*. These two proteins are secreted by all *M. tuberculosis* and pathogenic *M. bovis* strains. Because these proteins are absent from all Bacille Calmette-Guérin (BCG) vaccine strains and from commonly encountered nontuberculous mycobacteria, QuantiFERON is more specific for *M. tuberculosis*.[59]

The most recent guidelines and recommendations for treatment of latent tuberculosis in adolescents were published in 2004.[60] The recommended regimen is a 9-month course of isoniazid, and directly observed therapy (DOT) should be considered in high-risk social situations. With DOT, isoniazid may be given 2–3 times weekly. Rifampin alone has been used for the treatment of latent tuberculosis in adolescents when the patient is unable to tolerate or found to be resistant to isoniazid.

For adolescents specifically, few data exist for guiding recommendations about tuberculosis prevention. Adolescents probably differ from younger children in clinical manifestations of tuberculosis and in social issues related to treatment, but more research is needed in this area.

*Viral Causes of Adolescent Pneumonia*

Viruses make up the majority of cases of lower respiratory infection in preschool-age children and continue to cause a significant amount of disease in adolescents.[61] Influenza virus is most frequently associated with outbreaks resulting in medical consultation and increased mortality, and morbidity is most common in children and young adults.[62] As evidenced by the most recent H1N1 influenza virus epidemic, adolescents and young adults may be disproportionately hospitalized and affected by influenza disease.[63] A recent update from the CDC's *Morbidity and Mortality Weekly Report* reported 236 pediatric deaths secondary to H1N1 occurring between August 30, 2009, and January 9, 2010.[64] Of these 236 deaths, a total of 43 (18.2%) were among children aged <2 years, 26 (11.0%) were among children aged 2–4 years, 87 (36.9%) were among children aged 5–11 years, and 80 (33.9%) were among children aged 12–17 years. This recent H1N1 experience reiterates the concern that influenza outbreaks pose an increased risk to the adolescent population.

Other viral causes of pneumonia in adolescents include human metapneumovirus, parainfluenza viruses, adenoviruses, rhinoviruses, and enteroviruses. Coronavirus caused significant concern around the globe in 2003, causing the severe respiratory distress syndrome.[65] More recently, a member of the *Parvoviridae* family, human bocavirus, has been linked with respiratory tract disease in children.[66] Significant illness is usually found in children under the age of 12 months.

*Diagnosis of Viral Pneumonia*

Viruses are best identified by tissue culture or by detection of viral products in respiratory secretions. Combined real-time PCR is a highly sensitive and specific detection method when obtained properly. Nasopharyngeal washes or aspirates are the most sensitive specimens for PCR, as they contain infected epithelial cells. Many respiratory PCR panels are available for rapid diagnosis of multiple respiratory viruses, including influenza virus. In general, these studies are not recommended under most circumstances, as the results do not usually affect initial management decisions.[16]

## Prevention

Good hand-washing and good personal hygiene are important preventative measures for any infection spread by droplet or contact transmission. Limiting exposure to infected individuals and reducing exposure to cigarette smoke are also helpful.

*Immunization*

After their primary vaccination series, adolescents should be protected from pneumonia caused by *Haemophilus influenzae*, pertussis (see Chapter 4), and *S. pneumoniae*. The heptavalent pneumococcal vaccine has dramatically decreased the incidence of invasive pneumococcal disease, despite increasing rates of empyema hospitalizations.[30,38] Because viruses are often the direct cause of pneumonia, immunization against influenza is particularly helpful, especially in adolescents.

## CONCLUSION

Even in this age of immunizations and antibiotic treatment, pneumonia continues to have a significant impact on adolescent health. Mortality fortunately remains low, but pneumonia is associated with significant morbidity at considerable cost to our health care system. As we continue to combat this formidable illness, continued education and innovation is necessary to face each new challenge.

## REFERENCES

1. Niederman MS, McCombs JS, Unger AN, Kumar A, Popovian R. The cost of treating community-acquired pneumonia. *Clin Ther*. 1998;20(4):820–837
2. Murphy TF, Henderson FW, Clyde WA Jr, Collier AM, Denny FW. Pneumonia: an eleven-year study in a pediatric practice. *Am J Epidemiol*. 1981;113(1):12–21

3. Durbin WJ, Stille C. Pneumonia. *Pediatr Rev.* 2008;29(5):147-158
4. Garau J, Baquero F, Perez-Trallero E, et al. Factors impacting on length of stay and mortality of community-acquired pneumonia. *Clin Microbiol Infect.* 2008;14(4):322-329
5. Tanski SE, Prokhorov AV, Klein JD. Youth and tobacco. *Minerva Pediatrica.* 2004;56(6):553-565
6. Juven T, Mertsola J, Waris M, et al. Etiology of community-acquired pneumonia in 254 hospitalized children. *Pediatr Infect Dis J.* 2000;19(4):293-298
7. Michelow IC, Olsen K, Lozano J, et al. Epidemiology and clinical characteristics of community-acquired pneumonia in hospitalized children. *Pediatrics.* 2004;113(4):701-707
8. Sazawal S, Black RE. Effect of pneumonia case management on mortality in neonates, infants, and preschool children: a meta-analysis of community-based trials. *Lancet Infect Dis.* 2003;3(9):547-556
9. Palafox M, Guiscafre H, Reyes H, Munoz O, Martinez H. Diagnostic value of tachypnoea in pneumonia defined radiologically. *Arch Dis Childhood.* 2000;82(1):41-45
10. Shah S, Bachur R, Kim D, Neuman MI. Lack of predictive value of tachypnea in the diagnosis of pneumonia in children. *Pediatr Infect Dis J.* 2010;29(5):406-409
11. Smyth A, Carty H, Hart CA. Clinical predictors of hypoxaemia in children with pneumonia. *Ann Trop Paediatr.* 1998;18(1):31-40
12. Mathews B, Shah S, Cleveland RH, Lee EY, Bachur RG, Neuman MI. Clinical predictors of pneumonia among children with wheezing. *Pediatrics.* 2009;124(1):e29-e36
13. Donnelly LF. Practical issues concerning imaging of pulmonary infection in children. *J Thorac Imaging.* 2001;16(4):238-250
14. Mahabee-Gittens EM, Grupp-Phelan J, Brody AS, et al. Identifying children with pneumonia in the emergency department. *Clin Pediatrics.* 2005;44(5);427-435
15. Swingler GH, Zwarenstein M. Chest radiograph in acute respiratory infections. *Cochrane Database Syst Rev.* 2008(1):CD001268
16. Community Acquired Pneumonia Guideline Team. Evidence-based care guideline for medical management of Community Acquired Pneumonia in children 60 days to 17 years of age. Cincinnati, OH: Cincinnati Children's Hospital Medical Center; 2005:Guideline 14:1-16
17. Don M, Valent F, Korppi M, Canciani M. Differentiation of bacterial and viral community-acquired pneumonia in children. *Pediatr Int.* 2009;51(1):91-96
18. Kennedy M, Bates DW, Wright SB, Ruiz R, Wolfe RE, Shapiro NI. Do emergency department blood cultures change practice in patients with pneumonia? *Ann Emer Med.* 2005;46(5);393-400
19. Long SS, Pickering LK, Prober CG. *Principles and practice of pediatric infectious diseases.* 3rd ed. Philadelphia, PA: Churchill Livingstone; 2008
20. Wubbel L, Muniz L, Ahmed A, et al. Etiology and treatment of community-acquired pneumonia in ambulatory children. *Pediatric Infect Dis J.* 1999;18(2):98-104
21. Atkinson M, Yanney M, Stephenson T, Smyth A. Effective treatment strategies for paediatric community-acquired pneumonia. *Expert Opin Pharmacother.* 2007;8(8):1091-1101
22. McIntosh K. Community-acquired pneumonia in children. *N Engl J Med.* 2002;346(6):429-437
23. Jantausch BA, Deville J, Adler S, et al. Linezolid for the treatment of children with bacteremia or nosocomial pneumonia caused by resistant gram-positive bacterial pathogens. *Pediatr Infect Dis J.* 2003;22(9 Suppl):S164-S171
24. Bradley JS, Arguedas A, Blumer JL, Saez-Llorens X, Melkote R, Noel GJ. Comparative study of levofloxacin in the treatment of children with community-acquired pneumonia. *Pediatr Infect Dis J.* 2007;26(10):868-878
25. Clark JE, Hammal D, Spencer D, Hampton F. Children with pneumonia: how do they present and how are they managed? *Arch Dis Childhood.* 2007;92(5):394-398
26. Tan TQ, Mason EO Jr, Wald ER, et al. Clinical characteristics of children with complicated pneumonia caused by Streptococcus pneumoniae. *Pediatrics.* 2002;110(1 Pt 1):1-6
27. Byington CL, Spencer LY, Johnson TA, et al. An epidemiological investigation of a sustained high rate of pediatric parapneumonic empyema: risk factors and microbiological associations. *Clin Infect Dis.* 2002;34(4):434-440

28. Alfaro C, Fergie J, Purcell K. Emergence of community-acquired methicillin-resistant Staphylococcus aureus in complicated parapneumonic effusions. *Pediatr Infect Dis J.* 2005;24(3):274–276
29. Baranwal AK, Singh M, Marwaha RK, Kumar L. Empyema thoracis: a 10-year comparative review of hospitalised children from south Asia. *Arch Disease Childhood.* 2003;88(11):1009–1014
30. Li ST, Tancredi DJ. Empyema hospitalizations increased in US children despite pneumococcal conjugate vaccine. *Pediatrics.* 2010;125(1):26–33
31. Balfour-Lynn IM, Abrahamson E, Cohen G, et al. BTS guidelines for the management of pleural infection in children. *Thorax.* 2005;60 Suppl 1:i1–i21
32. Kurian J, Levin TL, Han BK, Taragin BH, Weinstein S. Comparison of ultrasound and CT in the evaluation of pneumonia complicated by parapneumonic effusion in children. *AJR Am J Roentgenol.* 2009;193(6);1648–1654
33. Kurt BA, Winterhalter KM, Connors RH, Betz BW, Winters JW. Therapy of parapneumonic effusions in children: video-assisted thoracoscopic surgery versus conventional thoracostomy drainage. *Pediatrics.* 2006;118(3);e547–e553
34. Li ST, Gates RL. Primary operative management for pediatric empyema: decreases in hospital length of stay and charges in a national sample. *Arch Pediatr Adolesc Med.* 2008;162(1):44–48
35. Shah SS, DiCristina CM, Bell LM, Ten Have T, Metlay JP. Primary early thoracoscopy and reduction in length of hospital stay and additional procedures among children with complicated pneumonia: results of a multicenter retrospective cohort study. *Arch Pediatr Adolesc Med.* 2008;162(7):675–681
36. Avansino JR, Goldman B, Sawin RS, Flum DR. Primary operative versus nonoperative therapy for pediatric empyema: a meta-analysis. *Pediatrics.* 2005;115(6):1652–1659
37. World Health Organization. Challenges in global immunization and the Global Immunization Vision and Strategy 2006–2015. Releve epidemiologique hebdomadaire/Section d'hygiene du Secretariat de la Societe des Nations. *Weekly Epidemiological Record/Health Section of the Secretariat of the League of Nations* 2006;81(19):190–195
38. Pilishvili T, Lexau C, Farley MM, et al. Sustained reductions in invasive pneumococcal disease in the era of conjugate vaccine. *J Infect Dis.* 2010;201(1):32–41
39. Whitney CG, Farley MM, Hadler J, et al. Decline in invasive pneumococcal disease after the introduction of protein-polysaccharide conjugate vaccine. *N Engl J Med.* 2003;348(18):1737–1746
40. Saha SK, Darmstadt GL, Baqui AH, et al. Identification of serotype in culture negative pneumococcal meningitis using sequential multiplex PCR: implication for surveillance and vaccine design. *PloS One.* 2008;3(10):e3576
41. Casado Flores J, Nieto Moro M, Berron S, Jimenez R, Casal J. Usefulness of pneumococcal antigen detection in pleural effusion for the rapid diagnosis of infection by Streptococcus pneumoniae. *Eur J Pediatr.* 2010;169(5):581–584
42. Centers of Disease Control and Prevention. Licensure of a 13-valent pneumococcal conjugate vaccine (PCV13) and recommendations for use among children - Advisory Committee on Immunization Practices (ACIP), 2010. *MMWR.* 2010;59(9):258–261
43. Korppi M, Heiskanen-Kosma T, Kleemola M. Incidence of community-acquired pneumonia in children caused by Mycoplasma pneumoniae: serological results of a prospective, population-based study in primary health care. *Respirology (Carlton, Vic.)* 2004;9(1):109–114
44. Esposito S, Bosis S, Cavagna R, et al. Characteristics of Streptococcus pneumoniae and atypical bacterial infections in children 2–5 years of age with community-acquired pneumonia. *Clin Infect Dis.* 2002;35(11);1345–1352
45. Aldous MB, Grayston JT, Wang SP, Foy HM. Seroepidemiology of Chlamydia pneumoniae TWAR infection in Seattle families, 1966–1979. *J Infect Dis.* 1992;166(3):646–649
46. Cassell GH, Cole BC. Mycoplasmas as agents of human disease. *N Engl J Med.* 1981;304(2):80–89
47. Blasi F, Tarsia P, Aliberti S, Cosentini R, Allegra L. Chlamydia pneumoniae and Mycoplasma pneumoniae. *Semin Respir Crit Care Med.* 2005;26(6):617–624

48. Vervloet LA, Marguet C, Camargos PA. Infection by Mycoplasma pneumoniae and its importance as an etiological agent in childhood community-acquired pneumonias. *Braz J Infect Dis.* 2007;11(5):507–514
49. Loens K, Beck T, Ursi D, et al. Evaluation of different nucleic acid amplification techniques for the detection of *M. pneumoniae, C. pneumoniae* and *Legionella spp.* in respiratory specimens from patients with community-acquired pneumonia. *J Microbiol Meth.* 2008;73(3);257–262
50. Moran GJ, Krishnadasan A, Gorwitz RJ, et al. Methicillin-resistant S. aureus infections among patients in the emergency department. *N Engl J Med.* 2006;355(7);666–674
51. Gonzalez BE, Hulten KG, Dishop MK, et al. Pulmonary manifestations in children with invasive community-acquired Staphylococcus aureus infection. *Clin Infect Dis.* 2005;41(5);583–590
52. Mongkolrattanothai K, Aldag JC, Mankin P, Gray BM. Epidemiology of community-onset Staphylococcus aureus infections in pediatric patients: an experience at a Children's Hospital in central Illinois. *BMC Infect Dis.* 2009;9:112
53. Reed C, Kallen AJ, Patton M, et al. Infection with community-onset Staphylococcus aureus and influenza virus in hospitalized children. *Pediatr Infect Dis J.* 2009;28(7);572–576
54. Frieden TR, Sterling TR, Munsiff SS, Watt CJ, Dye C. Tuberculosis. *Lancet.* 2003;362(9387): 887–899
55. Dye C, Watt CJ, Bleed DM, Hosseini SM, Raviglione MC. Evolution of tuberculosis control and prospects for reducing tuberculosis incidence, prevalence, and deaths globally. *JAMA.* 2005; 293(22):2767–2775
56. Liu Y, Weinberg MS, Ortega LS, Painter JA, Maloney SA. Overseas screening for tuberculosis in U.S.-bound immigrants and refugees. *N Engl J Med.* 2009;360(23);2406–2415
57. Wright A, Zignol M, Van Deun A, et al. Epidemiology of antituberculosis drug resistance 2002–07: an updated analysis of the Global Project on Anti-Tuberculosis Drug Resistance Surveillance. *Lancet.* 2009;373(9678);1861–1873
58. Alves dos Santos JW, Torres A, Michel GT, et al. Non-infectious and unusual infectious mimics of community-acquired pneumonia. *Respir Med.* 2004;98(6);488–494
59. Mazurek GH, Jereb J, Lobue P, Iademarco MF, Metchock B, Vernon A. Guidelines for using the QuantiFERON-TB Gold test for detecting Mycobacterium tuberculosis infection, United States. *MMWR Recomm Rep.* 2005;54(RR-15):49–55
60. Pediatric Tuberculosis Collaborative Group. Targeted tuberculin skin testing and treatment of latent tuberculosis infection in children and adolescents. *Pediatrics.* 2004;114:1175–1201
61. Henrickson KJ, Hoover S, Kehl KS, Hua W. National disease burden of respiratory viruses detected in children by polymerase chain reaction. *Pediatr Infect Dis J.* 2004;23(1 Suppl):S11–S18
62. Monto AS. Occurrence of respiratory virus: time, place and person. *Pediatr Infect Dis J.* 2004;23(1 Suppl):S58–S64
63. Louie JK, Acosta M, Winter K, et al. Factors associated with death or hospitalization due to pandemic 2009 influenza A(H1N1) infection in California. *JAMA.* 2009;302(17):1896–1902
64. Centers for Disease Control and Prevention. Update: influenza activity — United States, August 30, 2009–January 9, 2010. *MMWR.* 2010;59(2):38–43
65. Cooke FJ, Shapiro DS. Global outbreak of severe acute respiratory syndrome (SARS). *Int J Infect Dis.* 2003;7(2);80–85
66. Bastien N, Brandt K, Dust K, Ward D, Li Y. Human bocavirus infection, *Canada. Emerg Infect Dis.* 2006;12(5);848–850

# Pertussis in Adolescents and Its Prevention Using Tdap Vaccination

ChrisAnna Marie Mink, MD*[a], Sylvia Hsin-Hue Yeh, MD[a]

[a]Department of Pediatrics, Harbor-UCLA Medical Center 1124 W. Carson Street, Torrance, CA 90502

Pertussis (whooping cough) is a highly communicable respiratory disease of global importance. The World Health Organization (WHO) estimates that worldwide 20 to 40 million cases of pertussis occur annually, with over 90% occurring in developing nations where they have limited vaccinations. In industrialized nations with widespread use of pertussis vaccines, a dramatic decline in the overall number of pertussis cases has been observed; however, the incidence of disease in young infants, adolescents, and adults has significantly increased over the past 2 decades. Although infants <12 months of age, especially those <6 months, suffer the highest morbidity and mortality, pertussis may also cause significant morbidity in older age groups. Additionally, adolescents and adults are often identified as the source case of infection in young children. To improve protection against pertussis across a wider age spectrum, new vaccines and new vaccination policies are needed. With recent availability of reduced-dose acellular pertussis vaccines combined with diphtheria and tetanus toxoids (Tdap), immunization of older age groups is now possible. Ideally, use of Tdap boosters will afford better control of disease in adolescents and adults, leading to less pertussis in the community and lower risk for infection for all age groups.

## EPIDEMIOLOGY

*Bordetella pertussis*, a strictly human pathogen, is the most commonly recognized causative agent of whooping cough. In the prevaccine era, pertussis was a significant cause of childhood disease and infant mortality in the United States. Routine childhood vaccination led to a reduction in disease incidence from an average of 150 reported cases per 100 000 persons between 1922 and 1940 to all-time low of 0.5 per 100 000 in 1976 (Fig. 1).[1] In most countries, including the United States, pertussis is endemic, with 3- to 5-year epidemic cycles superimposed on the endemic rate. These epidemic cycles have been attributed to accumulation of a significant pool of

---

*Corresponding author.
*E-mail address*: cmink@labiomed.org (C. M. Mink).

Copyright © 2010 American Academy of Pediatrics. All rights reserved. ISSN 1934-4287

## Pertussis—United States, 1940-2007

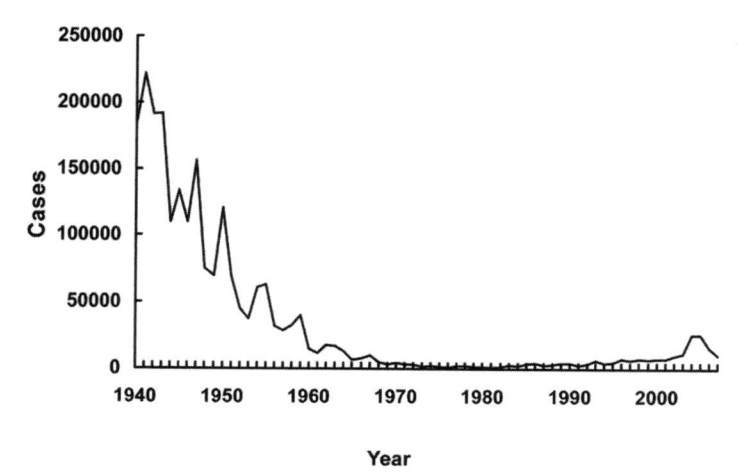

Fig 1. Epidemiology of pertussis in the United States, 1940–2007. (From: Centers for Disease Control and Prevention. Advisory Committee on Immunization Practices Vaccines for Children. Available at: www.cdc.gov/vaccines/programs/vfc/downloads/resolutions/1003hepb.pdf. Accessed June 25, 2010.)

susceptible individuals and have not been significantly altered in the postvaccination era, suggesting continuing circulation of *B. pertussis*.

Before widespread vaccinations in the United States, 85% of pertussis cases occurred in children ages 1–9 years, with only 10% of cases reported in infants.[2] Placentally acquired maternal antibodies likely provided protection for very young infants. With routine use of pertussis vaccines in infancy and early childhood in the United States, as well as other countries with high vaccine uptake, the burden of pertussis shifted from a disease of middle childhood to one primarily affecting young infants (who are too young to be immunized) and older children, adolescents and adults (who have waning immunity). Immunity elicited by pertussis vaccines is of short duration (~5–10 years); with decreased natural exposure to the organism, adults have decreased immunity and lower passive antibodies for transfer to infants. These factors contribute to the observed shift in age groups affected by pertussis.

Pertussis in older age groups is not a new phenomenon. One of the earliest reports of pertussis in adults was in 1902.[3] In 1934, Mannerstedt described pertussis in adults, including some individuals who had a history of pertussis during childhood.[4] This article was one of the first to suggest that immunity to *B. pertussis*, even after natural infection, was not lifelong.

Pertussis vaccines composed of whole killed cells of *B. pertussis* were first developed in the early 1900s and introduced into widespread use in 1940s.

Starting in 1948 in the United States, these whole-cell pertussis (wP) vaccines were combined with diphtheria and tetanus toxoids (DTwP) and were widely used. The wP vaccines were over 75% effective in reducing clinical disease in recipients, with an ensuing shift in the predominant age groups afflicted with pertussis. From the 1950s through the 1970s, few reports of adult pertussis are in the literature, with some notable exceptions of outbreaks in hospitals and other child-associated institutions.[5]

During the 1970s, with the decreasing number of clinical cases of pertussis in children, concerns about real and perceived adverse events associated with the whole-cell pertussis vaccine were growing. This led to two important consequences: 1) a decline in the acceptance of wP vaccinations and 2) an impetus for development of less reactogenic pertussis vaccines. In Japan, decreased acceptance of wP vaccines led to a 20-fold rise in reported pertussis cases. Subsequently, acellular pertussis (aP) vaccines containing more purified pertussis components were developed. Introduction of aP vaccines in Japan led to a decline in pertussis cases and attracted interest from other countries, including the United States. The first acellular vaccines were introduced in the United States for the preschool boosters in 1991 and for infant use in 1996, but no vaccines were available for individuals over 7 years old.[6]

In the 1980s, an increasing number of pertussis cases in adolescents and adults were reported. At that time, there were also increasing clinical recognition of atypical pertussis and improved capabilities for obtaining laboratory confirmation of pertussis. With both of these changes, it was difficult to know if the increasing disease rate in older individuals was a true increase or related to improved case identification. This debate continues, though both are likely factors. A true increase in adolescent disease is plausible as vaccine-induced immunity wanes, and this age group is less likely to have natural boosting of their immunity in the postvaccine era.

From 1996 through 2005, the annual number of reported pertussis cases increased from ~7800 to 25 616. Even with the rising number of cases, it is estimated that pertussis cases are significantly underreported. The Centers for Disease Control and Prevention estimates that at best one-third of pertussis cases are reported.[7] Although the incidence remained highest among infants younger than 12 months (~50 per 100 000), the rates reported in adolescents 10–19 years of age also rose (Fig. 2).[8,9] In 2002, 24% of all reported cases were among infants younger than 1 year of age and ~33% of cases were reported among adolescents and adults. From 2001 to 2003, the rate among adolescents 10–19 years old increased from 5.5 per 100 000 to 10.9. In 2004 and 2005, ~60% of reported cases (a total of 7,347 cases in 2005) were among persons 11 years of age and older.[10] During 2000 to 2006 in the United States, 27% of the reported 103 940 cases of pertussis occurred in individuals 15–39 years of age.

## Reported Pertussis by Age Group, 1990-2007

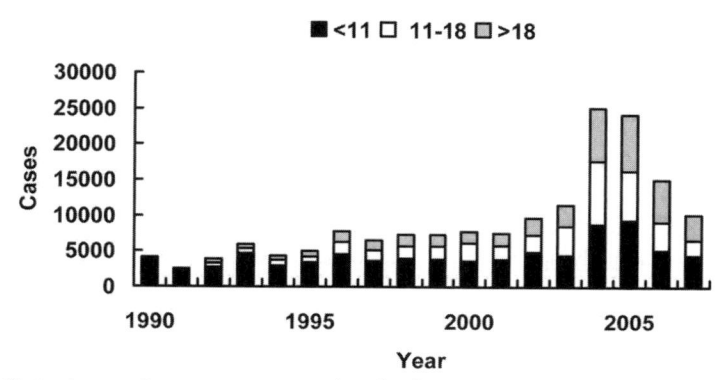

■ <11   □ 11-18   ▨ >18

Fig 2. Pertussis cases in age groups reported to the Centers for Disease Control and Prevention. (From: Centers for Disease Control and Prevention. Epidemiology and prevention of vaccine-preventable diseases. The Pink Book: Course Textbook (11th ed.). Available at: http://www.cdc.gov/vaccines/pubs/pinkbook/downloads/pert.pdf. Accessed February 21, 2010.)

Using seroprevalance studies, a peak in pertussis antibodies was observed in the 4- to 6-year-old age groups (correlating with the receipt of the fifth booster dose of DTaP), followed by a decline in titers among elementary school age groups. Another peak in antibodies was observed in teens 13–17 years of age.[11] The National Health and Nutrition Examination Survey seroprevalence study showed antibody peaks in similar age groups, with the addition of a peak in the 40- to 45-year-old adults (possibly the parents of the teenage group).[12] During the time of these studies, pertussis vaccines were not routinely given to children over 7 years old, so the peaks in the older age groups reflect an immune response from natural exposure to *B. pertussis*.

The true incidence of pertussis disease in adolescents and adults is unclear. Results of a prospective trial of a reduced dose acellular pertussis vaccine in adolescents and adults suggest that ~1 million cases of pertussis occur annually in persons over 15 years.[13] In investigations of coughing illnesses in adolescents and adults, ~20–30% of the illnesses were attributable to pertussis. Many of these cases are considered to be mild or atypical, and were not recognized clinically but were identified using serology.[14–17]

Adolescent and adult contacts are most often identified as the source of infection for young infants. In ~75% of infant pertussis cases, adolescent and adult household contacts, and most commonly the mother (~34%), were the source of infection. These adult contacts often had mild or unrecognized disease, and were not identified until after evaluation of the infant index case.[5,9,18,19]

## CLINICAL PRESENTATION

### Etiology

*Bordetella pertussis* is a small Gram-negative coccobacillus that attaches to the respiratory epithelium of humans. *B. pertussis* produces several virulence factors, but it is unknown which factor(s) contribute to the clinical symptoms or elicit a protective immune response. Many of the virulence factors have been identified and purified, and are components of the acellular pertussis vaccines. The four factors that have primarily been used in aP vaccines are pertussis toxin (PT), filamentous hemagglutinin (FHA), pertactin (PRN), and fimbriae (FIM). PT has a number of biological activities, including lymphocytosis induction, histamine sensitization, and adjuvancy; however, the role in clinical disease remains unknown. An immune response to PT affords some protection against clinical pertussis, but immunity to disease may be present in the absence of antibodies to PT.[6,11,12] FHA, PRN, and FIM antigens all have a role in adhesion of the bacteria to the host cells, and antibodies to these antigens may have a role in protection. Other biologically active components of *B. pertussis* include adenylate cyclase, tracheal cytotoxin, lipooligosaccharide, dermonecrotic toxin, and possibly others.

### Symptoms

*B. pertussis* is spread person-to-person via respiratory droplets. After an incubation period averaging 7–10 days, the onset of symptoms begins. The clinical illness is divided into three stages: catarrhal (lasting 1–2 weeks), paroxysmal (2–6 weeks), and convalescent (weeks to months) (Fig. 3). In the catarrhal stage, the onset of symptoms is insidious, presenting similarly to a minor upper respiratory infection with nonspecific cough. However, instead of abating, the cough may become progressive or persistent. Fever is usually minimal throughout the course of the illness. Infected individuals are most contagious during the catarrhal stage, and individuals with mild symptoms may transmit the infection. Most individuals are contagious for 14–21 days after the onset of symptoms, but transmissibility may be longer in immunocompromised hosts.

During the paroxysmal stage, the cough is the hallmark feature either due to its persistence or its distinguishing characteristics. In classic pertussis, most often seen in toddlers and young children, the cough occurs in attacks or paroxysms and may be followed by a forced inspiratory effort causing a whooping sound. The inspiratory whoop is generally absent in very young infants and in older children, teens, and adults. Complications of pertussis occur most often during this stage and include death (0.2%), malnutrition, respiratory events (eg, pneumonia, pneumothorax or apnea), central nervous system events (eg, seizures and encephalopathy) and pressure-related events (eg, conjunctival hemorrhages, epistaxis, hernia, and urinary incontinence).[6,8] In the United States in the past decade, ~10 deaths per year are attributable to pertussis and most occur among infants too young to be vaccinated or unvaccinated children.[20–22]

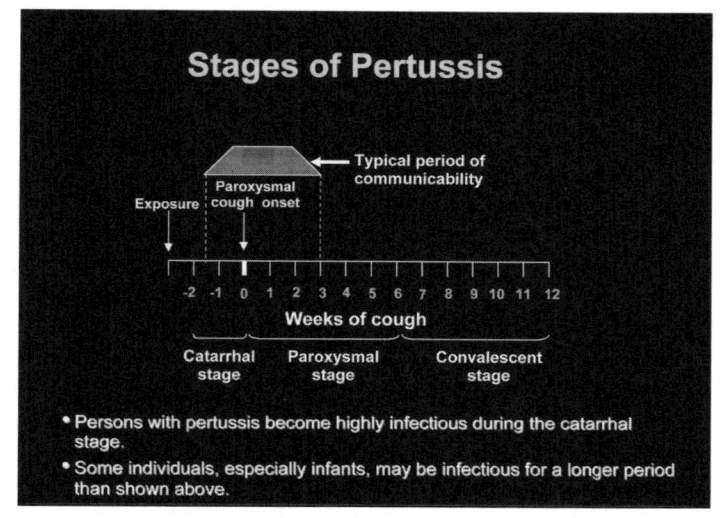

Fig 3. Stages and communicability of pertussis. (From: Adapted from Bisgard K. Chapter 1: Background. In Centers for Disease Control and Prevention, ed. *Guidelines for the Control of Pertussis Outbreaks*. Available at: http://www.cdc.gov/vaccines/pubs/pertussis-guide/guide.htm. Accessed February 21, 2010.)

## Symptoms in Adolescents and Adults

In adolescents and adults, the disease is often milder than is observed in infants and children, but may have a wide spectrum from unrecognized, mildly symptomatic disease to classic whooping cough (Fig. 4). Yih et al reported that 83%

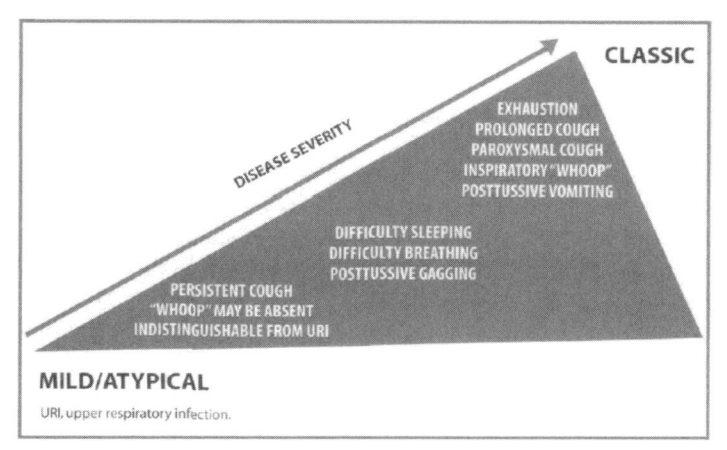

Fig 4. Schematic of adolescent pertussis disease. (From: Marchant C. Pertussis in adolescents: controlling outbreaks through vaccination. *Contemporary Pediatrics*. Philadelphia, PA: GlaxoSmith Kline; July 2007.)

of teens had paroxysmal cough and 41% had cough for >4 weeks at the time of diagnosis.[23]

In older age groups, pertussis may be characterized by a prolonged cough (3 months or longer), posttussive vomiting, and lethargy, as well as other complications and hospitalization. The diagnosis of pertussis may not be entertained in older individuals, leading to multiple medical visits. Although complications occur more frequently in young infants, they can occur in any age group. From 1997–2000, 3.5% of pertussis hospitalizations were in adults over 20 years old.[20] Other complications observed in adolescents and adults include syncope, precipitation of angina, rib fractures, and secondary respiratory infections.[6,17] In between coughing spells, the individual may appear well. Some older individuals undergo extensive medical evaluations, such as bronchoscopy, for chronic cough. The illness may be associated with significant costs for medical care, missed school or work days, and costs to the public health system for case investigation and management. Purdy et al estimated the total cost (direct and indirect) of pertussis to be $17 billion (2002 values) over 10 years based on incidence data from the CDC for infants and prospective studies in adults. For individuals over 10 years of age, 88% of the costs were indirect, related to missed school/work days and missed recreational activities.[24] As the number of cases is significantly underreported, the true cost of pertussis is difficult to determine and further studies are needed.

## DIAGNOSIS

In all age groups, pertussis is a clinical diagnosis and a high index of suspicion is essential for making the diagnosis. When the classic features of whooping cough are present, the diagnosis may be readily considered. However, the spectrum of illness is quite varied and frequently not classic; this is especially true for adolescents, adults, and individuals who have had previous pertussis immunizations.

### Clinical Case Definition

In June 1997, the Council of State and Territorial Epidemiologists defined a clinical case of pertussis as a cough illness lasting at least 2 weeks with one of the following: paroxysms of coughing, inspiratory "whoop," or posttussive vomiting; and without other apparent cause (as reported by a health care professional).[25]

*Laboratory Criteria for Diagnosis*

Laboratory criteria for diagnosis include isolation of *B. pertussis* from a clinical specimen or positive polymerase chain reaction (PCR) assay for *B. pertussis* DNA.

## Case Classifications

*Probable*: Meets the clinical case definition, but is not laboratory confirmed, and is not epidemiologically linked to a laboratory-confirmed case.

*Confirmed*: A case of acute cough illness of any duration with a positive culture for *B. pertussis,* a case that meets the clinical case definition and is confirmed by PCR, or a case that meets the clinical definition and is epidemiologically linked directly to a case confirmed by either culture or PCR.

## Laboratory Studies

*Bacterial Culture* All persons with suspected pertussis should have a nasopharyngeal (NP) aspirate or swab obtained from the posterior nasopharynx for culture. Growth of *B. pertussis* is considered to be the "gold standard" for diagnosing pertussis. For *B. pertussis*, NP aspirates yield similar or higher rates of recovery than NP swabs. If swabs are use, NP sampling should be performed by experienced personnel using Dacron or rayon swabs, as shown in Fig. 5. NP specimens should be plated directly onto selective culture medium (Bordet-Gengou or Regan-Lowe Charcoal Agar) or placed in transport medium. The organism is fastidious and slow growing, usually requiring at least 3–5 days. Additionally, although growth on culture is 100% specific, the sensitivity may be quite low. Recovery of *B. pertussis* in culture may be decreased by examining an inadequate NP sample, host factors (including prolonged duration of symptoms,

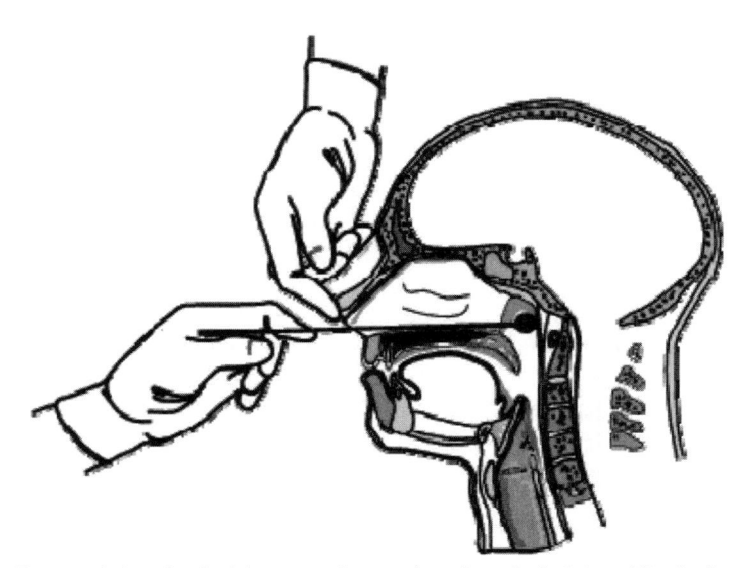

Fig 5. Proper technique for obtaining a nasopharyngeal specimen for isolation of *Bordetella pertussis*. (From: Centers for Disease Control and Prevention. Manual for the Surveillance of Vaccine-Preventable Diseases. Available at: http://www.cdc.gov/vaccines/pubs/surv-manual. Accessed March 1, 2010.)

previous immunizations or antibiotics) or laboratory factors (challenges of growth and identification of tiny, fastidious bacteria in a busy clinical microbiology lab).[6,17,22,26–29]

*Direct Fluorescent Antibody* Direct fluorescent antibody (DFA) assay is also available for testing NP samples, but suffers from variable sensitivity and specificity. Therefore, in most settings outside of a research laboratory, the DFA is not a reliable test and is not recommended. The CDC recommends that if the DFA is used, it should be used alongside culture or PCR.[22,26]

*Polymerase Chain Reaction* PCR is an amplified molecular testing tool that often detects DNA sequences of pertussis toxin (PT). The same NP sample can be used for culture and PCR; however, calcium alginate swabs cannot be used to collect specimens for PCR. When compared with culture, PCR has demonstrated higher sensitivity, as well as a more rapid turnaround time.[16,22,30,31] Given the greater sensitivity and rapidity of PCR as compared with culture, it is gaining favor for diagnosing pertussis. However, PCR suffers from decreased specificity, limited availability, and lack of assay standardization. Although many commercial laboratories offer PCR testing for *B. pertussis*, no U.S. Food and Drug Administration (FDA)-approved assays are available.

*Serology* Similar to PCR, there are no standardized serologic assays available. The most widely available assay is an enzyme-linked immunosorbent assay for antibodies to purified antigens of *B. pertussis*. These assays are most frequently performed in a research setting or public health laboratory. Additionally, there is no established serologic correlate of immunity or serologic marker of acute infection, making interpretation of results difficult. Serologic testing may be most useful when simultaneous testing of acute and convalescent serum samples is performed; however, fold-rise in titers may not be observed if the first sample is obtained late in the illness. The Massachusetts Department of Public Health has been successful in using single-point serologic testing for identifying pertussis cases, most notably in adolescents and adults.[32]

Interestingly, although no serologic marker of infection has been identified, serology has proven invaluable in investigating and understanding the spectrum of pertussis disease.[5,6,11,12,14,26,32,33] In household contact studies and serologic epidemiologic investigations, evaluation of antibodies to pertussis antigens has identified atypical and previously unrecognized cases of pertussis. This is especially true for adolescents and adults, as well as individuals that have been previously immunized.

*Other Laboratory Findings* In classic pertussis, leukocytosis and lymphocytosis are the characteristic hematologic findings noted during the paroxysmal phase. These abnormalities are typically absent in adolescents and adults. The degree of leukocytosis can exceed 50 000 cells/mm$^3$, and the absolute lymphocyte count may exceed 10 000 cells/mm$^3$. Hypoglycemia has been reported in young infants, which may be related to their inability to eat due to coughing or possibly secondary to toxins produced by *B. pertussis*. Chest radiographs may be normal or may have subtle abnormalities such as peribronchial cuffing, perihilar infiltrates, or atelectasis. Pulmonary consolidation, due to *B. pertussis* or secondary bacterial infections, occurs in 20% of hospitalized patents.

**Differential Diagnosis**

Other *Bordetella* species, notably *B. parapertussis*, can cause respiratory infections in humans, but is generally milder. Clinical whooping cough may be caused by other organisms, including *Chlamydia pneumoniae*, *Chlamydia trachomatis*, *Mycoplasma pneumonia*, and viral agents (eg, adenovirus and respiratory syncytial virus).[34] Other diagnostic considerations for prolonged coughing illnesses include sinusitis, tuberculosis, reactive airway disease, severe gastro-esophogeal reflux, and foreign body aspiration.

**TREATMENT**

The mainstay of therapy is supportive care. Maintaining adequate hydration and nutrition are challenging for infants and young children with pertussis, but less problematic for adolescents and adults. For infants, more intensive monitoring and supportive care may be needed, including hospitalization, parenteral nutrition, and oxygen supplementation. In the older age groups, coughing may cause disturbed sleep and decreased daytime productivity; however, no specific therapies are available. In general, use of cough suppressants is discouraged in all age groups, as cough is the main mechanism for airway protection. Treatment with bronchodilators or steroids has not been clearly proven beneficial.

**Antibiotic Therapy**

Prompt treatment may ameliorate symptoms and limit spread of the infection. Thus, antibiotic therapy should be initiated based on a high degree of clinical suspicion, even without laboratory confirmation. Antibiotic treatment is recommended for all infected individuals, regardless of their age or immunization status. The duration of symptoms before treatment seems to be an important factor for the impact of antibiotics. Initiation of effective antibiotics within the first 7 days of symptoms may decrease the severity of symptoms.[35] After 21 days of symptoms, antibiotics may still decrease spread to contacts, but are unlikely to alter the clinical course of the infected individual.[36] Unfortunately, most individuals, especially teens and adults, do not seek medical care until the paroxysmal phase, when there is less likelihood of successful laboratory confirmation or impact of treatment on the clinical course.

The antibiotics of choice are macrolides, including erythromycin, clarithromycin, and azithromycin. Erythromycin should be taken for 14 days, clarithromycin for 7 days, and azithromycin for 5 days. For individuals over the age of 8 years, doxycycline is an alternative antibiotic choice and for adults over 18 years of age, fluoroquinolones may be considered. Doxycyline and the fluoroquinolones are not routinely recommended for use in young children due to potential toxicities; however, in some settings these agents may be considered after weighing risks and benefits. Although it has excellent in vitro activity, trimethoprim-sulfamethoxazole has not been systematically evaluated and its clinical efficacy is largely unproven; however, it may be considered as an alternative agent for individuals over 6 weeks of age who cannot tolerate macrolides. The β-lactam antibiotics have variable activity against *B. pertussis* and are not recommended.[6,34]

## PREVENTION

### Antibiotic Prophylaxis

Chemoprophylaxis is recommended for all household contacts and other close contacts regardless of age or immunization status (as vaccinations are not 100% protective). The antibiotic regimens for prophylaxis are the same as those recommended for a treatment course. Prompt use of antibiotic prophylaxis may limit the development of secondary cases.[34]

After exposure, close contacts younger than 7 years or 10 years and older who are unimmunized or under immunized should receive a pertussis-containing vaccine according to the recommended schedule. In health care settings, exposed, unprotected individuals should receive prompt prophylaxis, including antibiotics and immunization (if indicated), similar to the recommendations for household and other close contacts.[9,34,40,41]

### Active Immunization

In most industrialized nations, higher dose aP combined with higher dose diphtheria toxoid and tetanus toxoid vaccines (DTaP) are given to infants, with boosters given to toddlers or preschool children. In the United States, the primary pertussis vaccination series is given to infants at 2, 4, 6, and 12–18 months of age, with a booster at 4 to 6 years of age. Several DTaP vaccine formulations are licensed in the United States for use for the primary series in children younger than 7 years old. Although licensed vaccines differ in their formulation, their efficacy appears to be similar.[34] At this time, no pertussis-containing vaccines are licensed for use in children ages 7–9 years of age.

In general, at least 3 doses of pertussis vaccines are needed before a significant immune response is observed in infants. After 3 doses, the efficacy of DTaP vaccination is 80% or greater. Immunization of infants as young as 1 month is recommended during pertussis epidemics in a community, but this is not routinely done as the immune responses observed may not be as robust. The fourth dose is given at least 6 months after the third dose, and the fifth dose is recommended between 4 and 6 years of age.

Two reduced-dose acellular pertussis (ap) combined with reduced-dose diphtheria toxoid and standard-dose tetanus toxoid vaccines (Tdap) were licensed in the United States by the FDA for adolescents and adults in 2005.[36,37] Adacel was licensed for a single booster dose in individuals 11–64 years of age who had previously received their childhood pertussis vaccinations. Adacel contains PT, FHA, PRN, and fimbriae types 2 and 3 and is comparable to the Sanofi Pasteur infant DTaP vaccine, Daptacel, though it has a reduced dose of PT. Boostrix, the Tdap produced by GlaxoSmithKline, was licensed for booster use in adolescents 10–18 years of age, and in 2008 was approved for adults through 64 years old of age. Boostrix contains three pertussis antigens (PT, FHA, and PRN) in reduced quantity compared with the pediatric formulation of DTaP (Infanrix). Adacel had been in use in adolescents in some areas of Canada since 1999, providing supporting safety and some effectiveness data. Following introduction of an adolescent booster dose, pertussis incidence in the Northwest Territories decreased from 7.9 per 100 000 in the late 1990s to 0.2 per 100 000 in 2004.[39]

The primary objective of using Tdap vaccines is to protect the vaccinated adolescent or adult. The additional objective is to reduce the reservoir of *B. pertussis* in the community and thus potentially reduce the incidence of pertussis in other age groups, most notably very young infants, who have the highest morbidity and mortality. A few studies have been performed to estimate the cost savings of implementing Tdap vaccinations. Purdy et al estimated that universal vaccination of everyone ≥10 years of age in the United States with an aP vaccine could prevent 1.3–6.5 million pertussis cases for a cost savings of $1.6–8.4 billion per decade, not including vaccine costs.[24] The Advisory Committee for Immunization Practices of the CDC estimated that vaccinating adolescents one time would prevent 31 000 cases of pertussis at a cost of $44 million with a savings of $11 million (2005 values), which is considered to be within reasonable expense from the societal prospective in the United States.[5,40]

The CDC and American Academy of Pediatrics (AAP) recommend that adolescents 11 through 18 years of age should receive one dose of Tdap instead of Td for booster immunization against diphtheria, tetanus, and pertussis. The current platform for delivery is during a health maintenance visit at 11–12 years of age. For teens 11–18 years of age who have already received a Td booster, an interval of at least 2 years is recommended before receipt of Tdap. A shorter interval may be considered when the risks of possible vaccine local or systemic reactions are outweighed by the potential benefits, such as in the settings of close contact with an infant, exposure to a pertussis case or during an outbreak. Additional populations in whom administration of Tdap should be considered include health care workers, especially those caring for children, and pregnant or postpartum women to help protect the vaccinee, as well as the infant. The AAP recommends for pregnant women for whom Tdap or Td is indicated, administration in the second or third trimester (and ideally before 36 weeks gestation) is preferred to decrease the risk of a perceived association of an adverse pregnancy event with the vaccination. At this time, there is no evidence of associated adverse pregnancy outcomes and receipt of an inactivated bacterial vaccine or toxoid.[34,41,42] The CDC also recommends a single dose of Tdap for adults over the age of 18 years to replace one decennial Td booster.[41]

Both U.S.-licensed Tdap vaccines appear to be associated with similar or slightly higher rates of local and systemic reactions as Td boosters. Local reactions are common, including pain at the injection site (~75% of recipients), redness (~20%), and swelling (~20%). Severe local reactions occur in ≤6% of vaccinees. In prelicensure trials, systemic reactions, including fever, headache, and feeling tired, occurred at slightly higher rates in Tdap than Td recipients. However, severe systemic reactions were reported by ≤4% of Tdap vaccinees.[9,34,37,38,43] Syncope following all immunizations, including Tdap, appears to occur more commonly in adolescents and young adults than in other age groups, and poses the risk of injury. Vaccinees should be observed for 15 minutes after immunization.

**Contraindications, Precautions, and Deferral of Tdap in Adolescents**

*Contraindications* Contraindications for use of Tdap include history of immediate anaphylactic reaction to any components of the vaccines and history of encephalopathy within 7 days of receipt of a pertussis vaccine.[9,34,41]

*Precautions* A history of Guillan-Barre syndrome within 6 weeks of receipt of a tetanus-containing vaccine is a precaution. Additionally, a history of a progressive neurologic disorder, uncontrolled seizure disorder, or progressive encephalopathy is considered precautions to receipt of a Tdap vaccine. These precautions are related to the pertussis component of the vaccine. If a decision is made to withhold pertussis vaccination, Td can be used instead of Tdap.

*Deferral* General recommendations for deferral of any active immunization should also be observed for use of Tdap. These include a moderate or severe acute illness with or without fever, until the acute illness resolves. Additionally, deferral of Tdap should be considered for at least 10 years after a severe Arthus reaction following receipt of any vaccine containing tetanus toxoid or diphtheria toxoid.

*Vaccine Delivery* The most effective methods to deliver vaccines to adolescents are not yet clearly defined. In 2008, the National Immunization Survey–Teens reported that the vaccination coverage rate for teens 13–17 years of age was <41% for Tdap and <35% for 2 childhood doses of varicella vaccine. These data suggest that availability of new vaccines is not enough, but programs that assure delivery must also be developed.[43] Tdap is only one of several vaccinations that have recently become available and/or routinely recommended for use in adolescents, including meningococcal conjugate vaccine, human papillomavirus vaccine, and influenza vaccines.

The health care visit at age 11–12 years is optimal for children who have a medical home, but does not capture all children. Other venues for administering vaccines need to be explored. Possibilities include school-based immunization clinics, athletic team venues, after-school programs, and other teen-centered group activities. In 2009, Daley et al reported success of a school-based clinic system and noted that there are over 2000 such programs already operating in the United States.[44] For older adolescents, possible vaccine check points may include employment applications, issuance of driver's licenses, college entrance, and military service.

In the United States, infant and childhood pertussis vaccinations have succeeded in reducing the overall burden of disease; however, the shift in disease to young infants, adolescents, and adults, as well as the global burden of pertussis, suggest the need for different preventative strategies. With increasing public awareness and availability of Tdap vaccines, there has never been a more opportune time for mounting new defenses against *B. pertussis*. Nor has there been a more exciting time for incorporating other immunizations, as well as increasing all preventative care, for adolescents and adults.

## REFERENCES

1. The Centers for Disease Control and Prevention. The epidemiology of pertussis. Available at: www.cdc.gov/vaccines/programs/vfc/downloads/resolutions/1003hepb.pdf. Accessed March 1, 2010
2. Cherry JD. The epidemiology of pertussis and pertussis immunization in the United Kingdom and the United States: a comparative study. *Curr Prob Pediatr.* 1984;14:1–78
3. Laring JS, Hay M. Whooping-cough: its prevalence and mortality in Aberdeen. *Public Health.* 1902;14:584–598
4. Mannerstedt G. Pertussis in aults. *J Pediatr.* 1934;5:596–600
5. Yeh S, Mink CM. Shift in the epidemiology of pertussis infection: an indication for pertussis vaccine boosters for adults? *Drugs.* 2006;66(6);731–741
6. Hewlitt E. *Bordetella* species. In: Mandell GL, Bennett JE, Dolin R, eds. *Mandell, Douglas and Bennett's Principles and Practice of Infectious Diseases* (6th ed.). Philadelphia, PA: Elsevier; 2005:2701–2708
7. Sutter RW, Cochi SL. Pertussis hospitalizations and mortality in the United States, 1985–1988. Evaluation of the completeness of national reporting. *JAMA.* 1992;267:386–391
8. Marchant C. Pertussis in adolescents: controlling outbreaks through vaccination. *Contemporary Pediatrics.* Philadelphia, PA: GlaxoSmith Kline; July 2007
9. Centers for Disease Control and Prevention. Preventing tetanus, diphtheria, and pertussis among adolescents: Use of tetanus toxoid, reduced diphtheria toxoid, and acellular pertussis vaccine. Recommendations of the Advisory Committee on Immunization Practices (ACIP). *MMWR* 2006;55(RR 03);1–34

10. Centers for Disease Control and Prevention. Epidemiology and prevention of vaccine-preventable diseases. The Pink Book: Course Textbook (11th ed.). Available at http://www.cdc.gov/vaccines/pubs/pinkbook/downloads/pert.pdf. Accessed February 21, 2010
11. Cattaneo LA, Reed GW, Haase DH, Willis MJ, Edwards KM. The seroepidemiology of *Bordetella pertussis* infections: a study of persons 1–65 years. *J Infect Dis*. 1996;173:1265–1269
12. Baughman AL, Bisgard KM, Edwards KM, et al. Establishment of diagnostic cutoff points for levels of serum antibodies to pertussis toxin, filamentous hemagglutinin and fimbriae in adolescents and adults in the United States. *Clin Diagn Lab Immunol*. 2004;11:1045–1053
13. Ward JL, Cherry JD, Chang SJ, et al. Efficacy of an acellular pertussis vaccine among adolescents and adults. *N Engl J Med*. 2005;353:1555–1563
14. Brooks DA, Clover R. Pertussis infection in the United States: Role for vaccination of adolescents and adults. *J Am Board Fam Med*. 19(6):603–611
15. Cherry JD. The epidemiology of pertussis: a comparison of the epidemiology of the disease pertussis with the epidemiology of Bordetella pertussis infection. *Pediatrics*. 2005;115:1422–1427
16. Jackson LA, Cherry JD, Wang SP, Grayson ST. Frequency of serologic evidence of *Bordetella* infections and mixed infections with other respiratory pathogens in university students with cough illness. *Clin Infect Dis*. 2000;31:3–6
17. von Koenig CH, Haloerin S, Riffleman M, Guisso N. Pertussis in adults and infants. *Lancet Infect Dis*. 2002;2:744–750
18. Deen JL, Mink CM, Cherry JD, et al. A household contact study of Bordetella pertussis infections. *Clin Infect Dis*. 1995;21:1211–1219
19. Bisgard Km, Pascaul FB, Ehresmann KR, et al. Infant pertussis, who was the source? *Pediatr Infect Dis*. 2004;23:985–989
20. Centers for Disease Control and Prevention. Pertussis—United States, 2001–2003. *MMWR* 2005;54(50):1283–1286
21. Haberling DL, Holman RC, Paddock CD, Murphy TV. Infant and maternal risk factors for pertussis–related infant mortality in the United States 1999 to 2004. *Pediatr Infect Dis*. 2009;28(3):194–198
22. Centers for Disease Control and Prevention. Manual for the Surveillance of Vaccine-Preventable Diseases. Available at: http://www.cdc.gov/vaccines/pubs/surv-manual. Accessed March 1, 2010
23. Yih WK, Lett SM, des Vignes FN, Garrison KM, Sipe PL, Marchant CM. The increasing incidence of pertussis in Massachusetts adolescents and adults, 1989–1998. *J Infect Dis*. 2000;182:1409–1416
24. Purdy KW, Hay JW, Botteman MF, et al. Evaluation of strategies for use of acellular pertussis vaccines in adolescents and adults: a cost-benefit analysis. *Clin Infect Dis*. 2004;39:20–28
25. Council of State and Territorial Epidemiologists. CSTE Position Statement 1997-ID-9: Public health surveillance, control and prevention of pertussis. CSTE, 1997. Available at: http://www.cste.org/ps/1997/1997-id-09.htm. Accessed March 1, 2010
26. Murphy T, Bisgard K, Sanden G. Diagnosis and laboratory methods. Available at: http://www.cdc.gov/vaccines/pubs/pertussis-guide/downloads/_DRAFT_chapter2_amended.pdf. Accessed June 25, 2010
27. Hallander HO, Reizenstein E, Renemar B, Rasmuson G, Mardin L, Olin P. Comparison of nasopharyngeal aspirates with swabs for culture of *Bordetella* pertussis. *J Clin Microbiol*. 1993;31:50–52
28. Halperin SA, Bortolussi R, Wort AJ. Evaluation of culture, immunofluorescence, and serology for the diagnosis of pertussis. *J Clin Microbiol*. 1989;7:752–757
29. Hoppe JE, Weiss A. Recovery of *Bordetella* pertussis from four kinds of swabs. *Eur J Clin Microbiol*. 1987;6:203–205
30. Koidl C, Bozic M, Burmeister A, Hess M, Marth E, Kessler HH. Detection and differentiation of *Bordetella* spp. by real-time PCR. *J Clin Microbiol*. 2007;45:347–350
31. Qin X, Galanakis E, Martin ET, Englund JA. Multi-target polymerase chain reaction for diagnosis of pertussis and its clinical implications. *J Clin Microbiol*. 2007;45:506–511

32. Marchant CD, Loughlin AM, Lett SM, Todd CW, Wetterlow LH, Bicchieri R, et al. Pertussis in Massachusetts, 1981–1991: incidence, serologic diagnosis, and vaccine effectiveness. *J Infect Dis*. 1994;169:1297–1305
33. Poynten M, Hanlon M, Irwig L, Gilbert GL. Serologic diagnosis of pertussis: Evaluation of IgA against whole cel and specific Bordetella pertussis antigens as markers of recent infection. *Epidemiol Infect* 2002;128:161–167
34. American Academy of Pediatrics. Pertussis (whooping cough). In: Pickering LK, Baker CJ, Kimberlin DW, Long SS, eds. *Red Book: 2009 Report of the Committee on Infectious Diseases* (28th ed.). Elk Grove Village, IL: American Academy of Pediatrics; 2009;504–519
35. Guris D. Treatment and prophylaxis. In: *National Immunization Program Guidelines for Control of Pertussis Outbreaks*. Atlanta: Centers for Disease Control and Prevention; 2003
36. Rilitta H. The effect of early erythromycin treatment on the infectiousness of whooping cough patients. *Acta Pediatrica*. 2008;200:10–12
37. Mink CM. FDA clinical briefing document for Tdap from Aventis Pasteur, 2005. Available at: http://www.fda.gov/ohrms/dockets/ac/05/briefing/2005-4097B1_4a.pdf. Accessed March 1, 2010
38. Swartz A. FDA clinical briefing document: GlaxoSmith Kline (GSK) Biologics Tdap, 2005. Available at: http://www.fda.gov/ohrms/dockets/ac/05/briefing/2005-4097B1_1.pdf. Accessed March 1, 2010
39. Kandola K, Lea A, Santos M. Pertussis rates in Northwest Territories after introducing adult formulation acellular vaccine (abstract). *Can J Infect Dis Med Microbiol*. 2004;15:351
40. Centers for Disease Control and Prevention National Immunization Program. Record of the meeting of the Advisory Committee on Immunization Practices, 2005. Available at: http://www.cdc.gov/nip/ACIP/minutes.acip-min-feb05.pdf. Accessed March 1, 2010
41. Centers for Disease Control and Prevention. Preventing tetanus, diphtheria, and pertussis among adults: Use of tetanus toxoid, reduced diphtheria toxoid, and acellular pertussis vaccine. Recommendations of the Advisory Committee on Immunization Practices (ACIP) recommendations of the ACIP, supported by the Healthcare Infection Control Practices Advisory Committee (HICPAC) for use of Tdap among healthcare personnel. *MMWR*. 2006;55 (RR17):1–33
42. Centers for Disease Control and Prevention. Prevention of pertussis, tetanus and diphtheria among pregnant and postpartum women and their infants. Recommendations of the Advisory Committee on Immunization Practices (ACIP). *MMWR*. 2008;57(04):1–47
43. Centers for Disease Control and Prevention. National, state and local area vaccination coverage among adolescents aged 13–17 years—United States, 2008. *MMWR*. 2009;58(36):997–1001
44. Daley MF, Curtis CR, Pyranowski J, et al. Adolescent immunization delivery in school-based health centers: a national survey. *J Adolesc Health*. 2009;45(5);445–452
45. Bisgard K. Chapter 1: Background. In Centers for Disease Control and Prevention, ed. *Guidelines for the Control of Pertussis Outbreaks*. Available at http://www.cdc.gov/vaccines/pubs/pertussis-guide/guide.htm. Accessed February 21, 2010

# Influenza

Rebecca C. Brady, MD*

*Division of Pediatric Infectious Diseases, Department of Pediatrics, Cincinnati Children's Hospital Medical Center, 3333 Burnet Avenue, Cincinnati, OH 45229*

Influenza is an acute, highly contagious, febrile respiratory illness that occurs in epidemics of varying severity almost every winter. The causative viruses infect the respiratory tract and produce prominent fever, malaise, myalgias, and cough. Patients with asthma, cardiac disease, or compromised immunity may develop pneumonia or other complications. In the United States, an average of more than 200 000 hospitalizations and 36 000 deaths are associated with influenza each year.[1-3] Between April and mid-December 2009, the Centers for Disease Control and Prevention (CDC) estimates that between 173 000 and 362 000 novel H1N1 influenza-related hospitalizations occurred with an estimated 7880 to 16 460 deaths.[4]

## Virology

Influenza viruses belong to the family Orthomyxoviridae.[5] They are single-stranded RNA viruses with a segmented genome and a lipid envelope. Influenza viruses are classified as A, B, or C on the basis of major antigenic differences.[6] Influenza A and B viruses are responsible for seasonal epidemics, whereas influenza C virus predominantly causes mild upper respiratory infections.[7] Influenza A viruses primarily infect aquatic birds and sometimes other animals, including swine, cats, and dogs.[8] In contrast, influenza B and C viruses are principally human pathogens.[9]

Influenza A viruses are further classified into subtypes on the basis of their 2 surface glycoproteins: the hemagglutinin (HA) and the neuraminidase (NA). These surface glycoproteins are the major targets of the protective host immune response.[10,11] There are 16 HA and 9 NA subtypes that circulate in nature, but only 3 HA subtypes (H1, H2, and H3) and 2 NA subtypes (N1 and N2) are known to cause widespread disease in humans.[12] The standard convention for the nomenclature of influenza viruses specifies the type, host (for strains of animal origin), geographic source, strain number, and year of isolation, followed by the HA and NA subtypes in the case of

---

*Corresponding author.
*E-mail address*: rebecca.brady@cchmc.org (R. C. Brady).

Copyright © 2010 American Academy of Pediatrics. All rights reserved. ISSN 1934-4287

influenza A viruses.[13] Examples are A/Uruguay/716/2007 (H3N2) and A/goose/Guangdong/1/96 (H5N1).

Changes in the HA and NA glycoproteins largely account for why influenza continues to be a major epidemic disease of humans. During virus replication, point mutations in the RNA segments coding the HA and/or NA may lead to amino acid substitutions in antigenic sites on these proteins.[14] These small antigenic changes (antigenic drift) occur frequently and lead to almost yearly epidemics. Immunologic selection favors the new variant over the old because antibodies directed against the old virus may not recognize and neutralize the new variant.[15]

New influenza A virus subtypes may also arise by antigenic shift. When two influenza A viruses simultaneously infect a single cell, reassortment of their RNA segments may occur. The resultant "new" virus may have HA (or HA and NA) glycoproteins new to humans. Much of the population will lack immunity to the "new" virus; therefore, worldwide epidemics or pandemics may develop.[16] The genetics of the virus responsible for the 2009 pandemic revealed a quadruple reassortant with genes from the influenza of pigs in Europe, Asia, and North America plus genes from avian strains and from human strains.[17,18]

Infrequently, avian strains may be directly transmitted to humans without prior reassortment in an intermediate host.[5] Recent examples include avian influenza viruses of the H5N1, H7N7, and H9N2 subtypes.[19-21] Their spread has been limited because person-to-person transmission appears to occur rarely.[22]

**Epidemiology**

Epidemics of influenza typically occur annually during the winter months in temperate climates. Usually a single strain of influenza prevails but occasionally two different influenza A subtypes (H1N1 and H3N2) or influenza A and B viruses may circulate simultaneously.[5] In a given community, influenza spreads first among children in school. Schoolchildren have the highest attack rates for infection each year, ranging from 30 to 50 per 100 children.[23] The peak of influenza illness in children is soon followed by illness in adults. In a prospective study of 313 schoolchildren, influenza accounted for an excess of 28 illness episodes and 63 missed school days per 100 children, 22 secondary illnesses in families, and 20 days of missed parental work per 100 children.[24]

Influenza viruses are also the most important causes of acute respiratory tract illnesses leading to hospitalization of schoolchildren. Among those aged 10-19 years, influenza accounts for a hospitalization rate of 3 to 4 per 10 000.[25] Those with high-risk medical conditions including asthma, cardiac disease, and neuromuscular disorders have a significantly higher rate of hospitalization.[26]

Approximately 90% of deaths from seasonal influenza occur among persons aged 65 years or older.[1] Among children, the highest mortality rate is for infants younger than 6 months of age.[9,26] In 2003–2004, a total of 153 influenza-associated deaths were reported among children in the United States.[26] Thirty-three percent had underlying conditions recognized to increase the risk of developing influenza-related complications, 20% had other chronic conditions, and 47% had been previously healthy.

Pandemic influenza may differ from seasonal influenza in certain features as was evident in 2009. The 2009 pandemic began in April and continued its spread worldwide throughout the warmer months.[18] Although pandemic influenza infects much of the population by definition, the virulence of the infecting strain and host factors influence the burden of disease.[27] The 1918 pandemic was notable for its high mortality among young, healthy adults.[28] In comparison, the 2009 pandemic has caused milder disease, but the frequency and severity of infection have been greatest in those younger than 24 years.[29] Pregnant women, especially those in the second and third trimesters, have had an increased risk of severe or fatal illness.[30] Obesity may also be a risk factor for severe disease.[31] People 65 years and older have had the lowest rates of 2009 H1N1 influenza disease.[4]

**Pathogenesis and Host Immune Response**

Influenza is transmitted from person to person primarily by inhalation of airborne droplets produced by coughing or sneezing.[32] Spread may also occur via contact with respiratory droplet-contaminated surfaces. Influenza virus attaches to sialic acid receptors on respiratory epithelial cells via its HA, enters these cells by endocytosis, and begins to replicate.[5] Peak virus replication occurs 1–3 days after inoculation.[9] Virus shedding continues for 6–8 days in adults but may persist into the second week in young children.[33] Inflammation and death of the respiratory epithelial cells ensue. Infection may extend to involve the smaller airways such as the bronchioles and alveoli of the lungs. Epithelial cell recovery follows, but complete restoration of ciliary function and mucus production may take ~2 weeks.[9]

In humans, influenza infection remains, for practical purposes, limited to the respiratory tract.[5] The release of inflammatory mediators by the infected respiratory epithelial cells and responding lymphocytes is likely responsible for the systemic manifestations of influenza.[34]

Influenza infection induces both mucosal and systemic antibody responses, as well as cytotoxic T-cell responses. Nasal HA-specific immunoglobulin (Ig) A antibodies provide an early protective response, but persist for only a short period.[7] Serum IgM, IgA, and IgG antibodies to the HA and NA glycoproteins appear within 2 weeks of inoculation of virus.[35] Antibodies to HA are necessary for virus neutralization, and those to NA reduce virus replication.[5,9] Cytotoxic T lymphocyte responses are important in mediating recovery from influenza infection.

The host immune response to influenza provides resistance to reinfection with the homologous virus for many years.[5,36] In addition, some cross-protection within a subtype is present. However, such immunity is limited by antigenic variations in the HA and NA.

## Clinical Manifestations

### Uncomplicated Influenza

The symptoms and signs of classic influenza in older children and adolescents are presented in Table 1.[37] Fever up to 40°C (104°F), chills, headache, myalgia, and malaise develop suddenly.[12] Dry cough and rhinitis are also early manifestations. Pharyngitis is nonexudative and ocular symptoms may include tearing and burning. The average duration of fever is 3 days. Most children and adolescents with influenza recover fully within 7 days.

### Complications of Influenza

The most frequent complications of influenza are bacterial infections of the respiratory tract, specifically otitis media, pneumonia, and sinusitis.[23,38] The

Table 1
Relative frequency of symptoms and signs during classic influenza in older children and adolescents

| Symptoms | Occurrence |
| --- | --- |
| Chilly sensation | ++++ |
| Cough | +++ |
| Headache | +++ |
| Sore throat | +++ |
| Prostration | ++ |
| Nasal stuffiness | ++ |
| Dizziness | + |
| Eye irritation or pain | + |
| Vomiting | + |
| Myalgia | + |
| **Signs** | |
| Fever | ++++ |
| Pharyngitis | +++ |
| Conjunctivitis (mild) | ++ |
| Rhinitis | ++ |
| Cervical adenitis | + |
| Pulmonary rales, wheezes, or rhonchi | + |

++++, 76–100%; +++, 51–75%; ++, 26–50%; +, 1–25%.
From: Cherry JD. Influenza viral infections. In: Vaughan V, McKay R, Behrman R, eds. *Nelson Textbook of Pediatrics.* 14th ed. Philadelphia, PA: Saunders;1987:675–678.

incidence of these complications in community studies of children is ~10%, with otitis media being most frequent.[39]

*Pulmonary Complications*

Secondary bacterial pneumonias are characterized by a recrudescence of fever in association with increased cough, sputum production, and pleuritic chest pain. *Streptococcus pneumoniae*, *Staphylococcus aureus*, and group A streptococci are the most commonly identified bacterial pathogens.[9] In recent years, severe, necrotizing pneumonitis and empyema due to community-acquired methicillin-resistant *S. aureus* have been increasingly reported as complications of influenza among previously healthy individuals.[40]

Primary influenza viral pneumonia begins as typical influenza, but is followed by a rapid progression of fever, cough, dyspnea, and cyanosis.[5] It is uncommon during epidemics but has been the major manifestation of patients with H5N1 illness.[41] It has also been reported among previously healthy children, adolescents, and adults infected with the 2009 pandemic virus.[31] Patients may develop the adult respiratory distress syndrome. Mortality is high and at autopsy, diffuse hemorrhagic pneumonia, and hyaline membranes lining the alveoli have been noted.[5]

Influenza may lead to exacerbations of chronic pulmonary diseases including asthma and cystic fibrosis.[42,43] Superinfection with *S. aureus* has also been associated with bacterial tracheitis and toxic shock syndrome.[44,45]

*Myositis*

Children and adolescents may develop acute pain and tenderness in the calf muscles that is severe enough to limit walking as the respiratory symptoms of influenza are waning. This complication occurs more commonly following influenza B infection than following influenza A.[46] No neurologic changes are evident. Serum creatine kinase levels are transiently elevated. Complete recovery usually occurs in 3 to 4 days.[9]

*Central Nervous System Complications*

Encephalitis, encephalopathy, transverse myelitis, and Guillain-Barré syndrome are unusual complications of influenza infection.[5] Cases of acute necrotizing encephalopathy have been reported in association with influenza infection in young children in recent years, most often in Japan.[47] These children present with sudden onset of fever and convulsions and progress rapidly to coma. Magnetic resonance imaging demonstrates bilateral thalamic necrosis and brainstem involvement. Affected children often die within a few days. Survivors are usually severely neurologically damaged. The pathogenesis has not been elucidated.

*Reye Syndrome*

Reye syndrome (encephalopathy and fatty degeneration of the liver) is uncommon and occurs almost exclusively in children who have received aspirin for influenza and other febrile viral illnesses.[5] Children present with a change in mental status occurring several days into their illness course. They may progress to obtundation, seizures, and respiratory arrest. Elevation of the blood ammonia level is the most frequent laboratory abnormality. Cerebrospinal fluid protein and cell counts are normal.

**Diagnosis**

The CDC defines an influenza-like illness as an individual with a fever 100°F or higher, as well as cough and/or sore throat in the absence of a known cause other than influenza.[48] Because it is not practical to test every patient with these signs and symptoms for influenza, the CDC recommends that such patients be managed as cases of influenza when influenza is known to be present in the local area. The CDC has a triage algorithm for children ≤18 years with influenza-like illness.[49]

During an influenza outbreak, cough and fever are the best predictors of influenza in mainly unvaccinated adults and adolescents who had influenza-like illness symptoms, with a positive predictive value of 79% and a sensitivity of 64% for laboratory-confirmed influenza.[50] The triad of cough, headache, and pharyngitis during a community outbreak of influenza as a predictor of influenza in children had a sensitivity of 80%, specificity of 78%, likelihood ratio of 3.7, and posttest probability of 77%.[51] When influenza is circulating in the local community, the diagnosis should be considered when an adolescent presents with the sudden onset of fever and a dry cough.

Laboratory testing for influenza is recommended when the result will be used to guide patient care. Examples include decisions on initiation of antiviral or antibiotic treatments, impact on other diagnostic testing, and infection control practices.[52] Interpretation of test results depends on the pretest probability that the patient has influenza based on signs and symptoms and the epidemiology of influenza in the community. The sensitivity and specificity of the test must also be considered.

Commercial rapid influenza diagnostic tests can be performed at the point of care and provide results in 10–30 minutes. They are based on antigen detection by enzyme immunoassay or neuraminidase detection. Their performance depends on patient age, sample type, duration of illness, and type of virus. For older children, adolescents, and adults, nasopharyngeal aspirates and swabs should be collected as close to illness onset as possible, preferably within 5 days of illness onset. In children, rapid tests are 70–90% sensitive and >90% specific for the detection of seasonal influenza.[53,54] Their positive predictive value is greatest during influenza season, and negative predictive value is greatest outside of influenza season.

Reverse-transcriptase polymerase chain reaction (RT-PCR) is currently the most sensitive and specific laboratory test for influenza.[52] Results are generally available within 4–6 hours after specimen submission. RT-PCR is useful for confirming negative test results from rapid influenza diagnostic tests and for quickly differentiating between influenza types and subtypes. It is the preferred test when there is concern for H5N1 or the 2009 pandemic H1N1 influenza.[52,55] Some laboratories offer it in a multiplex format to test for other respiratory viruses.

Viral isolation in standard cell culture may take 3–10 days, so it is not useful for timely clinical management decisions.[52] It is most useful for public health surveillance purposes to define strain characteristics, including antigenic comparison to influenza vaccine strains and antiviral susceptibility. It may also allow for the detection of other respiratory viruses.

Updated information regarding influenza testing methods is available on the CDC's seasonal flu web site.[55]

**Management**

Most individuals with uncomplicated influenza require only symptomatic treatment including acetaminophen or ibuprofen for fever, myalgia, and headache.[7] Salicylates should be avoided because of the potential for the development of Reye syndrome.

Specific antiviral therapy is available for influenza (Table 2). It should be considered for adolescents who have suspected or confirmed influenza and require hospitalization; present with evidence of lower respiratory tract infection or clinical deterioration; are pregnant or are up to 2 weeks postpartum; have chronic medical or immunosuppressive conditions; or are younger than 19 years of age and are receiving long-term aspirin therapy.[56]

Table 2
Antiviral medications for the treatment and prophylaxis of influenza in adolescents

| Antiviral Agent | Treatment | Chemoprophylaxis |
| --- | --- | --- |
| Amantadine | 100 mg twice daily | 100 mg twice daily |
| Rimantadine | 100 mg twice daily | 100 mg twice daily |
| Oseltamivir | 75 mg twice daily | 75 mg once daily |
| Zanamivir | Two 5-mg inhalations twice daily | Two 5-mg inhalations once daily |

From: American Academy of Pediatrics, Committee on Infectious Diseases. Policy statement—recommendations for the prevention and treatment of influenza in children, 2009–2010. *Pediatrics.* 2009;124:1216–1226.

During outbreaks, the CDC's web site has updated recommendations for the use of antiviral medications.[57] These medications can reduce the severity and duration of influenza illness and can reduce the risk of influenza-related complications. These benefits are greatest when therapy is initiated within the first 2 days of illness.

Two classes of antiviral medications are effective in the treatment of influenza.[5] These two classes are the tricyclic amines (amantadine and rimantadine) and the neuraminidase inhibitors (oseltamivir and zanamivir). The tricyclic amines act by blocking the function of an ion channel on the viral envelope and are only effective against certain strains of influenza A. The neuraminidase inhibitors decrease the release of influenza virus from infected cells and are active against most influenza A and B viruses. Recently circulating H3N2 strains and the 2009 pandemic H1N1 virus are sensitive to neuraminidase inhibitors but resistant to tricyclic amines.[27,58] Seasonal H1N1 strains have become resistant to oseltamivir but remain sensitive to amantadine and rimantadine. All of these strains remain sensitive to zanamivir. The CDC provides periodic updates to guide antiviral use[57] as well as weekly surveillance reports that include the geographic distribution of prevailing strains.[59]

Table 2 provides a list of antiviral medications for the treatment and prophylaxis of influenza in adolescents. The recommended duration of treatment for each of these drugs is 5 days. Amantadine may be associated with central nervous system (CNS) adverse effects, including agitation and tremors.[60] Individuals who have epilepsy may experience an increase in seizures. These CNS effects are less prominent with rimantadine. The major adverse effects of oseltamivir, which is only available as oral preparations, are nausea and vomiting.[61] Zanamivir is delivered with a breath-activated inhaler and should be used cautiously in those with a history of asthma because it may induce bronchospasm.[62]

In October 2009, the U.S. Food and Drug Administration issued an Emergency Use Authorization of the unapproved drug, peramivir, an intravenous neuraminidase inhibitor, for the treatment of severely ill, hospitalized patients with known or suspected 2009 H1N1 influenza who cannot tolerate other antiviral agents.[63]

**Prevention**

*Vaccines*

Influenza vaccines are the most effective measure available for the prevention of influenza. They are generally formulated as trivalent preparations, containing one example each of influenza A (H1N1) virus, A (H3N2) virus, and influenza B virus that are anticipated to circulate in the coming winter. The American Academy of Pediatrics and the Advisory Committee on Immunization Practices (ACIP) recently expanded recommendations for influenza vaccination in the

United States to include all children aged 6 months to 18 years of age as long as no specific contraindication exists.[58] Currently, 2 types of influenza vaccines are licensed in the United States—the inactivated vaccine administered by intramuscular injection and the live attenuated influenza vaccine (LAIV) given by nasal spray.

Trivalent inactivated influenza vaccine (TIV) is a split-virus vaccine made up of inactivated, disrupted virus particles. It does not contain live virus, and therefore cannot produce an active virus infection. It may be administered to people 6 months of age and older, including those with chronic medical conditions. The most common adverse effects are soreness at the injection site and fever. Fever is much less frequent in adolescents and adults than in younger children. Mild systemic symptoms, such as malaise, headache, and muscle aches, may occur within the first 1–2 days and usually resolve without treatment.

LAIV is a vaccine containing live, cold-adapted reassortant viruses that replicate more efficiently at the lower temperatures of the upper respiratory tract than the original wild-type virus.[5] The goal of administering LAIV by nasal spray is to induce a mucosal immune response that may more closely mimic the response induced by natural influenza infection.[64] Additionally, certain patients may prefer the nasal, rather than the intramuscular, route of administration.

LAIV is only licensed for use in healthy individuals 2–49 years of age.[58] Children and adolescents who have underlying medical conditions that are associated with an increased risk for complications from influenza (Table 3) should receive TIV, not LAIV. LAIV should not be administered to individuals with nasal congestion if the amount of congestion is anticipated to impede the

Table 3
Medical conditions associated with an increased risk of complications from influenza

Asthma or other chronic pulmonary diseases, including cystic fibrosis
Hemodynamically significant cardiac disease
Immunosuppressive disorders or therapy
Human immunodeficiency virus infection
Sickle cell anemia and other hemoglobinopathies
Diseases that require long-term aspirin therapy, including juvenile idiopathic arthritis or Kawasaki disease
Chronic renal dysfunction
Chronic metabolic disease, including diabetes mellitus
Pregnancy during influenza season
Any condition that may compromise respiratory function or handling of secretions or can increase the risk for aspiration, such as cognitive dysfunction, spinal cord injuries, seizure disorders, or other neuromuscular disorders

From: Centers for Disease Control and Prevention. Updated interim recommendations for the use of antiviral medications in the treatment and prevention of influenza for the 2009–2010 season. Available at: http://www.cdc.gov/h1n1flu/recommendations.htm. Accessed January 27, 2010.

Table 4
Comparison of influenza vaccines

| Vaccine Characteristic | Trivalent Inactivated Influenza Vaccine | Live Attenuated Influenza Vaccine |
| --- | --- | --- |
| Type of vaccine | Killed virus | Live virus |
| Product composition | Inactivated split virus | Attenuated, cold-adapted |
| Viral strains | A(H1N1), A(H3N2), B | A(H1N1), A(H3N2), B |
| Route of administration | Intramuscularly | Intranasally |
| Frequency of administration | Annually | Annually |
| Approved age and risk groups | Persons ≥6 months | Healthy persons 2–49 years |

From: American Academy of Pediatrics, Committee on Infectious Diseases. Policy statement—recommendations for the prevention and treatment of influenza in children, 2009–2010. *Pediatrics*. 2009;124:1216–1226.

delivery of vaccine to the nasal mucosa. LAIV may produce mild symptoms related to attenuated influenza virus infection.

Because both TIV and LAIV are grown in eggs, neither should be administered to anyone with known allergic reactions (ie, hives, angioedema, allergic asthma, and systemic anaphylaxis) to chicken and egg proteins. Table 4 provides a comparison of TIV with LAIV. Both TIV and LAIV can be administered simultaneously with other vaccines. If LAIV is not given concurrently with a live virus vaccine such as varicella, then the 2 live virus vaccines should be separated by at least 4 weeks.

Both types of influenza vaccines are cost effective for the prevention of influenza among children, adolescents, and their families when circulating and vaccine strains are closely matched. A study among children 5–18 years of age in the 2003–2004 season when the circulating H3N2 strain was not well matched to the vaccine strain suggested that LAIV, in comparison to TIV, provided better protection against influenza-positive illness.[65] Since current data comparing the effectiveness of these 2 vaccines are limited, additional studies are warranted.

The emergence of the 2009 H1N1 pandemic influenza virus had not been predicted[18] and therefore, a separate monovalent vaccine had to be manufactured and distributed quickly. Inactivated and live attenuated vaccines were manufactured using processes similar to those used for production of seasonal influenza vaccines. The ACIP[66] recommended that all individuals 6 months to 24 years of age receive the 2009 H1N1 vaccine. One dose of either the inactivated or LAIV preparation of the 2009 H1N1 vaccine was indicated for healthy persons 10–18 years of age. Those with underlying medical conditions that placed them at increased risk for complications from influenza were only eligible to receive the TIV preparation. The effectiveness of this vaccine will need to be monitored throughout the remainder of the 2009–2010 influenza season.

Table 5
Indications for considering influenza postexposure antiviral chemoprophylaxis

- Individuals who are at high risk of developing complications from influenza for whom influenza vaccination is contraindicated
- Individuals who are at high risk of developing complications from influenza whose response to vaccine may be inadequate such as those who are immunocompromised
- Individuals who are at high risk of developing complications from influenza during the 2 weeks after receipt of influenza vaccine if influenza virus is already circulating in the community
- Individuals who are at high risk of developing complications from influenza when the circulating strains of influenza virus in the community are not matched with the vaccine strains
- Family members or health care providers who are unimmunized and are likely to have ongoing, close exposure to unimmunized individuals who are at high risk of developing complications from influenza
- Control of influenza outbreaks for unimmunized staff and children in a closed institutional setting (eg, group homes) with individuals who are at high risk of developing complications from influenza

From: Centers for Disease Control and Prevention. Updated interim recommendations for the use of antiviral medications in the treatment and prevention of influenza for the 2009–2010 season. Available at: http://www.cdc.gov/h1n1flu/recommendations.htm. Accessed January 27, 2010; and American Academy of Pediatrics, Committee on Infectious Diseases. Policy statement—recommendations for the prevention and treatment of influenza in children, 2009–2010. *Pediatrics*. 2009;124:1216–1226.

*Chemoprophylaxis*

Antiviral prophylaxis is not a substitute for vaccination but may be beneficial in select circumstances. Table 5 lists situations in which chemoprophylaxis should be considered.[56] For these recommendations, the infectious period for influenza is defined as one day before symptoms begin until 24 hours after fever resolves. The doses of antiviral agents for prophylaxis of influenza in adolescents are shown in Table 2. The duration of prophylaxis depends on the specific setting; durations of 14 days after immunization or 7–10 days for postexposure prophylaxis are appropriate. The CDC's web site[57] may be consulted for updates regarding influenza chemoprophylaxis. Antiviral agents may interfere with response to LAIV but not TIV.

**Infection control**

Increased media attention to prevention of influenza transmission in the community was observed in 2009. Cough etiquette and hand hygiene were emphasized. In past years, patients hospitalized with suspected or known influenza were managed with droplet precautions for the duration of illness.[32] With the unique situation in 2009, the CDC advised additional precautions including a fit-tested disposable N95 respirator when in close contact with patients who were suspected or proven to have 2009 H1N1 pandemic influenza.[67]

## CONCLUSIONS

The 2009 influenza pandemic served as a reminder of the global impact of this virus. Primary care clinics and emergency departments evaluated record numbers of patients. Hospitalizations and deaths were noted among previously healthy children, adolescents, and young adults. Renewed interest was dedicated to laboratory testing and vaccine development. Many questions remain to be answered, but we will be better prepared for future influenza epidemics and pandemics.

## REFERENCES

1. Thompson WW, Shay DK, Weintraub E, et al. Mortality associated with influenza and respiratory syncytial virus in the United States. *JAMA*. 2003;289:179–186
2. Thompson WW, Shay DK, Weintraub E, et al. Influenza-associated hospitalizations in the United States. *JAMA*. 2004;292:1333–1340
3. Thompson WW, Weintraub E, Dhankhar P, et al. Estimates of US influenza-associated deaths made using four different methods. *Influenza Other Respi Viruses*. 2009;3:37–49
4. Centers for Disease Control and Prevention. CDC estimates of 2009 H1N1 influenza cases, hospitalizations and deaths in the United States, April-December 12, 2009. Available at: http://www.cdc.gov/h1n1flu/estimates_2009_h1n1.htm. Accessed January 27, 2010
5. Treanor JJ. Influenza viruses, including avian influenza and swine influenza. In: Mandell GL, Bennett JE, Dolin R, eds. *Principles and Practice of Infectious Diseases*. 7th ed. Philadelphia, PA: Churchill Livingstone; 2010:2265–2288
6. Palese P, Shaw ML. Orthomyxoviridae: the viruses and their replication. In: Knipe DM, Howley PM, eds. *Field's Virology*. 5th ed. Philadelphia, PA: Lippincott Williams & Wilkins; 2007:1647–1690
7. Wright P. Influenza viruses. In: Kliegman RM, Behrman RE, Jenson HB, Stanton BF, eds. *Nelson Textbook of Pediatrics*. 18th ed. Philadelphia, PA: Saunders Elsevier; 2007:1384–1386
8. Webster RG, Bean WJ, Gorman OT, Chambers TM, Kawaoka Y. Evolution and ecology of influenza A viruses. *Microbiol Rev*. 1992;56:152–179
9. Subbarao K. Influenza viruses. In: Long SS, Pickering LK, Prober CG, eds. *Principles and Practice of Pediatric Infectious Diseases*. 3th ed. Philadelphia, PA: Churchill Livingstone; 2008:1130–1138
10. Murphy BR, Kasel JA, Chanock RM. Association of serum anti-neuraminidase antibody with resistance to influenza in man. *N Engl J Med*. 1972;286:1329–1332
11. Virelizier JL. Host defenses against influenza virus: the role of anti-hemagglutinin antibody. *J Immunol*. 1975;115:434–439
12. Hayden FG. Influenza. In: Goldman L, Ausiello D, eds. *Cecil Medicine*. 23rd ed. Philadelphia, PA: Saunders Elsevier; 2007:2464–2470
13. Chanock RH, Cockburn WC, Davenport FM, et al. A revised system of influenza virus nomenclature: a report of the WHO study group on classification. *Virology*. 1972;47:854–856
14. Wilson IA, Cox NJ. Structural basis of immune recognition of influenza virus hemagglutinin. *Annu Rev Immunol*. 1990;8:737–771
15. Webster RG, Laver WG, Air GM, Ward C, Gerhard W, van Wyke KL. The mechanism of antigenic drift in influenza viruses: analysis of Hong Kong (H3N2) variants with monoclonal antibodies to the hemagglutinin molecule. *Ann N Y Acad Sci*. 1980;354:142–161
16. Cox NJ, Subbarao K. Influenza. *Lancet*. 1999;354:1277–1282
17. Trifonov V, Khiabanian H, Rabadan R. Geographic dependence, surveillance, and origins of the 2009 influenza A (H1N1) virus. *N Engl J Med*. 2009;361:115–119
18. Fisher MC. Novel H1N1 pandemic: when pigs fly. *Pediatr Infect Dis J*. 2009;28:911–914

19. Subbarao K, Klimov A, Katz J, et al. Characterization of an avian influenza A (H5N1) virus isolated from a child with a fatal respiratory illness. *Science.* 1998;279:393–396
20. Fouchier RA, Schneeberger PM, Rozendaal FW, et al. Avian influenza A virus (H7N7) associated with human conjunctivitis and a fatal case of acute respiratory distress syndrome. *Proc Natl Acad Sci U S A.* 2004;101:1356–1361
21. Peiris M, Yuen K, Leung CW, et al. Human infection with H9N2. *Lancet.* 1999;354:916–917
22. Katz JM, Lim W, Bridges CB, et al. Antibody response in individuals infected with avian influenza A (H5N1) viruses and detection of anti-H5 antibody among household and social contacts. *J Infect Dis.* 1999;180:1763–1770
23. Glezen WP. Influenza viruses. In: Feigin RD, Cherry JD, Demmler-Harrison GJ, Kaplan SL, eds. *Feigin & Cherry's Textbook of Pediatric Infectious Diseases.* 6th ed. Philadelphia, PA: Saunders Elsevier; 2009:2395–2413
24. Neuzil KM, Hohlbein C, Zhu Y. Illness among schoolchildren during influenza season: effect on school absenteeism, parental absenteeism from work, and secondary illness in families. *Arch Pediatr Adolesc Med.* 2002;156:986–991
25. Glezen WP, Decker M, Perrotta DM. Survey of underlying conditions of persons hospitalized with acute respiratory disease during influenza epidemics in Houston, 1978–1981. *Am Rev Respir Dis.* 1987;136:550–555
26. Bhat N, Wright JG, Broder KR, et al. Influenza-associated deaths among children in the United States, 2003–2004. *N Engl J Med.* 2005;353:2559–2567
27. Hessen MT. Influenza. *Ann Intern Med.* 2009;151:ITC5.1–5.16
28. Glezen WP. Emerging infections: pandemic influenza. *Epidemiol Rev.* 1996;18:64–76
29. Centers for Disease Control and Prevention. 2009 H1N1 early outbreak and disease characteristics. Available at: http://www.cdc.gov/h1n1flu/surveillanceqa.htm. Accessed January 27, 2010
30. Louie JK, Acosta M, Jamieson DJ, Honein MA, for the California Pandemic (H1N1) Working Group. Severe 2009 H1N1 influenza in pregnant and postpartum women in California. *N Engl J Med.* 2010;362:27–35
31. Jain S, Kamimoto L, Bramley AM, et al. Hospitalized patients with 2009 H1N1 influenza in the United States, April-June 2009. *N Engl J Med.* 2009;361:1935–1944
32. American Academy of Pediatrics. Influenza. In: Pickering LK, Baker CJ, Long SS, Kimberlin DW, eds. *Red Book: 2009 Report of the Committee on Infectious Diseases.* 28th ed. Elk Grove Village, IL: American Academy of Pediatrics; 2009:400–412
33. Frank AL, Taber LH, Wells CR, Wells JM, Glezen WP, Paredes A. Patterns of shedding of myxoviruses and paramyxoviruses in children. *J Infect Dis.* 1981;144:433–441
34. Hayden FG, Fritz R, Lobo MC, Alvord W, Strober W, Straus SE. Local and systemic cytokine responses during experimental human influenza A virus infection. Relation to symptom formation and host defense. *J Clin Invest.* 1998;101:643–649
35. Murphy BR, Nelson DL, Wright PF, Tierney EL, Phelan MA, Chanock RM. Secretory and systemic immunological response in children infected with live attenuated influenza A virus vaccines. *Infect Immun.* 1982;36:1102–1108
36. Couch RB, Kasel JA. Immunity to influenza in man. *Annu Rev Microbiol.* 1983;37:529–549
37. Cherry JD. Influenza viral infections. In: Vaughan V, McKay R, Behrman R, eds. *Nelson Textbook of Pediatrics.* 14th ed. Philadelphia, PA: Saunders; 1987:675–678
38. Mogabgab WJ. The complications of influenza. *Med Clin North Am.* 1963;47:1191–1199
39. Jordan WS, Denny FW, Badger GF, et al. A study of illness in a group of Cleveland families. XVII. The occurrence of Asian influenza. *Am J Hyg.* 1958;68:190–212
40. Finelli L, Fiore A, Dhara R, et al. Influenza-associated pediatric mortality in the United States: increase of *Staphylococcus aureus* coinfection. *Pediatrics.* 2008;122:805–811
41. The Writing Committee of the World Health Organization (WHO) Consultation on Human Influenza A/H5. Avian influenza A (H5N1) infection in humans. *N Engl J Med.* 2005;353:1374–1385
42. Ferson MJ, Morton JR, Robertson PW. Impact of influenza on morbidity in children with cystic fibrosis. *J Paediatr Child Health.* 1991;27:308–311

43. Glezen WP. Asthma, influenza, and vaccination. *J Allergy Clin Immunol.* 2006;118:1199–1206
44. Sperber SJ, Francis JB. Toxic shock during an influenza outbreak. *JAMA.* 1987;257:1086–1087
45. Troendle JF, Demmler GJ, Glezen WP, Finegold M, Romano MJ. Fatal influenza B virus pneumonia in pediatric patients. *Pediatr Infect Dis J.* 1992;11:117–121
46. Middleton PJ, Alexander RM, Szymanski MT. Severe myositis during recovery from influenza. *Lancet.* 1970;2:533–535
47. Shinjoh M, Bamba M, Jozaki K, Takahashi E, Koinuma G, Sugaya N. Influenza A-associated encephalopathy with bilateral thalamic necrosis in Japan. *Clin Infect Dis.* 2000;31:611–613
48. Centers for Disease Control and Prevention. Flu activity and surveillance. Available at: http://www.cdc.gov/flu/weekly/fluactivity.htm. Accessed January 27, 2010
49. Centers for Disease Control and Prevention. 2009–2010 influenza season triage algorithm for children (≤18 years) with influenza-like illness. Available at: http://www.cdc.gov/h1n1flu/clinicians/pdf/childalgorithm.pdf. Accessed January 27, 2010
50. Monto AS, Gravenstein S, Elliott M, Colopy M, Schweinle J. Clinical signs and symptoms predicting influenza infection. *Arch Intern Med.* 2000;160:3243–3247
51. Friedman MJ, Attia MW. Clinical predictors of influenza in children. *Arch Pediatr Adolesc Med.* 2004;158:391–394
52. Harper SA, Bradley JS, Englund JA, et al. Expert Panel of the Infectious Diseases Society of America. Seasonal influenza in adults and children: diagnosis, treatment, chemoprophylaxis, and institutional outbreak management—clinical practice guidelines of the Infectious Diseases Society of America. *Clin Infect Dis.* 2009;48:1003–1032
53. Uyeki TM. Influenza diagnosis and treatment in children: a review of studies on clinically useful tests and antiviral treatment for influenza. *Pediatr Infect Dis J.* 2003;22:164–177
54. Hurt AC, Alexander R, Hibbert J, Deed N, Barr IG. Performance of six influenza rapid tests in detecting human influenza in clinical specimens. *J Clin Virol.* 2007;39:132–135
55. Centers for Disease Control and Prevention. Influenza symptoms and laboratory diagnostic procedures. Available at: http://www.cdc.gov/flu/professionals/diagnosis/labprocedures.htm. Accessed January 27, 2010
56. Centers for Disease Control and Prevention. Updated interim recommendations for the use of antiviral medications in the treatment and prevention of influenza for the 2009–2010 season. Available at: http://www.cdc.gov/h1n1flu/recommendations.htm. Accessed January 27, 2010
57. Centers for Disease Control and Prevention. Seasonal influenza. Information for health professionals. Available at: http://www.cdc.gov/flu/professionals/index.htm. Accessed January 27, 2010
58. American Academy of Pediatrics, Committee on Infectious Diseases. Policy statement—recommendations for the prevention and treatment of influenza in children, 2009–2010. *Pediatrics.* 2009;124:1216–1226
59. Centers for Disease Control and Prevention. Fluview. A weekly influenza surveillance report prepared by the Influenza Division. Available at: http://www.cdc.gov/flu/weekly. Accessed January 27, 2010
60. Hayden FG, Gwaltney JM, Van de Castle RL, Adams KF, Giordani B. Comparative toxicity of amantadine hydrochloride and rimantadine hydrochloride in healthy adults. *Antimicrob Agents Chemother.* 1981;19:226–233
61. Moscona A. Neuraminidase inhibitors for influenza. *N Engl J Med.* 2005;353:1363–1373
62. Glezen WP. Clinical practice. Prevention and treatment of seasonal influenza. *N Engl J Med.* 2008;359:2579–2585
63. Centers for Disease Control and Prevention. H1N1 Flu. Emergency Use Authorization (EUA) of medical products and devices. Available at http://www.cdc.gov/h1n1flu/eua. Accessed January 27, 2010
64. Johnson PR, Feldman S, Thompson JM, Mahoney JD, Wright PF. Immunity to influenza A infection in young children: a comparison of natural infection, live cold-adapted vaccine, and inactivated vaccine. *J Infect Dis.* 1986;154:121–127

65. Piedra PA, Gaglani MJ, Kozinetz CA, et al. Trivalent live attenuated intranasal influenza vaccine administered during the 2003–2004 influenza type A (H3N2) outbreak provided immediate, direct, and indirect protection in children. *Pediatrics*. 2007;120:e553–e564
66. National Center for Immunization and Respiratory Diseases, Centers for Disease Control and Prevention. Use of influenza A (H1N1) 2009 monovalent vaccine. Recommendations of the Advisory Committee on Immunization Practices (ACIP), 2009. *MMWR*. 2009;58:1–8
67. Centers for Disease Control and Prevention. H1N1 flu: infection control. Available at: http://www.cdc.gov/h1n1flu/infection control. Accessed January 27, 2010

# Epstein-Barr Virus, Cytomegalovirus, and Infectious Mononucleosis

### Terrill Bravender, MD, MPH*

*Department of Adolescent Medicine, Nationwide Children's Hospital, Associate Professor of Clinical Pediatrics, The Ohio State University College of Medicine, Columbus, OH 43210*

The clinical syndrome of what we now understand as infectious mononucleosis (IM) was described in the late 1800s as "glandular fever," but the term IM was first used formally in 1920.[1] The term was based on the similarities noted in the peripheral blood smears of six college students with glandular fever: lymphocytosis with atypically abundant cytoplasm in many of their mononuclear cells.[2] Even before the causative agent was discovered, it was noted that serum from patients with IM caused sheep erythrocytes to agglutinate[3] and this property forms the basis of the heterophile antibody diagnostic tests used today. The fact that heterophile antibody tests for the diagnosis of IM were even discovered is a tribute to a combination of scientific observation and serendipity. In the 1920s, it was noted that anti-sheep erythrocyte antibodies develop following serum sickness. Physicians at Yale University studying rheumatic fever noted the clinical similarities between rheumatic fever and serum sickness, and began examining the sera of rheumatic fever patients for heterophile antibodies. Although the researchers were disappointed at the lack of heterophile antibodies in the rheumatic fever patients, they did note very high antibody levels in the serum of a single control patient. One of the investigators ran out of time while processing this particular sample and placed the test in the refrigerator overnight, leading to cold-enhanced agglutination. The donor of the control serum was then identified as a medical student who happened to be suffering from symptoms of IM.[1] Subsequent to these observations, the first article describing the heterophile antibody test for the diagnosis was IM was published in 1932.[4] A simplified test for heterophile antibodies was developed in the late 1960s[5] and continues in use today as "monospot" tests.

In 1964, Epstein, Achong, and Barr first described EBV in Burkitt's lymphoma samples using electron microcopy.[6] Four years later, the association between Epstein-Barr virus infection and IM was discovered when a research assistant

---

*Corresponding author.
*E-mail address*: bravender.1@osu.edu (T. Bravender).

who worked with EBV developed the symptoms of IM.[7] It has been proposed that the term IM should be used specifically for EBV infection associated illness and that similar clinical illnesses caused by other organisms should be referred to as "mononucleosis-like illnesses" (MLI).[8] However, because there is often little clinical value in differentiating IM from MLI, such differential terminology tends to be inconsistently applied.

**Epstein-Barr Virus**

*Virology*

Humans and a few other primates are the only known reservoirs of EBV, which is a fragile, enveloped herpesvirus. The virus cannot survive for long outside of a host. Because of this, transmission occurs primarily from direct exposure to oropharyngeal secretions, most often saliva, hence its reputation among adolescents as "the kissing disease." After exposure, the virus infects oral epithelial cells then spreads to B lymphocytes, which spread the infection throughout the lymphoreticular system. There is polyclonal B-cell proliferation with a significant T-cell response. The atypical T cells that are frequently seen on peripheral blood smears are mainly CD8 cytotoxic or suppressor cells. This immune response accounts for many of the clinical manifestations of IM, including lympadenopathy and hepatosplenomegaly.[9] During the acute phase of the illness, a large number of B lymphocytes are infected, but they are all resting memory cells; these circulating cells do not proliferate and thus have no oncogenic potential.[10] Over the next 3–4 months, the number of infected cells falls, but such cells continue to circulate indefinitely even in healthy, asymptomatic individuals.[11] The virus remains in the body for life, and 60–100% of normal asymptomatic individuals who are seropositive for EBV shed the virus intermittently in an unpredictable fashion.[12] Over time, EBV infection of B cells may lead to cell transformation and establishment of lymphoblastoid cell lines. This transformation occurs very quickly in vitro, demonstrating the critical role that host immunity plays in containing latent infection.[13]

*Epidemiology*

Between 30% and 40% of adolescents who contract EBV will develop symptoms of IM.[14] About half of children have been exposed to EBV before the age of 5 years, and over 90% of adults have evidence of past EBV infection.[15] Infection in early childhood is usually asymptomatic; it is thought that in many underdeveloped nations, this is the most frequent time of transmission. In the United States and other developed countries, infants and young children are not as frequently exposed to EBV. Instead, the virus is frequently encountered during the adolescent or young adult years, often resulting in clinical symptoms of IM.[16] IM occurs less frequently in African-American youth than in white youth; this may be because African-American children are more likely to live in more densely-populated environments and acquire EBV infection young enough to have subclinical infections.[17] An infected individual will transmit EBV to about half of susceptible household contacts, and repeated exposure may induce higher levels of asymptomatic viral shedding in seropositive household members.[18] EBV infection occurs throughout the year and does not demonstrate consistent seasonal peaks.[19] Despite the fact that multiple different strains of EBV exist, it appears that a single episode of IM confers lifelong immunity. Indeed, less than 10% of individuals with IM are infected with a single strain of EBV; the vast majority of patients are infected with multiple strains at the same time.[20]

*Clinical Syndrome*

Classic IM is common in adolescents and young adults. Yet even in these populations, most EBV infections are asymptomatic or associated with mild nonspecific symptoms such as malaise, fever, and decreased appetite. In those who develop clinical IM, there is an incubation period lasting 4–7 weeks, after which time there may be a 3- to 5-day prodrome of malaise, fatigue, headache, decreased appetite, and myalgias. The prodrome is followed by worsening signs and symptoms as the immune response mounts.[9] The traditional triad of IM includes: 1) fever, lymphadenopathy, and pharyngitis; 2) lymphocytosis with atypical lymphocytes; and 3) heterophile or EBV-specific antibody response.[17]

The differential diagnosis of EBV-seronegative mononucleosis-like illnesses is quite extensive,[9] and may include infection with cytomegalovirus (CMV) (which is covered in detail later), human herpesvirus 6 (HHV-6), group A streptococcus, *Mycoplasma pneumoniae*, acute human immunodeficiency virus (HIV) infection, adenovirus, herpes simplex virus (HSV), *Steptococcus pyogenese*, *Toxoplama gondii*, or pharyngitis caused by other viruses. Less common causes that may need to be considered include leukemia or a lymphoproliferative disorder, viral hepatitis, rubella, or diphtheria.

*Laboratory Evaluation*

The classic test for EBV-associated IM is the presence of heterophile antibodies, which detect immunoglobulin M (IgM) antibodies. The IgM antibodies detected are induced by EBV infection and cross-react with unrelated antigens, typically sheep, horse, or bovine erythrocytes. When compared with EBV-specific serologies, rapid test kits for heterophile antibodies have sensitivities ranging from 78% to 84% and specificities ranging from 89% to 100%.[21] These tests are simple to perform, relatively inexpensive, and have high sensitivity and specificity.[22] Sensitivity is lower (<50%) in children under the age of 12 years,[23] and younger children with EBV may not demonstrate the classic symptoms of IM. By age 4, about 80% of children with IM will have heterophile antibodies, and up to 90% of adolescents with IM will be positive at some point during the illness.[24]

The sensitivity of heterophile antibody tests is also lower during the first week of illness.[25] Levels of heterophile antibodies peak between 2 and 5 weeks into the illness, and low levels may be detected up to a year later.[8] About 10% of adolescents with EBV-associated IM will remain heterophile antibody negative, but may be diagnosed by the detection of IgM antibodies against EBV viral capsid antigen (VCA).[26] Both IgM and IgG VCA antibodies peak at about 3–4 weeks after the onset of clinical symptoms. VCA-IgM levels decline rapidly, and are undetectable by 3 months. VCA-IgG levels also decline somewhat, but are detectable for life. Anti-early antigen (EA) antibodies are seen in between 70% and 90% of patients. Anti-EA antibodies are produced very early in the infection and persist for 1–2 months, but as many as 30% of patients will have persistently high EA titers. Finally, antibodies against Epstein-Barr nuclear antigen (EBNA) develop 2–3 months after the acute infection and persist indefinitely.[9] Table 1 summarizes specific EBV antibody tests and their relationship to clinical illness.

The traditional laboratory diagnostic criteria for IM include a relative lymphocytosis (comprising >50% of the white blood cell (WBC) differential), as well as atypical lymphocytes comprising at least 10% of the WBC differential.[27] Brigden and colleagues found that 86% of patients with the lymphocytosis described were heterophile-antibody positive.[28] They also noted that patients who were heterophile-antibody positive had significantly higher total WBC counts and lower platelet counts than IM patients who were antibody negative. Mild thrombocytopenia (with platelet counts in the range of $100–140 \times 10^5/L$), mild granulocytopenia, and a mild hemolytic anemia associated with cold ag-

Table 1
Serologic patterns of Epstein-Barr virus associated infectious mononucleosis

| Antigen-Antibody | Stage of Illness | | | | |
|---|---|---|---|---|---|
| | Susceptible | Acute Primary Infection | Recent Past Infection | Remote Past Infection | Reactivation |
| Heterophile antibody | — | + | + | — | +/− |
| VCA-IgM | — | + | — | — | — |
| VCA-IgG | — | ++ | + | + | +++ |
| Anti-EA | — | + | +/− | — | + |
| Anti-EBNA | — | — | — | + | +/− |

VCA, viral capsid antigen; EA, early antigen; EBNA, Epstein-Barr nuclear antigen; Ig, immunoglobulin.
From: Bravender T, Walter EB. Infectious respiratory illnesses. In: Neinstein LS, Gordon CM, Katzman DK, Rosen DS, Woods ER, eds. Adolescent Healthcare: A Practical Guide. 5th ed. Philadelphia, PA: Lippincott Williams & Wilkins; 2008:413–426; and Gerber MA, Shapiro ED, Ryan RW, Bell GL. Evaluations of enzyme-linked immunosorbent assay procedure for determining specific Epstein-Barr virus serology and of rapid test kits for diagnosis for infectious mononucleosis. J Clin Microbiol. 1996;34(12):3240–3241.

glutinins occur in up to 3% of patients.[29] Rarely, a more severe hemolytic anemia may be seen.[30]

Evidence of a mild hepatitis is so common that entirely normal findings from liver chemistries may suggest a diagnosis other than EBV infection.[9] The liver function test abnormalities peak during the second or third week of symptoms, and resolve by the end of the fourth week. Transaminase levels may be as high as 2–3 times normal, and alkaline phosphatase and lactate dehydrogenase levels may also be elevated. Bilirubin may be slightly elevated in the range of 1 to 3 mg/dL in as many as 15% of patients.[31] More severe hyperbilirubinemia due to cholestatic jaundice is extremely rare, but may be complicated by an associated hemolytic anemia.[30]

*Acute Complications*

Although the vast majority of IM cases are self-limited and mild, there are a few specific and potentially serious complications that can be associated with the infection. Splenic rupture has been reported to occur in as many as 0.1–0.2% of cases of IM, with only about half of these cases associated with physical trauma or sports participation.[32] Patients with splenic rupture typically develop abrupt onset of left upper quadrant abdominal pain radiating to the left shoulder (Kehr's sign).[33] Patients may then experience generalized abdominal pain, pleuritic chest pain, and signs and symptoms of hypovolemia. Occasionally, the onset is insidious, without any history of Kehr's sign. There have been case reports of iatrogenic splenic rupture as a result of deep palpitation during abdominal examinations.[34] Because there is no correlation between splenic rupture and clinical severity or laboratory findings, all patients with IM should be considered at risk.[35] The greatest risk for splenic rupture is between the 4th and 21st days of the illness. Given the dramatic risk of morbidity and mortality associated with splenic rupture, all patients with IM should refrain from all physical activity for a minimum of 4 weeks after the onset of symptoms. This is unlikely to cause hardship for most athletes, as their other clinical symptoms are likely to persist at least this long, and they will be unlikely to feel well enough to participate in vigorous physical activities. It has been traditionally recommended that athletes refrain from participating in contact sports a longer period of time, but there is no evidence to support any specific time period beyond 4 weeks. The likelihood of splenic rupture decreases as more time progresses, and decisions about returning to play should be made on a case-by-case basis. Although ultrasound may be used to assess splenomegaly, there is significant variability in normal spleen size.[36,37] Because of this, single measurements are unlikely to provide any useful data, and splenic imaging is not recommended.[35]

Airway obstruction is an uncommon but potentially life-threatening complication that is related to lymphoid hyperplasia and mucosal edema. This typically occurs 1 week after the onset of symptoms and tends to be more common in younger teens. Corticosteroids have been used with varying degrees of success in an attempt to reduce the edema and hypertrophy. In more severe cases, acute tonsillectomy may be indicated, and an emergency situation may even require endotracheal intubation or tracheostomy.[38]

Coinfection with group A β-hemolytic streptococci (GAS) was once believed to be quite common. It was thought that EBV infection allows the streptococci to adhere to epithelial cell membranes, and older studies reported coinfection in up to one-third of patients with IM. However, only ~4% of those with IM are coinfected with GAS, which is about the same as the asymptomatic rate of streptococcal colonization in the general population.[39] One should use caution when treating a comorbid streptococcal pharyngitis due to the rash that often occurs in patients with EBV infection who are exposed to amoxicillin or ampicillin.[40] Rashes on the face, neck, trunk, extremities, and often the palms and soles occur in 70–100% of patients with IM who are exposed to an amino-penicillin.[41] This pruritic rash usually does not present until the patient has been on the medication for at least 5 days, and may last as long as a week. The exact mechanism of the rash is unknown, and it is unclear whether patients who develop the IM-associated drug rash remain sensitive to the inciting drug.[42] Patients with suspected streptococcal pharyngitis should not be treated with amoxicillin, but may use oral penicillin, which is less likely to result in a rash.

There are a variety of rare but well-described neurologic complications associated with EBV infection, including Guillain-Barre syndrome, cranial nerve palsy, optic neuritis, peripheral neuropathy, cerebellar ataxia, and transverse myelitis.[43] Patients may develop encephalitis,[44] including symptoms of the "Alice in Wonderland" syndrome. This is an encephalopathy that involves defects in the perception of size, shape, color, and spatial relationships of objects known as metamorphopsia.[45] Genital ulcerations caused by EBV have been reported,[46] and may develop before the development of IM symptoms. It has been suggested that EBV may play a role in chronic autoimmune diseases such as systemic lupus erythematosus[47] and multiple sclerosis.[48] However, it remains unclear what, if any, role EBV plays in these disorders, and the ubiquity of EBV exposure has limited research in this area.

*Management*

The vast majority of patients with IM will only require supportive, symptomatic care. The most important intervention is to encourage the adolescent to get adequate rest during the acute phase of illness. The adolescent (and parents) should be counseled that this acute phase typically lasts 1–2 weeks, but the associated fatigue may last 2–4 weeks, or occasionally even longer. Many patients require up to 2 months to achieve complete recovery.[49] About 1 in 10 patients with IM report persistent fatigue 6 months after the onset of symptoms.[50] Because there have been a few case reports of Reye syndrome associated with IM,[51] the use of aspirin should be avoided. Other nonsteroidal anti-inflammatory agents or acetaminophen may be used as needed for fever and pain. Patients may find oral intake difficult due to their pharyngitis, and they should be counseled regarding the importance of maintaining adequate hydration.

In the rare instances of a coinfection with group A streptococcus or *Mycoplasma pneumoniae*, appropriate antibiotic therapy should be initiated. Otherwise, antibiotics serve no purpose and their use should be avoided. Antiviral agents such as acyclovir are not indicated. Although the use of acyclovir may reduce viral shedding, it does not impact the severity or duration of the clinical syndrome. Similarly, routine treatment with corticosteroids is not indicated.[52] Despite their lack of effectiveness and abundant recommendations to avoid their use, corticosteroids are prescribed frequently for IM. Their use is only indicated in patients with pharyngeal edema that is significant enough to threaten respiratory compromise.[53] An EBV vaccine has shown some promise in decreasing the risk of IM in EBV-seronegative young adults,[54] but the potential public health impact is, as of yet, unknown.

*Chronic and Latent Infection*

Virtually all patients with EBV-associated IM develop lifelong immunity to reinfection, and remain asymptomatic from the latent infection. Very rarely, patients will develop persistent, chronic EBV infection associated with very high titers of EBV antibodies.[55] In addition to high antibody levels, it has been proposed that the diagnostic criteria for chronic EBV infection should include all of the following: 1) clinical symptoms lasting >6 months; 2) persistent histologic evidence of end-organ disease, such as hepatitis, pneumonitis, or uveitis; and 3) evidence of EBV antigen or DNA in tissue.[56] Despite some clinical similarities between chronic fatigue syndrome (CFS) and chronic EBV infection, there is little evidence that EBV causes CFS. A positive EBV IgG test in a patient with CFS does not imply a causal relationship, and given how common EBV infection is in the general population, it appears that EBV is likely an innocent bystander.[57]

Latent EBV resides primarily in the B lymphocyte pool, and to a lesser degree in epithelial cells. This, combined with EBV's ability to alter cellular gene transcription, is likely the basis for EBV's association with a variety of lymphoid and epithelial cancers.[58] In equatorial Africa, Burkitt's lymphoma is associated with malaria, and 90% of these tumors are also associated with EBV infection. In contrast, in the United States, only ~20% of Bukitt's lymphomas are associated with EBV.[55] Hodgkin's lymphoma, nasopharyngeal carcinoma, and gastric carcinoma are also linked to EBV infection.[59] Those with impaired immune function are at greatest risk. For example, those with HIV are at elevated risk for primary central nervous system lymphoma and diffuse large B-cell lymphoma. In patients who have received both solid organ and bone marrow transplants, EBV infection is implicated in posttransplant lymphoproliferative disorders.[60] In the rare genetic disorder X-linked lymphoproliferative syndrome, affected males are unable to control the EBV infection, and in one registry of such patients, over half died of IM.[61] Finally, infection of host T cells with EBV may be associated with hemophagocytic syndrome resulting in severe pancytopenia and hepatitis.[62]

## Cytomegalovirus Infection

### Virology

Human cytomegalovirus (CMV) was first isolated from salivary gland tissue in 1956 and was initially referred to as "salivary gland virus."[63] A mononucleosis-like illness associated with CMV infection was first described in 1965,[64] and soon after transmission via blood transfusion was noted.[65] CMV is a member of the herpes family, and is the largest virus that infects humans. Because the virus is so large and codes for so many proteins, the exact mechanism of infection has been difficult to elucidate. The incubation period for infection is not precisely known, but is likely between 1 and 2 months.[66] Like other herpes viruses, CMV infection remains latent after acute infection and may be reactivated, particularly if there is an alteration in host immunity.[67] Although the exact mechanisms of latency and reactivation are unknown, CMV downregulates cell surface markers, which likely helps the virus avoid the host immune system.[68] Once infection is established, the virus may be harbored in a variety of body tissues, including polymorphonuclear cells, T lymphocytes, pulmonary secretions, vascular endothelial cells, renal epithelial cells, and salivary glands.[69] When host immunity is impaired, such as in HIV infection or due to chemotherapeutic agents, reactivation of latent disease may occur, resulting in severe end-organ damage. In addition to primary infection in naïve hosts and reactivation in immunocompromised hosts, some seropositive individuals may develop secondary infections with different strains of CMV.[70] Previous concerns regarding CMV-induced cancers[71] were likely overstated, and the virus does not share the oncogenic potential of EBV.[69]

### Epidemiology

It has been estimated that between 1% and 2% of the population in the United States is infected annually, and nearly everyone has been infected by age 70. Children who attend day care centers are likely to contract CMV earlier in life. Although the risk may be lower in home-based child care settings,[72] ~20% of preschool children and as many as 70% of toddlers in day care excrete CMV,[73] and these children may pose a risk for seronegative adults who care for them.[74] Despite the frequent excretion of CMV by children, nosocomial transmission rarely occurs. This may be because person-to-person transmission requires prolonged, intimate contact as might occur among family members, among children together for long periods in day care, and in sexual activity. CMV is excreted in all bodily fluids except tears. These include breast milk, urine, saliva, and cervical and vaginal secretions; the highest concentration is found in semen. The assumption of sexual transmission is supported by the fact that seroconversion to CMV may be associated with increased sexual activity in adolescents, and men who have sex with men have been shown to have very high rates of CMV infection.[69]

*Clinical Manifestations*

Infected newborns are most likely to be seriously affected by CMV infection, as are those who are immunocompromised. Detailed discussions of these at-risk groups are beyond the scope of this review. The vast majority of CMV infections in immunocompetent adolescents are asymptomatic. However, acute CMV infection may result in a mononucleosis syndrome consisting of fever, lymphadenopathy, and atypical lymphocytosis. As many as 20% of patients with mononucleosis will have CMV,[75] and CMV should be considered in patients with IM who have negative heterophile antibody tests.[76] The clinical disease is likely to be indistinguishable from IM caused by EBV, although CMV infection may not result in the same severity of lymphadenopathy, splenomegaly, or pharyngitis.[77] Wreghitt and colleagues examined serum samples that had been drawn from 7630 patients who had presented with fever, malaise, lymphadenopathy, jaundice, hepatitis, or sweats.[78] Of these patients, 124 (1.63%) had CMV-specific IgM levels >300 U/mL and were negative for EBV, hepatitis A, hepatitis B core antigen, and *Toxoplasma gondii* IgM antibodies. The most common symptoms were malaise (67%), fever (46%), and sweats (46%), and 69% had abnormal liver function tests. Of the 124 patients studied, only 4 were <20 years of age. The most common laboratory abnormalities seen in primary CMV infection include mild elevation of liver function tests to between 2 and 5 times the normal values. Patients may have normal total white blood cell counts, but are likely to have a relative leukocytosis.[79]

*Complications and Prevention*

The vast majority of immunocompetent patients will require nothing more than supportive care, similar to that recommended for EBV-associated IM. Reactivation of latent CMV used to be a potentially devastating complication of HIV infection, but the introduction of highly active antiretroviral therapy (HAART) in the mid-1990s dramatically reduced the risks for CMV disease in HIV-positive patients.[80] CMV remains a potentially serious complication in other immunocompromised states, particularly in patients who have received solid organ transplants, in whom approximately three-quarters are affected by CMV disease.[81] Potentially devastating CMV pneumonia, retinitis, encephalitis, hepatitis, or even widespread multiorgan involvement are exceedingly rare in otherwise healthy patients, but have been reported. Eddleston et al reviewed 34 cases in the medical literature, 7 of whom were 21 years old or younger.[82] Given the rarity of these cases, evidence for appropriate treatment is lacking, but severe end-organ involvement likely merits treatment with antiviral medications such as ganciclovir or foscarnet, as one would treat an immunocompromised patient.

The most significant public-health impact of CMV infection remains congenital transmission of the virus by seronegative pregnant women.[83] The cost of caring for children with congenital CMV is approximately $2 billion annually, or about $300 000 per child per year.[84] Because of this, in 1999, the Institute of Medicine ranked CMV vaccine as having the highest priority for development. Recently, the first phase II trial of a CMV vaccine demonstrating benefits for seronegative women was published.[85] Although promising, one should keep in mind that the primary outcome for such a vaccine is maternal-fetal transmission of CMV, not prevention of primary disease in otherwise healthy patients.[86]

## CONCLUSIONS

Infections with both EBV and CMV are common in adolescents, and many infections are asymptomatic. The vast majority of cases of IM are caused by acute EBV infection, and many of those patients with IM who are EBV-negative will have symptoms attributable to acute CMV infection. In adolescents, there is a wide range of clinical manifestations for these infections, and providers should maintain a high index of suspicion in any teen with fever, lymphadenopathy, pharyngitis, and fatigue. There are a variety of potentially serious effects seen with EBV infection, but most patients will require only supportive care. Despite the persistent fatigue that patients may observe following acute EBV infection, there is little evidence to support a role for EBV as the etiologic agent in chronic fatigue. Although CMV infection in adolescents is usually self-limited and benign, congenital CMV infection continues to have a serious public health impact, which has lead to ongoing vaccine research.

## REFERENCES

1. Evans AS. The history of infectious mononucleosis. *Am J Med Sci*. 1974;267(3):189–195
2. Sprunt TP, Evans FA. Mononucleosis leukocytosis in reaction to acute infections (infectious mononucleosis). *Johns Hopkins Hospital Bulletin*. 1920;31:410
3. Davidsohn I. Serologic diagnosis of infectious mononucleosis. *JAMA*. 1937;108:289–295
4. Paul JR, Burnell WW. The presence of heterophile antibodies in infectious mononucleosis. *Am J Med Sci*. 1932;183:90–104
5. Basson V, Sharp AA. Monospot: a differential slide test for infectious mononucleosis. *J Clin Pathol*. 1969;22:324–325
6. Epstein MA, Achong BG, Barr YM. Virus particles in cultured lymphoblasts from Burkitt's lymphoma. *Lancet*. 1964;1(7335):702–703
7. Henle G, Henle W, Diehl V. Relation of Burkitt's tumor-associated herpes-ytpe virus to infectious mononucleosis. *Proc Natl Acad Sci U S A*. 1968;59(1):94–101
8. Hurt C, Tammaro D. Diagnostic evaluation of mononucleosis-like illnesses. *Am J Med*. 2007; 120(10);e1–e8
9. Bravender T, Walter EB. Infectious respiratory illnesses. In: Neinstein LS, Gordon CM, Katzman DK, Rosen DS, Woods ER, eds. *Adolescent Healthcare: A Practical Guide*. 5th ed. Philadelphia, PA: Lippincott Williams & Wilkins; 2008:413–426

10. Thorley-Lawson DA, Gross A. Persistence of the Epstein-Barr virus and the origins of associated lymphomas. *N Engl J Med.* 2004;350(13);1328–1337
11. Miyashita EM, Yang B, Lam KM, Crawford DH, Thorley-Lawson DA. A novel form of Epstein-Barr virus latency in normal B cells in vivo. *Cell.* 1995;80(4):593–601
12. Hadinoto V, Shapiro M, Sun CC, Thorley-Lawson DA. The dynamics of EBV shedding implicate a central role for epithelial cells in amplifying viral output. *Plos Pathogens.* 2009; 5(7):e1000496
13. Rowe M. Cell transformation induced by Epstein-Barr virus–living dangerously. *Sem Cancer Biol.* 2001;11(6):403–405
14. Fleisher G, Henle G, Lennette ET, Biggar RJ. Primary infection with Epstein-Barr virus in infants in the United States: clinical and serologic observations. *J Infect Dis.* 1979;139:553–558
15. Pereira MS, Blake JM, Macrae AD. EB virus antibody at different ages. *BMJ.* 1969;4:526–527
16. Nye FJ. Social class and infectious mononucleosis. *J Hygiene.* 1973;71:145–149
17. Johannsen EC, Kaye KM. Epstein-Barr virus (infectious mononucleosis, Epstein-Barr virus-associated malignant diseases, and other diseases. In: Mandell GL, Bennett JE, Dolin R, eds. *Mandell, Douglas, and Bennett's Principles and Practice of Infectious Diseases.* 7th ed. Philadelphia, PA: Churchill, Livingston; 2009:1989–2010
18. Sumaya CV, Ench Y. Epstein-Barr virus infections in families: the role of children with infectious mononucleosis. *J Infect Dis.* 1986;154(5):842–850
19. Henke CE, Kurland LT, Elveback LR. Infectious mononucleosis in Rochester, Minnesota, 1950 through 1969. *Am J Epidemiol.* 1973;98(6):483–490
20. Sitki-Green DL, Edwards RH, Covington MM, Raab-Traub N. Biology of Epstein-Barr virus during infectious mononucleosis. *J Infect Dis.* 2004;189(3):483–492
21. Gerber MA, Shapiro ED, Ryan RW, Bell GL. Evaluations of enzyme-linked immunosorbent assay procedure for determining specific Epstein-Barr virus serology and of rapid test kits for diagnosis for infectious mononucleosis. *J Clin Microbiol.* 1996;34(12):3240–3241
22. Bell AT, Fortune B. What test is the best for diagnosing infectious mononucleosis? *J Fam Pract.* 2006;55(9);799–802
23. Linderholm M, Bowman J, Juto P, Linde A. comparative evaluation of nine kits for rapid diagnosis of infectious mononucleosis and Epstein-Barr virus-specific serology. *J Clin Microbiol.* 1994;32:259–307
24. Sumaya CV, Ench Y. Epstein-Barr virus infectious mononucleosis in children. II. Heterophil antiboy and viral-specific responses. *Pediatrics.* 1985;75:1011–1019
25. Fleisher GR, Collins M, Fager S. Limitations of available tests for diagnosis of infectious mononucleosis. *J Clin Microbiol.* 1983;17(4):619–624
26. Henle W, Henle GE, Horwitz CA. Epstein-Barr virus specific diagnostic tests in infectious mononucleosis. *Human Pathol.* 1974;5:551–565
27. Hoagland RJ. The clinical manifestations of infectious mononucleosis: a report of two hundred cases. *Am J Med Sci.* 1960;240:55–63
28. Brigden ML, Au S, Thompson S, Brigden S, Doyle P, Tsaparas Y. Infectious mononucleosis in an outpatient population: diagnostic utility of 2 automated hematology analyzers and the sensitivity and specificity of Hoagland's criteria in heterophile-positive patients. *Arch Pathol Lab Med.* 1999;123(10):875–881
29. Horwitz CA, Moulds J, Henle W, et al. Cold agglutinins in infectious mononucleosis and heterophil-antibody-negative mononucleosis-like syndromes. *Blood.* 1977;50(2):195–202
30. Place E, Wenzel JE, Arumugam R, Belani K, Messinger Y. Successful plasmapheresis for extreme hyperbilirubinemia caused by acute Epstein-Barr virus. *J Pediatr Hematol Oncol.* 2007;29(5):323–326
31. Grotto I, Mimouni D, Huerta M, et al. Clinical and laboratory presentation of EBV positive infectious mononucleosis in young adults. *Epidemiol Infect.* 2003;131(1);683–689
32. Maki DG, Reich RM. infectious mononucleosis in the athlete. Diagnosis, complications, and management. *Am J Sports Med.* 1982;10:62–73
33. Rutkow IM. Rupture of the spleen in infectious mononucleosis: a critical review. *Arch Surg.* 1978;113(6):718–720

34. Smith EB, Custer RP. Rupture of the spleen in infectious mononucleosis: a clinicopathologic report of seven cases. *Blood.* 1946;1:317–333
35. Putukian M, O'Connor FG, Stricker PR, et al. Mononucleosis and athletic participation: an evidence-based subject review. *Clin J Sports Med.* 2008;18(4):309–315
36. Spielmann AL, DeLong DM, Kliewer MA. Sonographic evaluation of spleen size in tall healthy athletes. *Am J Roentgenol.* 2005;184:45–49
37. Hosey RG, Mattacola CG, Kriss V, Armsey T, Quarles JD, Jagger J. Ultrasound assessment of spleen size in collegiate athletes. *Br J Sports Med.* 2006;40(3);251–254
38. Chan SC, Dawes PJ. The management of severe infectious mononucleosis tonsillitis and upper airway obstruction. *J Laryngol Otol.* 2001;115(12):973–977
39. Collins M, Fleisher G, Fager SS. Incidence of beta hemolytic streptococcal pharyngitis in adolescents with infectious mononucleosis. *J Adolesc Health Care.* 1984;5(2):96–100
40. Leung AK, Rafaat M. Eruption associated with amoxicillin in a patient with infectious mononucleosis. *Int J Dermatol.* 2003;42(7);553–555
41. Pauzek ME. Making a rash diagnosis: amoxicillin therapy in infectious mononucleosis. *Indiana Med J.* 1990;83:330–331
42. Renn CN, Straff W, Dorfmuller A, Al-Masaoudi T, Merk HF, Sachs B. Amoxicillin-induced exanthema in young adults with infectious mononucleosis: demonstration of drug-specific lymphocyte reactivity. *Br J Dermatol.* 2002;147(6):1166–1170
43. Connelly KP, DeWitt LD. Neurologic complications of infectious mononucleosis. *Pediatr Neurol.* 1994;10(3):181–184
44. Doja A, Bitnun A, Ford Jones EL, et al. Pediatric Epstein-Barr virus-associated encephalitis: 10-year review. *J Child Neurol.* 2006;21(5);384–391
45. Liaw SB, Shen EY. Alice in Wonderland syndrome as a presenting symptom of EBV infection. *Pediatr Neurol.* 1991;7(6):464–466
46. Halvorsen JA, Brevig T, Aas T, Skar AG, Slevolden EM, Moi H. Genital ulcers as initial manifestation of Epstein-Barr virus infection: two new cases and a review of the literature. *Acta Dermato-Venereologica.* 2006;86(5);439–442
47. Harley JB, Harley ITW, Guthridge JM, James JA. The curiously suspicious: a role for Epstein-Barr virus in lupus. *Lupus.* 2006;15(11);768–777
48. Pohl D. Epstein-Barr virus and multiple sclerosis. *J Neurol Sci.* 2009;286(1–2):62–64
49. Rea TD, Russo JE, Katon W, Ashley RL, Buchwald DS. Prospective study of the natural history of infectious mononucleosis caused by Epstein-Barr virus. *J Am Board Fam Pract.* 2001;14(4); 234–242
50. White PD, Thomas JM, Amess J, et al. Incidence, risk and prognosis of acute and chronic fatigue syndromes and psychiatric disorders after glandular fever. *Br J Psychiatry.* 1998;173:475–481
51. Fleisher G, Schwartz J, Lennette E. Primary Epstein-Barr virus infection in association with Reye syndrome. *J Pediatrics.* 1980;97(6):935–937
52. Tynell E, Aurelius E, Brandell A, et al. Acyclovir and prednisolone treatment of acute infectious mononucleosis: a multicenter, double-blind, placebo-controlled study. *J Infect Dis.* 1996;174(2): 324–331
53. Thompson SK, Doerr TD, Hengerer AS. Infectious mononucleosis and corticosteroids: management practices and outcomes. *Arch Otolaryngol Head Neck Surg.* 2005;131:900–904
54. Sokal EM, Hoppenbrouwers K, Vandermeulen C, et al. Recombinant gp350 vaccine for infectious mononucleosis: a phase 2, randomized, double-bind, placeb-controlled trial to evaluate the safety, immunogenicity, and efficacy of an Epstein-Barr virus vaccine in healthy young adults. *J Infect Dis.* 2007;196(12):1749–1753
55. Cohen JI. Epstein-Barr virus infection. *N Engl J Med.* 2000;343(7):481–492
56. Strauss SE. The chronic mononucleosis syndrome. *J Infect Dis.* 1988;157(3):405–412
57. Marshall GS. Report of a workshop on the epidemiology, natural history, and pathogenesis of chronic fatigue syndrome in adolescents. *J Pediatrics.* 1999;134(4):395–405
58. Young LS, Rickinson AB. Epstein-Barr virus: 40 years on. *Nature Rev Cancer.* 2004;4:757–768
59. Hsu JL, Glaser SL. Epstein-Barr virus-associated malignancies: epidemiologic patterns and etiologic implications. *Crit Rev Oncol Hematol.* 2000;34:27–53

60. Carbone A, Gloghini A, Dotti G. EBV-associated lymphoproliferative disroders: classification and treatment. *Oncologist.* 2008;13(5):577–585
61. Grierson H, Purtilo DT. Epstein-Barr virus infections in males with the X-linked lymphoproliferative syndrome. *Ann Intern Med.* 1987;106:538–545
62. Kitazawa Y, Saito F, Nomura S, Ishii K, Kadota E. A case of hemophagocytic lymphohistiocytosis after the primary Epstein-Barr virus infection. *Clin Appl Thromb Hemost.* 2007;13(3); 323–328
63. Smith MG. Propagation in tissue cultures of a cytopathogenic virus from human salivary gland virus (SGV) disease. *Proc Soc Exp Biol Med.* 1956;92(2):424–430
64. Klemola E, Kaarianen L. Cytomegalovirus as a possible cause of a disease resembling infectious mononucleosis. *Br Med J.* 1965;2(5470):1099–1102
65. Kaarianen L, Klemola E, Paloheimo J. Rise of cytomegalovirus antibodies in an infectious-mononucleosis-like syndrome after transfusion. *Br Med J.* 1966;1(5498):1270–1272
66. Adler SP, Marshall B. Cytomegalovirus infections. *Pediatr Rev.* 2007;28(3):92–100
67. Drew WL. Cytomegalovirus infection in patients with AIDS. *Clin Infect Dis.* 1992;14(2):608–615
68. Beersma MF, Bijlmakers MJ, Ploegh HL. Human cytomegalovirus down-regulates HLA class I expression by reducing the stability of class I H chains. *J Immunol.* 1993;151(9): 4455–4464
69. Crumpacker CS, Zhang JL. Cytomegalovirus. In: Mandell GL, Bennett JE, Dolin R, eds. *Mandell, Douglas, and Bennett's Principles and Practice of Infectious Diseases.* 7th ed. Philadelphia, PA: Churchill, Livingston; 2009:1971–1987
70. Ross SA, Arora N, Novak Z, Fowler KB, Britt WJ, Boppana SB. Cytomegalovirus reinfections in healthy seroimmune women. *J Infect Dis.* 2010;201(3);386–389
71. Spector DH, Spector SA. The oncogenic potential of human cytomegalovirus. *Prog Med Virol.* 1984;29:45–89
72. Bale JF Jr, Zimmerman B, Dawson JD, Souza IE, Petheram SJ, Murph JR. Cytomegalovirus transmission in child care homes. *Arch Pediatr Adolesc Med.* 1999;153(1):75–79
73. Murph JR, Bale JF Jr, Murray JC, Stinski MF, Perlman S. Cytomegalovirus transmission in a Midwest day care center: possible relationship to child care practices. *J Pediatr.* 1986;109(1): 35–39
74. Murph JR, Baron JC, Brown CK, Ebelhack CL, Bale JF Jr. The occupational risk of cytomegalovirus infection among day-care providers. *JAMA.* 1991;265(5):603–608
75. Klemola E, Von Essen R, Henle G, Henle W. Infectious-mononucleosis-like disease with negative heterophil agglutination test. Clinical features in relation to Epstein-Barr virus and cytomegalovirus antibodies. *J Infect Dis.* 1970;121(6):608–614
76. Taylor GH. Cytomegalovirus. *Am Fam Physician.* 2003;67(3);519–524
77. Jordan MC, Rousseau W, Stewart JA, Noble GR, Chin TD. Spontaneous cytomegalovirus mononucleosis. Clinical and laboratory observations in nine cases. *Ann Intern Med.* 1973;79(2): 153–160
78. Wreghitt TG, Teare EL, Sule O, Devi R, Rice P. Cytomegalovirus infection in immunocompetent patients. *Clin Infect Dis.* 2003;37(12);1603–1606
79. Just-Nubling G, Korn S, Ludwig B, Stephan C, Doerr HW, Preiser W. Primary cytomegalovirus infection in an outpatient setting–laboratory markers and clinical aspects. *Infection.* 2003;31(5): 318–323
80. Springer KL, Weinberg A. Cytomegalovirus infection in the era of HAART: fewer reactivations and more immunity. *J Antimicrob Chemother.* 2004;54(3);582–586
81. Fisher RA. Cytomegalovirus infection and disease in the new era of immunosuppression following solid organ transplantation. *Transplant Infect Dis.* 2009;11(3);195–202
82. Eddleston M, Peacock S, Juniper M, Warrell DA. Severe cytomegalovirus infection in immunocompetent patients. *Clin Infect Dis.* 1997;24(1):52–56

83. Arvin AM, Fast P, Myers M, Plotkin S, Rabinovich R. Vaccine development to prevent cytomegalovirus disease: report from the National Vaccine Advisory Committee. *Clin Infect Dis.* 2004;39(2);233–239
84. Fowler KB, Stagno S, Pass RF, Britt WJ, Boll TJ, Alford CA. The outcome of congenital cytomegalovirus infection in relation to maternal antibody status. *N Engl J Med.* 1992;326(10): 663–667
85. Pass RF, Zhang C, Evans A, et al. Vaccine prevention of maternal cytomegalovirus infection. *N Engl J Med.* 2009;360(12);1191–1199
86. Griffiths PD. CMV vaccine trial endpoints. *J Clin Virol.* 2009;46(Suppl 4):S64–S67

# Viral Hepatitis A, B, and C: Grown-Up Issues

## Umid M. Sharapov*[a], Dale J. Hu[a]

[a]*Division of Viral Hepatitis, National Center for HIV?AIDS, VH, STD, and TB Prevention, Centers for Disease Control and Prevention, MS G-37, 1600 Clifton Road, Atlanta, Georgia 30333*

Viral hepatitis is a major global health problem associated with significant morbidity and mortality. Although there are five major and distinct human hepatitis viruses characterized to date—which are referred to as hepatitis A, B, C, D, and E, respectively—only hepatitis A, B, and C are epidemiologically and clinically relevant for adolescents in North America.[1] The clinical presentation of acute infection with each of these viruses is similar (Table 1); thus, diagnosis depends on the use of specific serologic markers and viral nucleic acids (Table 2). This review will provide data on the epidemiology, clinical symptoms, diagnosis, treatment, and prevention of each of these 3 viral infections along with points important or unique to adolescents.

## Hepatitis A

*Epidemiology*

Hepatitis A virus (HAV) is caused by a 27-nm RNA picornavirus, primarily transmitted by the fecal-oral route, by either person-to-person contact or consumption of contaminated food or water. After an average incubation period of 28 days (range 15–50 days), HAV results in infections ranging from asymptomatic to acute debilitating disease.[2] Although the virus is only viable on fomites, including produce, for about a week, HAV can survive in water and sewage for months. The virus can be killed by disinfection of surfaces with solutions containing bleach, quaternary ammonium, hydrochloric acid, glutaraldehyde, or formaldehyde or by heating the virus to 185°F (85°C) for 1 minute.[3–5]

In many developing countries, HAV infection is endemic, and most persons are infected during childhood and typically develop asymptomatic infections. In contrast, in developed countries, the prevalence of HAV is low and infection typically occurs among adolescents and adults, most commonly resulting in symptomatic disease.[6] Asymptomatic and nonjaundiced HAV-infected persons,

---

*Corresponding author.
*E-mail address*: usharapov@cdc.gov (U. M. Sharapov).

Copyright © 2010 American Academy of Pediatrics. All rights reserved. ISSN 1934-4287

Table 1
Symptoms of acute viral hepatitis

Malaise
- Anorexia
- Nausea
- Abdominal pain
- Jaundice
- Dark urine
- Fever, rash, arthralgias
- Pruritus

The clinical symptoms of acute viral hepatitis caused by the various hepatitis viruses are similar. Serologic and molecular tests are necessary to establish a diagnosis.

especially children, are an important source of HAV transmission as they are able to pass the infection without knowing they are ill.[7] In the United States, international travel is the most frequently reported risk factor among patients contracting HAV, but nearly 70% of cases have no specific risk factor identified. Among children and adolescents <15 years of age, the most frequently reported risk factors include household contact with a hepatitis A patient, and international travel.[1] International adoption has been a recently recognized risk for acquiring HAV and has led the American Academy of Pediatrics (AAP) and the Advisory Committee on Immunization Practices (ACIP) to update its recommendations for use of hepatitis A vaccine.[8,9]

Common source outbreaks are unusual causes of HAV infection in the United States. When they do occur, an infected food handler or an infected food source is commonly identified.[10] Between 1992 and 2000 among 38 881 adults with hepatitis A, 8% were identified as food handlers, including 13% of the 3292 adolescents aged 16–19.[11]

While viral shedding in the stool can last up to 6 months, the period of contagiousness is highest during the 2-week period before onset of jaundice or elevation of liver enzymes, when concentration of virus in the stool is highest.[12,13]

*Clinical Manifestations*

Symptomatic HAV infection typically has an abrupt onset that can include fever, malaise, anorexia, nausea, abdominal discomfort, dark urine, and jaundice. The likelihood of developing a symptomatic HAV infection is directly related to age, with only 30% of children under 6 years of age having symptomatic infections, rising to 70% among older children, adolescents, and adults.[14–16] Symptomatic HAV infections last on average 2 months; however, prolonged or relapsing disease for up to 6 months can occur.[17] Persons with underlying chronic disease are at increased risk for acute liver failure from HAV infection.[18–20] The overall

Table 2
Markers of viral hepatitis infection

| | |
|---|---|
| Hepatitis A | |
| HAV | Hepatitis A virus, etiologic agent of hepatitis A, also known as infectious hepatitis; a picornavirus with a single serotype |
| Anti-HAV | Total antibody to HAV; detectable at onset of symptoms; lifetime persistence |
| IgM anti-HAV | IgM-class antibody indicating recent infection with HAV |
| Hepatitis B | |
| HBV | Hepatitis B virus; etiologic agent of hepatitis B, also known as serum hepatitis; agent also known as Dane particle |
| HBsAg | Hepatitis B surface antigen; produced in large quantities in serum both as whole virus and as smaller surface antigen particles; originally known as Australian antigen; several serotypes. Indicates present infection with HBV |
| HBeAg | Hepatitis B e antigen; soluble antigen that correlates with HBV replication and infectivity; conformational antigen of HBcAg |
| HBcAg | Hepatitis B core antigen; found within the core of the virus; no commercial test available |
| Anti-HBs | Antibody to hepatitis B surface antigen; indicates immune response to HBV infection, due either to passive acquisition, immune response to infection, or vaccination |
| Anti-HBc | Antibody to hepatitis B core antigen; indicates past or present infection with HBV; not present in vaccine-induced immunity |
| IgM anti-HBc | IgM-class antibody to HBcAg; indicates recent infection with HBV |
| Hepatitis C | |
| HCV | Hepatitis C virus; etiologic agent of most parenterally transmitted non-A, non-B hepatitis; single-stranded RNA virus classified in the family Flaviviridae |
| Anti-HCV | Antibody to hepatitis C virus; does not distinguish between acute and chronic infection. Detectable in 90% of patients with hepatitis C; interval between onset of disease and seroconversion may be prolonged |
| RIBA | Recombinant immunoblot assay; supplemental confirmatory test for anti-HCV screening assay |
| HCV RT-PCR | Reverse transcription polymerase chain reaction for hepatitic C virus; defects virus in blood and indicates present infection with HCV |

case-fatality ratio among patients with HAV infection is 0.3–0.6%, but reaches 1.8% among adults aged >50 years. HAV infection does not result in chronic infection.

*Diagnosis*

A diagnosis of HAV infection requires specific laboratory testing. Serum immunoglobulin (Ig) M against HAV is detectable 5–10 days before onset of symptoms. Serum IgG though does not appear until the convalescent phase of infection and remains detectable for the person's lifetime, providing long-term protection against the disease.[21–23] False-positive IgM anti-HAV results have been reported, prompting a recommendation to limit laboratory testing for acute HAV infection to persons with clinical symptoms of HAV or known exposure to the virus.[24,25] HAV can also be diagnosed by detection of viral RNA in the blood and/or stool; however, these tests are not widely available and typically used only in outbreak investigations.[26–28]

*Treatment*

As HAV infection is self-limited and does not result in chronic infection or chronic liver disease, treatment is supportive. Hospitalization may be necessary for patients who develop dehydration or fulminant hepatitis. Hepatotoxic medications and those metabolized by the liver should be used with caution. No specific restrictions on diet or activity are necessary but alcohol intake should be limited.

*Prevention*

General measures for the prevention of hepatitis A include the maintenance of good personal hygiene, washing of potentially contaminated foods and receipt of either immune globulin or hepatitis A vaccine.[29] Special education efforts should target populations at increased risk for developing HAV such as men who have sex with men (MSM), persons who use drugs, or persons with underlying liver disorders.

*Preexposure Prophylaxis*

Immunoglobulins (IG) are a sterile preparation of concentrated antibodies prepared from pooled human plasma processed by cold ethanol fractionation that provides passive protection against the infection.[30] Prophylactic administration of IG provides passive protection against HAV for up to 6 months and when given within 2 weeks of exposure to the virus is 80–90% effective in preventing the disease.[16]

Hepatitis A vaccines, which provide active protection against the virus, were first licensed in the United States in 1995–1996.[16] They are safe and highly effective in preventing infection with HAV. Vaccination programs have resulted in dramatic declines in HAV cases in the United States from 31 582 (national incidence 12.0 per 100 000 population) in 1995 to 2979 (national incidence 1.0 per 100 000 population) in 2007.[1]

Nearly all vaccine recipients develop protective antibody levels after one dose of vaccine with the second dose resulting in a high level of antibody production in all recipients.[31–35] Even 10 years after receiving vaccine, 99% of persons have protective antibody levels and disease has not been recorded among vaccinated people over 20 years after immunization.[36] In addition to the 2 monovalent

Table 3
Recommended doses of inactivated hepatitis A vaccine

| Vaccine | Age (yrs) | Dose | Volume (mL) | Dose Schedule (months)[a] |
|---|---|---|---|---|
| Havrix® | 1–18 | 720 EL.U. | 0.5 | 0, 6–12 |
|  | ≥19 | 1440 EL.U. | 1.0 | 0, 6–12 |
| Vaqta® | 1–18 | 25 U | 0.5 | 0, 6–18 |
|  | ≥19 | 50 U | 1.0 | 0, 6–18 |
| Twinrix®[b] | ≥18 | 720 EL.U. (HAV) 20 mcg (HBsAg) | 1.0 | 0, 1, 6 |

Use of trade names is for identification purposes only and does not imply endorsement by the US Public Health Service.
[a] 0 months represents timing of the initial dose; subsequent numbers represent months after the initial dose.
[b] Twinrix is a bivalent vaccine containing inactivated hepatitis A virus and recombinant surface antigen of the hepatitis B virus.
Adapted from: Prevention of hepatitis A through active or passive immunization: Recommendations of the Advisory Committee on Immunization Practices (ACIP). *MMWR.* 2006;55:RR-7.

preparations, a bivalent vaccine (combining hepatitis A and hepatitis B) is available for use in persons aged 18 years or older (Table 3).[37]

The AAP and ACIP first recommended use of hepatitis A vaccine in 1996 with updated recommendations in 1999 and 2006.[16,38,39] Currently, universal vaccination against HAV is recommended for children aged 1–18 years, as well as for high-risk groups including MSM, drug abusers, persons who have underlying liver disease, or persons who frequently travel to countries endemic for the virus.[16,40] Vaccinating adolescents and adults at risk for vaccine-preventable diseases has proven difficult since many people in these groups do not routinely visit health care providers for preventive health care, or they may not perceive themselves to be at high risk.[41,42] Overall immunization coverage rates for HAV are relatively low, but surveillance data demonstrate that even low coverage has resulted in a remarkable decrease in infection and suggest a strong herd immunity through active immunization of young children.[16]

*Postexposure Prophylaxis*

Postexposure prophylaxis (PEP) for hepatitis A has relied on administration of intramuscular Ig. However, a randomized, double-blind clinical trial in 2007 showed that hepatitis A vaccine provided protection equivalent to Ig when administered within 2 weeks of exposure.[43] The additional benefit of hepatitis A vaccine is the long-term protection it provides. Thus, PEP recommendations have been updated. For previously unvaccinated persons aged 1–40 years, a single dose of hepatitis A vaccine, within 2 weeks of exposure, is preferred to IG.[40] Efficacy of the vaccine administered >2 weeks after exposure has not been established. The second dose of vaccine should be administered according to the vaccine manufacturer's licensed schedule. Children <1 year of age, due to lack of efficacy of the vaccine, and adults aged >40 years, due to lack of data, should continue to receive a dose of IG.[40] Ig also should be used for immunocompromised persons, persons with chronic liver disease, and persons for whom vaccine is contraindicated.[40]

**Hepatitis B**

*Epidemiology*

Hepatitis B virus (HBV) is caused by a 42-nm double-shelled DNA virus of the *Hepadnaviridae* family.[44,45] An estimated 1.25 million persons in the United States are infected with HBV but worldwide estimates of infection exceed 350 million persons with 5 million new cases of acute HBV cases occurring annually, the majority living in Asia and the Western Pacific.[1,46,47] Between 1990 and 2007, the incidence of acute hepatitis B in the United States declined 82% from 8.5 per 100 000 to 1.5 per 100 000 population. An estimated 43 000 new infections occurred in 2007 after accounting for asymptomatic cases and underreporting of cases.[1] The greatest declines have occurred among persons aged <15 years (98%) and 15–24 years (93%). Most new HBV infections occur among adults, reflecting the low hepatitis B vaccine coverage for this group.[1,46]

Historically in the United States, males have nearly twice the prevalence of infection than females and non-Hispanic blacks have higher rates of infection than other racial/ethnic groups.[1] Common risk factors associated with acquisition of HBV include having multiple sexual partners (38%), sharing of equipment for injection drug use (15%), MSM (11%), recent surgery (12%), and sexual contact with persons known to have hepatitis B (6%).[1] In addition, continued immigration of persons from intermediate to high HBV prevalence countries makes hepatitis B an ongoing public health challenge.[46]

*Transmission*

High titers of HBV are present in blood; moderate titers are present in vaginal secretions, semen, and saliva.[48] As a result, HBV can be transmitted through blood exposure, sexually, vertically at the time of birth, and horizontally in a household (nonsexual transmission).[49–51] Persons with chronic hepatitis B infection are the main source of infection,[52] and persons with hepatitis B surface antigen (HBsAg) are infectious to both sexual and nonsexual contacts. People with detectable hepatitis B "e" antigen (HBeAg) in addition to HBsAg are considered highly infectious with HBV titers in blood up to $10^7$-$10^9$ virions/mL.[3,53] Indirect transmission of HBV from environmental surfaces without visible blood can occur due to the long viability of the virus on contaminated surfaces (for up to 7 days) and the relatively low inoculum needed for infection.[54,55]

Transmission to newborns and infants occurs predominantly through perinatal transmission from infected mothers and horizontal transmission from exposure to a person with hepatitis B in the household. Over 95% of perinatal transmission occurs at the time of birth.[56,57] The risk of perinatal transmission is 5–20% in infants born to HBsAg-positive mothers but rises to 70–90% if the mother is both HBsAg and HBeAg-positive.[58] Furthermore, in the absence of postexposure prophylaxis, an infant born to a mother positive for only HBsAg has a 10% risk of developing a chronic HBV infection but this risk rises to 90% if the mother is positive for both HBsAg and HBeAg.[56,59,60] Several studies have shown breastfeeding does not increase the risk for acquiring of HBV infection by the infant and thus need not be discontinued simply because a mother is infected with the virus.[61] The transmission rate of HBV to unvaccinated household members living with a chronically infected person is 14–60%, which is why vaccination is imperative for prevention.[62,63] The greatest risks for acquisition of HBV among adolescents mirror the adult risk factors of multiple sex partners, male homosexual activity, and injection drug use.[49]

*Clinical Manifestations*

Similar to hepatitis A, infection with HBV can be with or without symptoms. Elevation of serum alanine aminotransferase (ALT) levels is noted ~60 days after exposure with jaundice appearing an average of 90 days (range 60–150 days) after exposure.[64,65] The likelihood of developing a symptomatic HBV infection is age-dependent, with children under 10 years of age typically not displaying symptoms and even in adolescents and adults up to 50% of people may be asymptomatic.[66] Common symptoms of HBV infection include malaise, anorexia, nausea, vomiting, abdominal pain, and jaundice as well as less common extrahepatic symptoms, including arthralgias, arthritis, and skin rashes.[64,67] Symptoms of acute HBV infection generally last 2–4 weeks, but symptoms, particularly fatigue, may persist for months. Acute HBV infection rarely results in acute liver failure (<1%), but when it occurs it is frequently fatal.[68] Overall, the fatality rate of acute hepatitis B is 0.5%–1.5% with highest rates observed among adults aged >60 years.[49]

Hepatitis B may develop into a chronic infection but unlike acute infection, the risk is *inversely* related to patient age. Approximately 90% of infected infants develop chronic infection compared with 30% of children <5 years of age and <5% of persons aged ≥5 years. Chronic HBV infection can result in cirrhosis, liver failure, hepatocellular carcinoma (HCC), and death and is responsible for the majority of serious sequelae associated with HBV. Annually 4000–5000 deaths in the United States are attributed to HBV infection and worldwide 500 000 to 1.2 million deaths annually are due to the sequelae of chronic HBV infection as well as 60–80% of the cases of HCC.[69,70]

*Diagnosis*

As with other hepatitides, specific laboratory testing is necessary to establish the diagnosis of HBV infection. Widely available commercial diagnostic assays are used

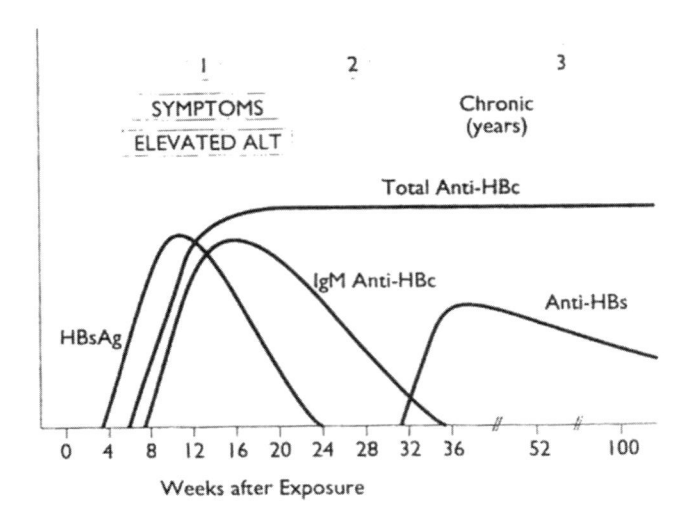

Fig 1. Typical serologic profile of acute HBV infection with recovery HBsAg usually appears 1–3 months after exposure. In acute HBV infection with recovery, HBsAg disappears within 6 months, whereas anti-HBs and total anti-HBc persists for lifetime.

to detect a combination of antigens and antibodies to determine the phase of HBV infection, and differentiate between acute and chronic infection (Fig. 1).[49,65]

Presence of HBsAg, first detectable ~30 days (range 6–60 days) after infection, is indicative of ongoing HBV infection and all persons with detectable HBsAg are considered contagious.[65] Occasionally HBsAg may be detectable for 2–3 weeks following hepatitis B vaccination but it is not clinically meaningful.[71,72] Antibody against the hepatitis B core antigen (anti-HBc) appears shortly after HBsAg and persists for life. In persons who recover from infection, HBsAg and HBeAg may persist for several months, and then gradually become undetectable. Subsequently, antibody to HBsAg (anti-HBs) develops, indicating recovery with long-term immunity to infection. Anti-HBs will also develop after receipt of the hepatitis B vaccine but in these cases, anti-HBc is not present as it is not a component of the vaccine. Occasionally, anti-HBc alone may be detected in the serum, typically representing an old resolved infection when anti-HBs has declined to undetectable levels.[50,73,74] Rarely, isolated detection of anti-HBc can occur during the "window phase" of acute infection between the disappearance of HBsAg and the appearance of anti-HBs. A last, very rare possibility occurs in

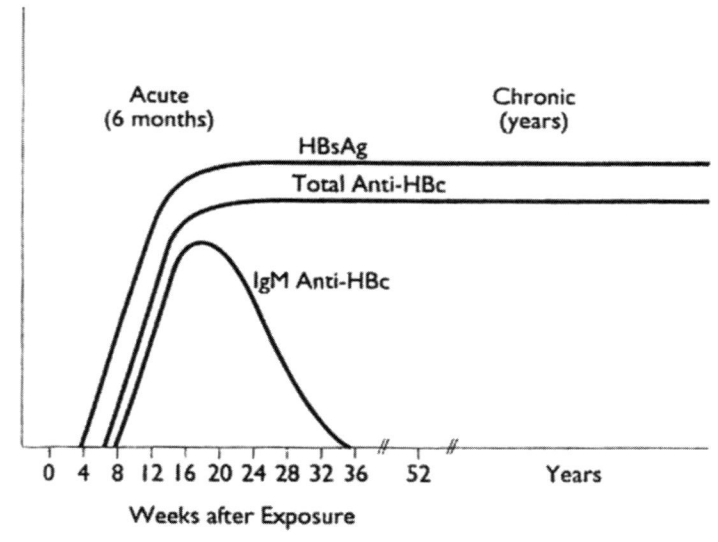

Fig 2. Typical serologic profile of acute HBV infection with progression to chronic infection HBsAg persists indefinitely and anti-HBs does not develop.

chronic infection with either extremely low levels of HBsAg or HBsAg mutations that make it undetectable by commercial serology.

Chronic HBV infection is typically diagnosed by detecting HBsAg on two serum specimens at least 6 months apart, or by the presence of HBsAg and IgG anti-HBc in the absence of IgM anti-HBc (Fig. 2, Table 4). Assessment of chronic HBV infection also should include testing and monitoring of HBV DNA as well as serum aminotransferases (ALT and AST) and possibly liver biopsy.[75] Detection of HBeAg in addition to HBsAg indicates the person is highly contagious as HBeAg is associated with active viral replication and higher circulating viral titers.[76]

Screening for HBsAg is recommended for all pregnant women in addition to infants born to HBsAg-positive mothers and people in any of the high risk groups previously discussed.[49,50,52,77] Knowledge of HBsAg positivity is important for minimizing spread of the virus but also has become important in deciding to initiate anti-HBV therapy.[52]

For persons with serologically confirmed HBV infection, serum HBV DNA load monitoring is important for treatment and prognostic reasons as the level of viral replication is predictive of the future risk of developing cirrhosis and HCC.[75,76,78] DNA evaluation can be further refined to enable genotypic or phenotypic analysis, which may by helpful for the selection of antiviral therapies for treatment of chronic HBV and predicting likelihood of disease progression.[78,79]

Table 4
Typical interpretation of serologic test results for hepatitis B virus infection

| HBsAg[a] | Serologic Marker | | Anti-HBs[d] | Interpretation |
|---|---|---|---|---|
| | Total Anti-HBc[b] | IgM[c] Anti-HBc | | |
| Negative[e] | Negative | Negative | Negative | Never infected |
| Positive[f,g] | Negative | Negative | Negative | Early acute infection; transient (up to 18 days) after vaccination |
| Positive | Positive | Positive | Negative | Acute infection |
| Negative | Positive | Positive | Positive or negative | Acute resolving infection |
| Negative | Positive | Negative | Positive | Recovered from past infection and immune |
| Positive | Positive | Negative | Negative | Chronic infection |
| Negative | Positive | Negative | Negative | False-positive (ie, susceptible); past infection; "low-level" chronic infection;[h] or passive transfer of anti-HBc to infant born to HBsAg-positive mother |
| Negative | Negative | Negative | Positive | Immune if concentration is ≥10 mlU/mL after vaccine series completion;[i] passive transfer after hepatitis B immune globulin administration |

[a] Hepatitis B surface antigen.
[b] Antibody to hepatitis B core antigen.
[c] Immunoglobulin M.
[d] Antibody to HBsAg.
[e] Negative test result.
[f] Postive test result.
[g] To ensure that an HBsAg-positive test result is not a false-positive, samples with reactive HBsAg results should be tested with a licensed neutralizing confirmatory test if recommended in the manufacturer's package insert.
[h] Persons positive only for anti-HBc are unlikely to be infectious except under unusual circumstances in which they are the source for direct percutaneous exposure of susceptible recipients to large quantities of virus (eg, blood transfusion or organ transplant).
[i] Milli-international units per milliliter.

## Treatment

Treatment of acute hepatitis B is typically supportive, although in the rare cases of fulminant acute hepatitis B, liver transplantation has been used successfully. Patients with chronic hepatitis B should be counseled to limit alcohol consumption and, if chronic liver disease is present, hepatitis A vaccination is recommended.[16,52,80] Patients with chronic HBV infection should receive long-term monitoring to assess disease progression and related complications plus the need for treatment. The goal of therapy is to prevent progression to cirrhosis, end-stage liver disease, and HCC. Success of treatment is based on shorter-term measures, such as low to undetectable hepatitis B viral load, drops in serum aminotransferase, and development of anti-HBeAg.[75,81,82]

Detailed discussion of specific therapies is beyond the scope of this paper. However, in brief it is important to know that seven agents (interferon alfa-2b, peginterferon alfa-2a, lamivudine, adefovir, entecavir, telbivudine, tenofovir) are approved for the treatment of chronic HBV infection in adults and other agents are in the process of development.[75] Therefore, patients with chronic HBV infections should be referred to an expert in the care of the disease to evaluate treatment options.[75,82–85]

*Prevention*

*Preexposure Prophylaxis*

Vaccination is the mainstay of prevention.[50] The first hepatitis B vaccine was licensed in the United States in 1981 and the vaccine has become part of the routine immunization schedule for infants and children in many countries. Several formulations of hepatitis B vaccine are available, but all use HBsAg as the antigen.[49,50] Single-antigen vaccines licensed in the United States are Recombivax HB (Merck & Co, Inc., Whitehouse Station, NJ) and Engerix-B (GlaxoSmithKline Biologicals, Rixensart, Belgium). Three combination vaccines are available: two vaccines—Comvax and Pediatrix—are used for vaccination of infants and young children, whereas Twinrix is licensed only for use in adults (Table 5).[49]

Hepatitis B vaccine is safe and highly effective. Three doses of vaccine induce protective levels of antibody in over 90% of recipients and a number of studies indicate protective immunity lasts 20 years or more.[50,86,87]

Over the past two decades, a comprehensive immunization strategy to eliminate HBV transmission in the United States has evolved.[49,50] The strategy focuses on 1) universal vaccination of infants beginning at birth, 2) prevention of perinatal HBV infection (through routine screening of all pregnant women for HBsAg and postexposure immunoprophylaxis of infants born to HBsAg-positive women or to women with unknown HBsAg status), 3) vaccination of all children and adolescents who were not vaccinated previously, and 4) vaccination of previously unvaccinated adults at risk for HBV infection.[49,50]

Hepatitis B vaccination programs targeting adolescents and adults at increased risk face many challenges, including inadequate resources allocations and poor preventive health care among persons with high-risk behaviors.[41] Sadly, when adolescents and young adults do enter the health care system,

Table 5
Recommended doses of currently licensed formulations of hepatitis B vaccine, by age group and vaccine type

| Age Group | Single-Antigen Vaccine ||||  Combination Vaccine ||||||
|---|---|---|---|---|---|---|---|---|---|---|
| | Recombivax HB || Engerix-B || Comvax || Pediarix || Twinrix ||
| | Dose (μg) | Vol (mL) | Dose (μg) | Vol (mL) | Dose (μg) | Vol (mL) | Dose (μg) | Vol (mL) | Dose (μg) | Vol (mL) |
| Infants (<1 year) | 5 | 0.5 | 10 | 0.5 | 5 | 0.5 | 10 | 0.5 | NA | NA |
| Children (1–10 years) | 5 | 0.5 | 10 | 0.5 | 5 | 0.5 | 10 | 0.5 | NA | NA |
| Adolescents | | | | | | | | | | |
| 11–15 years | 10[a] | 1 | NA | NA | NA | NA | NA | NA | NA | NA |
| 11–19 years | 5 | 0.5 | 10 | 0.5 | NA | NA | NA | NA | NA | NA |
| Adults (≥20 years) | 10 | 1 | 20 | 1 | NA | NA | NA | NA | 20 | 1 |
| Hemodialysis patients and other immuno compromised persons | | | | | | | | | | |
| <20 years[b] | 5 | 0.5 | 10 | 0.5 | NA | NA | NA | NA | NA | NA |
| ≥20 years | 40[c] | 1 | 40[d] | 2 | NA | NA | NA | NA | NA | NA |

Doses listed are recombinant hepatitis B surface antigen protein dose. Comvax, combined hepatitis B-*Haemophilus influenzae* type b conjugate vaccine, which cannot be administered at birth, before age 6 weeks, or after age 71 months; Pediarix, combined hepatitis B, diphtheria, tetanus, acellular pertussis adsorbed, inactivated poliovirus vaccine, which cannot be administered at birth, before age 6 weeks, or at age >7 years; Twinrix, combined hepatitis A and hepatitis B vaccine, which is recommended for persons aged ≥18 years who are at increased risk for both hepatitis B virus and hepatitis A virus infections.
[a] Adult formulation administered on a 2-dose schedule.
[b] Higher doses might be more immunogenic, but no specific recommendations have been made.
[c] Dialysis formulation administered on a 3-dose schedule at 0, 1, and 6 months.
[d] Two 1.0-mL doses administered at one site, on a 4-dose schedule at 0, 1, 2, and 6 months.
NA, not applicable.

they often do not receive adequate preventative measures. Among young adult MSM surveyed in 7 United States metropolitan areas during 1994–1998, only 9% had received hepatitis B vaccine although 9 out of 10 reported using a regular source of health care.[88] As another study demonstrated, 1 of 5 MSM who were unvaccinated against HBV acquired the infection by age 22—something that was preventable if they had been vaccinated during adolescence or earlier.[88]

However, even when vaccination is offered, it is not always accepted. Among users of sexually transmitted disease (STD) clinics in Alabama and California, only 14% of the susceptible target population received two doses of vaccine, and only 4% completed the three-dose series.[88,89] Nevertheless, even in high-risk and disenfranchised populations, with intense efforts, high vaccination coverage against HBV is possible.[90] Ensuring hepatitis B vaccine is available in settings frequented by high-risk populations such as STD clinics, correctional facilities (juvenile detention facilities, prisons, jails), drug treatment facilities, and community-based human immunodeficiency virus (HIV) prevention sites is vital if widespread protection against the infection is ever to be achieved.[91]

*Postexposure Prophylaxis*

Immediate, short-term (3–6 months), passive protection against HBV can be obtained through administration of hepatitis B immunoglobulin (HBIG). HBIG is usually administered in combination with hepatitis B vaccine to provide long-term protection.[49]

## Hepatitis C

*Epidemiology*

Hepatitis C virus (HCV), discovered in 1989, is an enveloped RNA virus of the Flaviviridae family; one of the leading causes of chronic liver diseases.[92] The incidence of hepatitis C peaked in the late 1980s and then steadily declined from 5.2 cases per 100 000 population in 1995 to 0.5 cases per 100 000 population in 2007 among persons aged 25–39 years.

Despite the decline in incidence, the prevalence of HCV infection in the United States remains substantial due to the propensity of the virus for establishing chronic infections. Approximately 1.8% of the US population, or 4 million persons, have been infected with HCV and ~3.2 million persons are chronically infected with the virus.[93] The highest prevalence of chronic disease is among persons aged 40–49 years, the majority of whom were presumably infected in the 1970s and 1980s when incidence was highest.[1,94] Each year in the United States, ~8000 people die from HCV infection and its complications. Although ~20% of persons infected with HCV clear the virus spontaneously, prior HCV infection does not protect against reinfection with the same or different genotype of the virus.

Initially HCV transmission was associated with blood transfusion. However, implementation of rigorous blood screening has made this mode of transmission rare and currently injection drug use is the most frequently reported risk factor for acquiring HCV with an estimated 40% of persons with a history of HCV infection reporting injection drug use.[1,94,95] HCV infection is acquired rapidly after initiation of injection drug use with HCV seroconversion rates of ~10–25 per 100 person years.[96–98] Based on data from National Health and Nutrition Examination Survey (1999–2002), a large epidemiologic study of persons in the United States conducted by the Centers for Disease Control and Prevention, of people reporting ever injecting drugs, 58% had been infected with HCV and 46% were chronically infected.[94] Limited epidemiologic data suggest use of noninjection (ie, snorted or smoked) cocaine also increases the risk of being infected with HCV but it is difficult to differentiate that risk from the risk associated with injecting drugs and sex with HCV-infected partners.[99,100]

Health-care-related transmission of HCV is rare in the United States but should be considered in persons with HCV infection without other risks factors. From 1998–2008, 16 health-care-related outbreaks of HCV infection due to lapses in infection control practices have been identified resulting in 275 persons becoming infected and another 58 000 persons estimated to have been exposed to the virus.[101]

The risk of progression of chronic HCV to cirrhosis is age related, with <5% of persons infected as juveniles or young adults developing cirrhosis compared with 10–20% among persons infected as older adults.[102] In addition, progression to cirrhosis is related to duration of HCV infection, HCV genotype, HIV coinfection, alcohol use, and male sex.[103–108] Of persons with chronic hepatitis C, HCC develops in 1% to 5% over a period of 20–30 years.[109–111]

*Clinical Manifestations*

Acute HCV infection is generally mild with 25% or less of people developing a recognized illness.[112–114] The incubation period ranges from 14–180 days (average 6–7 weeks), and the symptoms are indistinguishable from those of other types of viral hepatitis.[115–117]

Of persons infected as adolescents or young adults 50–60% will develop chronic HCV infection compared with 75–85% of persons infected over the age of 45 years.[102] The majority of persons with chronic HCV infection are asymptomatic, and ~30% have no evidence of liver disease.[118]

*Diagnosis*

Diagnosis of HCV relies on detection of either antibody to HCV (anti-HCV) or HCV RNA with detection of anti-HCV recommended as the initial screening test.[112,119,120] Persons with a positive anti-HCV test should have the result confirmed with a more specific assay (RIBA or reverse-transcriptase polymerase chain reaction for HCV RNA) (Fig. 3). The specificity of HCV EIA tests is high (≥99%). Even such a high specificity of the test does not enable high predictive positive value for a positive test: the proportion of false-positive results with HCV EIA among populations with low anti-HCV prevalence (<10%) can reach 35% (with range 15–60%).[120] Confirmed anti-HCV indicates past or current infection, whereas the presence of HCV RNA indicates current infection. If a chemiluminescence immunoassay (CIAs) is used for screening, no confirmatory testing is needed.

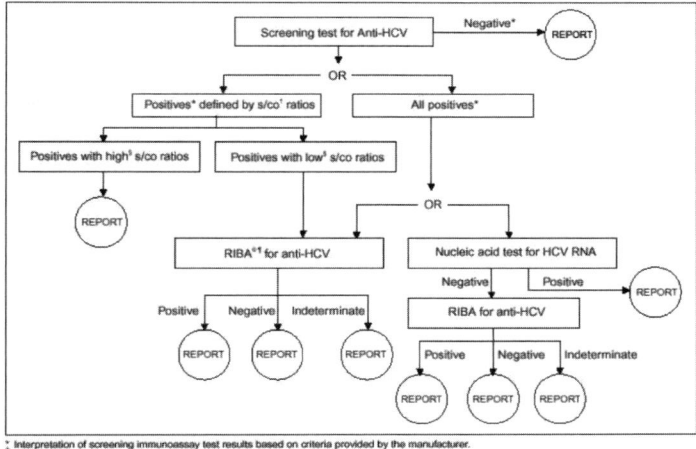

Fig 3. Laboratory algorithm for antibody to hepatitis C virus (Anti-HCV) testing and result reporting.

*Treatment*

The primary objective for treatment of HCV is attaining an undetectable serum HCV RNA level 6 months after cessation of therapy, termed a sustained virologic response,[121,122] Unlike HAV and HBV, treatment of HCV may be more effective when initiated during the period of acute infection both in eliminating the infection and in progression to chronic infection.[121] Although the standard combination of peginterferon alfa and ribavirin has resulted in sustained virologic response in many patients, a number of new therapies are currently being evaluated to further improve treatment outcomes and decrease side effects. In addition to adherence to specific therapies, limitation of alcohol consumption is important as alcohol can worsen the course and outcome of HCV infection, including poorer responses to therapy.[123]

Patients with chronic hepatitis C should be evaluated for severity of their liver disease, which may include a liver biopsy or noninvasive tests of fibrosis with treatment recommended for those at greatest risk of progression to cirrhosis.[121] Risks for disease progression include persistently elevated ALT levels; detectable HCV RNA; and portal or bridging fibrosis or at least moderate degrees of inflammation and necrosis on liver biopsy.

The current standard of care for chronic hepatitis uses a combination of pegylated interferon-α plus ribavirin.[121] The optimal duration of treatment is based on viral genotype with a 48-week period of treatment for patients with HCV genotype 1 but only 24 weeks for genotypes 2 and 3.[121]

Factors that predict a good therapeutic response include infection with genotype 2 and 3, low HCV viral load, no or minimal fibrosis on liver biopsy, female gender, aged <40 years at the time treatment is initiated, and white race.[121,124,125]

Administration of interferon-$\alpha$ is often accompanied by flu-like symptoms, but these diminish with continued treatment. Fatigue, bone marrow suppression, and neuropsychiatric symptoms including cognitive changes, irritability, and depression are other adverse events associated with interferon treatment. Ribavirin may cause hemolytic as well as teratogenic effects; therefore, pregnancy, or attempting to become pregnant, is an absolute contraindication for ribavirin use.

As therapy for hepatitis C is a rapidly changing area, clinicians are encouraged to refer patients to a specialist to ensure optimal therapeutic regimens are prescribed.[121]

*Prevention*

No effective vaccine to prevent HCV infection exists and it is unlikely one will be available in the near future. Therefore, prevention of HCV relies on education in an attempt to alter risk factors associated with contracting the infection. In patients already infected, education should be targeted to reduce risks for liver and other chronic diseases.[112]

As part of primary prevention activities, any health care professional providing care for adolescents should inquire about high-risk behaviors, including illicit drug use and high-risk sexual practices. Although all adolescents should be counseled about diseases associated with these risk factors, particular attention should be given to those who are actively undertaking such behaviors. Bringing educational messages to outreach settings, such as correctional institutions, drug treatment programs, and STD clinics, is another important means to combat the spread of the infection.[126]

## CONCLUSIONS

Viral hepatitis is the leading cause of liver cancer and the most common reason for liver transplantation. In the United States, an estimated 1.2 million Americans are living with chronic hepatitis B and 3.2 million are living with chronic hepatitis C. Many do not know they are infected. Each year, an estimated 25 000 persons become infected with hepatitis A; 43 000 with hepatitis B, and 17 000 with hepatitis C. Risky behaviors often initiated by people when they are teenagers and young adults may place them at risk for these infections. Safe and effective vaccines exist to prevent HAV and HBV infections. Early detection and treatment of hepatitis C may eliminate the virus or prevent progression to chronic infection.

# REFERENCES

1. Daniels D, Grytdal S, Wasley A. Surveillance for acute viral hepatitis—United States, 2007. *MMWR Surveill Summ.* 2009;58(3):1–27
2. Krugman S, Giles JP. Viral hepatitis. New light on an old disease. *JAMA.* 1970;212(6):1019–1029
3. Favero MS, Bond WW, Petersen NJ, et al. Detection methods for study of the stability of hepatitis B antigen on surfaces. *J Infect Dis.* 1974;129(2):210–212
4. Mbithi JN, Springthorpe VS, Sattar SA. Chemical disinfection of hepatitis A virus on environmental surfaces. *Appl Environ Microbiol.* 1990;56(11):3601–3604
5. Sattar SA, Jason T, Bidawid S, et al. Foodborne spread of hepatitis A: Recent studies on virus survival, transfer and inactivation. *Can J Infect Dis.* 2000;11(3);159–163
6. Green MS, Block C, Slater PE. Rise in the incidence of viral hepatitis in Israel despite improved socioeconomic conditions. *Rev Infect Dis.* 1989;11(3):464–469
7. Staes CJ, Schlenker TL, Risk I, et al. Sources of infection among persons with acute hepatitis A and no identified risk factors during a sustained community-wide outbreak. *Pediatrics.* 2000;106(4):E54
8. CDC. Updated recommendations from the Advisory Committee on Immunization Practices (ACIP) for use of hepatitis A vaccine in close contacts of newly arriving international adoptees. *MMWR Morb Mortal Wkly Rep.* 2009;58(36):1006–1007
9. Fischer GE, Teshale EH, Miller C, et al. Hepatitis A among international adoptees and their contacts. *Clin Infect Dis.* 2008;47(6);812–814
10. Greig JD, Todd EC, Bartleson CA, et al. Outbreaks where food workers have been implicated in the spread of foodborne disease. Part 1. Description of the problem, methods, and agents involved. *J Food Prot.* 2007;70(7);1752–1761
11. Bureau of Labor Statistics. Occupational outlook handbook: food and beverage serving and related workers. Available from: http://www.bls.gov/oco/ocos162.htm. Accessed February 6, 2009
12. Tassopoulos NC, Papaevangelou GJ, Ticehurst JR, et al. Fecal excretion of Greek strains of hepatitis A virus in patients with hepatitis A and in experimentally infected chimpanzees. *J Infect Dis.* 1986;154(2):231–237
13. Rosenblum LS, Villarino ME, Nainan OV, et al. Hepatitis A outbreak in a neonatal intensive care unit: risk factors for transmission and evidence of prolonged viral excretion among preterm infants. *J Infect Dis.* 1991;164(3):476–482
14. Hadler SC, Webster HM, Erben JJ, et al. Hepatitis A in day-care centers. A community-wide assessment. *N Engl J Med.* 1980;302(22):1222–1227
15. Lednar WM, Lemon SM, Kirkpatrick JW, et al. Frequency of illness associated with epidemic hepatitis A virus infections in adults. *Am J Epidemiol.* 1985;122(2):226–233
16. Fiore AE, Wasley A, Bell BP. Prevention of hepatitis A through active or passive immunization: recommendations of the Advisory Committee on Immunization Practices (ACIP). *MMWR Recomm Rep.* 2006;55(RR-7):1–23
17. Glikson M, Galun E, Oren R, et al. Relapsing hepatitis A. Review of 14 cases and literature survey. *Medicine.* 1992;71(1):14–23
18. Akriviadis EA, Redeker AG. Fulminant hepatitis A in intravenous drug users with chronic liver disease. *Ann Intern Med.* 1989;110(10):838–839
19. Willner IR, Uhl MD, Howard SC, et al. Serious hepatitis A: an analysis of patients hospitalized during an urban epidemic in the United States. *Ann Intern Med.* 1998;128(2):111–114
20. Vento S, Garofano T, Renzini C, et al. Fulminant hepatitis associated with hepatitis A virus superinfection in patients with chronic hepatitis C. *N Engl J Med.* 1998;338(5):286–290
21. Bower WA, Nainan OV, Han XH, et al. Duration of viremia in hepatitis A virus infection. *J Infect Dis.* 2000;182(1);12–17
22. Liaw YF, Yang CY, Chu CM, et al. Appearance and persistence of hepatitis A IgM antibody in acute clinical hepatitis A observed in an outbreak. *Infection.* 1986;14(4):156–158

23. Stapleton JT. Host immune response to hepatitis A virus. *J Infect Dis.* 1995;171 Suppl 1:S9–S14
24. Castrodale L, Fiore A, Schmidt T. Detection of immunoglobulin M antibody to hepatitis A virus in Alaska residents without other evidence of hepatitis. *Clin Infect Dis.* 2005;41(9);e86–e88
25. Centers for Disease Control and Prevention. Positive test results for acute hepatitis A virus infection among persons with no recent history of acute hepatitis–United States, 2002–2004. *MMWR Morb Mortal Wkly Rep.* 2005;54(18):453–456
26. Nainan O, Armstrong G, Han X-H, et al. Hepatitis a molecular epidemiology in the United States, 1996–1997: sources of infection and implications of vaccination policy. *J Infect Dis.* 2005;191(6);957–963
27. Amon JJ, Devasia R, Xia G, et al. Molecular epidemiology of foodborne hepatitis A outbreaks in the United States, 2003. *J Infect Dis.* 2005;192(8);1323–1330
28. Hutin YJ, Pool V, Cramer EH, et al. A multistate, foodborne outbreak of hepatitis A. National Hepatitis A Investigation Team. *N Engl J Med.* 1999;340(8):595–602
29. Fiore AE. Hepatitis A transmitted by food. *Clin Infect Dis.* 2004;38(5);705–715
30. Cohn EJ, Oncley JL, Strong LE, et al. Chemical, clinical, and immunological studies on the products of human plasma fractionation. I. The characterization of the protein fractions of human plamsa. *J Clin Invest.* 1944;23(4):417–432
31. Ashur Y, Adler R, Rowe M, et al. Comparison of immunogenicity of two hepatitis A vaccines–VAQTA and HAVRIX–in young adults. *Vaccine.* 1999;17(18):2290–2296
32. Chen XQ, Bulbul M, de Gast GC, et al. Immunogenicity of two versus three injections of inactivated hepatitis A vaccine in adults. *J Hepatol.* 1997;26(2):260–264
33. Clemens R, Safary A, Hepburn A, et al. Clinical experience with an inactivated hepatitis A vaccine. *J Infect Dis.* 1995;171 Suppl 1:S44–S49
34. McMahon BJ, Williams J, Bulkow L, et al. Immunogenicity of an inactivated hepatitis A vaccine in Alaska native children and native and non-native adults. *J Infect Dis.* 1995;171(3):676–679
35. Nalin DR, Kuter BJ, Brown L, et al. Worldwide experience with the CR326F-derived inactivated hepatitis A virus vaccine in pediatric and adult populations: an overview. *J Hepatol.* 1993;18 Suppl 2:S51–S55
36. Hammitt LL, Bulkow L, Hennessy TW, et al. Persistence of antibody to hepatitis A virus 10 years after vaccination among children and adults. *J Infect Dis.* 2008;198(12);1776–1782
37. Thoelen S, Van Damme P, Leentvaar-Kuypers A, et al. The first combined vaccine against hepatitis A and B: an overview. *Vaccine.* 1999;17(13–14):1657–1662
38. Centers for Disease Control and Prevention. Prevention of hepatitis A through active or passive immunization: Recommendations of the Advisory Committee on Immunization Practices (ACIP). *MMWR Recomm Rep.* 1996;45(RR-15):1–30
39. Centers for Disease Control and Prevention. Prevention of hepatitis A through active or passive immunization: Recommendations of the Advisory Committee on Immunization Practices (ACIP). *MMWR Recomm Rep.* 1999;48(RR-12):1–37
40. Centers for Disease Control and Prevention. Update. Prevention of hepatitis A after exposure to hepatitis A virus and in international travelers. Updated recommendations of the Advisory Committee on Immunization Practices (ACIP). *MMWR Morb Mortal Wkly Rep.* 2007;56(41):1080–1084
41. Handsfield HH. Hepatitis A and B immunization in persons being evaluated for sexually transmitted diseases. *Am J Med.* 2005;118 Suppl 10A:69S–74S
42. Centers for Disease Control and Prevention. Hepatitis A vaccination of men who have sex with men–Atlanta, Georgia, 1996–1997. *MMWR Morb Mortal Wkly Rep.* 1998;47(34):708–711
43. Victor JC, Monto AS, Surdina TY, et al. Hepatitis A vaccine versus immune globulin for postexposure prophylaxis. *N Engl J Med.* 2007;357(17);1685–1694
44. Block TM, Guo H, Guo JT. Molecular virology of hepatitis B virus for clinicians. *Clin Liver Dis.* 2007;11(4):685–706
45. Hollinger FB. Hepatitis B virus genetic diversity and its impact on diagnostic assays. *J Viral Hepat.* 2007;14 Suppl 1:11–15

46. Kim WR. Epidemiology of hepatitis B in the United States. *Hepatology.* 2009;49(5 Suppl): S28–34
47. Lavanchy D. Worldwide epidemiology of HBV infection, disease burden, and vaccine prevention. *J Clin Virol.* 2005;34 Suppl 1:S1–S3
48. Bond WW, Petersen NJ, Favero MS. Viral hepatitis B: aspects of environmental control. *Health Lab Sci.* 1977;14(4):235–252
49. Mast EE, Margolis HS, Fiore AE, et al. A comprehensive immunization strategy to eliminate transmission of hepatitis B virus infection in the United States: recommendations of the Advisory Committee on Immunization Practices (ACIP) part 1: immunization of infants, children, and adolescents. *MMWR Recomm Rep.* 2005;54(RR-16):1–31
50. Mast EE, Weinbaum CM, Fiore AE, et al. A comprehensive immunization strategy to eliminate transmission of hepatitis B virus infection in the United States: recommendations of the Advisory Committee on Immunization Practices (ACIP) Part II: immunization of adults. *MMWR Recomm Rep.* 2006;55(RR-16):1–33
51. Francis DP, Favero MS, Maynard JE. Transmission of hepatitis B virus. *Semin Liver Dis.* 1981;1(1):27–32
52. Weinbaum CM, Williams I, Mast EE, et al. Recommendations for identification and public health management of persons with chronic hepatitis B virus infection. *MMWR Recomm Rep.* 2008;57(RR-8):1–20
53. Biswas R, Tabor E, Hsia CC, et al. Comparative sensitivity of HBV NATs and HBsAg assays for detection of acute HBV infection. *Transfusion.* 2003;43(6);788–798
54. Alter MJ, Ahtone J, Maynard JE. Hepatitis B virus transmission associated with a multiple-dose vial in a hemodialysis unit. *Ann Intern Med.* 1983;99(3):330–333
55. Canter J, Mackey K, Good LS, et al. An outbreak of hepatitis B associated with jet injections in a weight reduction clinic. *Arch Intern Med.* 1990;150(9):1923–1927
56. Xu ZY, Liu CB, Francis DP, et al. Prevention of perinatal acquisition of hepatitis B virus carriage using vaccine: preliminary report of a randomized, double-blind placebo-controlled and comparative trial. *Pediatrics.* 1985;76(5):713–718
57. Wong VC, Ip HM, Reesink HW, et al. Prevention of the HBsAg carrier state in newborn infants of mothers who are chronic carriers of HBsAg and HBeAg by administration of hepatitis-B vaccine and hepatitis-B immunoglobulin. Double-blind randomised placebo-controlled study. *Lancet.* 1984;1(8383):921–926
58. Beasley RP, Trepo C, Stevens CE, et al. The e antigen and vertical transmission of hepatitis B surface antigen. *Am J Epidemiol.* 1977;105(2):94–98
59. Stevens CE, Neurath RA, Beasley RP, et al. HBeAg and anti-HBe detection by radioimmunoassay: correlation with vertical transmission of hepatitis B virus in Taiwan. *J Med Virol.* 1979;3(3):237–241
60. Stevens CE, Toy PT, Tong MJ, et al. Perinatal hepatitis B virus transmission in the United States. Prevention by passive-active immunization. *JAMA.* 1985;253(12):1740–1745
61. Beasley RP, Stevens CE, Shiao IS, et al. Evidence against breast-feeding as a mechanism for vertical transmission of hepatitis B. *Lancet.* 1975;2(7938):740–741
62. Steinberg SC, Alter HJ, Leventhal BG. The risk of hepatitis transmission to family contacts of leukemia patients. *J Pediatrics.* 1975;87(5):753–756
63. Nordenfelt E, Dahlquist E. HBsAg positive adopted children as a cause of intrafamilial spread of hepatitis B. *Scand J Infect Dis.* 1978;10(3):161–163
64. Krugman S, Overby LR, Mushahwar IK, et al. Viral hepatitis, type B. Studies on natural history and prevention re-examined. *N Engl J Med.* 1979;300(3):101–106
65. Hoofnagle JH, Di Bisceglie AM. Serologic diagnosis of acute and chronic viral hepatitis. *Semin Liver Dis.* 1991;11(2):73–83
66. McMahon BJ, Alward WL, Hall DB, et al. Acute hepatitis B virus infection: relation of age to the clinical expression of disease and subsequent development of the carrier state. *J Infect Dis.* 1985;151(4):599–603
67. Dienstag JL. Immunopathogenesis of the extrahepatic manifestations of hepatitis B virus infection. *Springer Semin Immunopathol.* 1981;3(4):461–472

68. Pappas SC. Fulminant viral hepatitis. *Gastroenterol Clin North Am.* 1995;24(1):161–173
69. Dienstag J. Hepatitis B virus infection. *N Engl J Med.* 2008;359(14):1486–1500
70. Parkin DM, Bray F, Ferlay J, et al. Estimating the world cancer burden: Globocan 2000. *Intl J Cancer.* 2001;94(2);153–156
71. Kloster B, Kramer R, Eastlund T, et al. Hepatitis B surface antigenemia in blood donors following vaccination. *Transfusion.* 1995;35(6):475–477
72. Lunn ER, Hoggarth BJ, Cook WJ. Prolonged hepatitis B surface antigenemia after vaccination. *Pediatrics.* 2000;105(6):E81
73. Hadler SC, Murphy BL, Schable CA, et al. Epidemiological analysis of the significance of low-positive test results for antibody to hepatitis B surface and core antigens. *J Clin Microbiol.* 1984;19(4):521–525
74. Lok AS, Lai CL, Wu PC. Prevalence of isolated antibody to hepatitis B core antigen in an area endemic for hepatitis B virus infection: implications in hepatitis B vaccination programs. *Hepatology.* 1988;8(4):766–770
75. Keeffe EB, Dieterich DT, Han SH, et al. A treatment algorithm for the management of chronic hepatitis B virus infection in the United States: 2008 update. *Clin Gastroenterol Hepatol.* 2008;6(12);1315–1341
76. Ganem D, Prince AM. Hepatitis B virus infection–natural history and clinical consequences. *N Engl J Med.* 2004;350(11);1118–1129
77. Centers for Disease Control and Prevention. Guidelines for prevention of transmission of human immunodeficiency virus and hepatitis B virus to health-care and public-safety workers. *MMWR Morb Mortal Wkly Rep.* 1989;38 Suppl 6:1–37
78. Valsamakis A. Molecular testing in the diagnosis and management of chronic hepatitis B. *Clin Microbiol Rev.* 2007;20(3):426–439
79. Keeffe EB, Dieterich DT, Pawlotsky JM, et al. Chronic hepatitis B: preventing, detecting, and managing viral resistance. *Clin Gastroenterol Hepatol.* 2008;6(3);268–274
80. Ikeda K, Saitoh S, Koida I, et al. A multivariate analysis of risk factors for hepatocellular carcinogenesis: a prospective observation of 795 patients with viral and alcoholic cirrhosis. *Hepatology.* 1993;18(1):47–53
81. European Association For The Study Of The LEASL Clinical Practice Guidelines. Management of chronic hepatitis B. *J Hepatol.* 2009;50(2);227–242
82. Liaw YF, Leung N, Kao JH, et al. Asian-Pacific consensus statement on the management of chronic hepatitis B: a 2008 update. *Hepatol Int.* 2008;2(3):263–283
83. Chen CJ, Yang HI, Iloeje UH. Hepatitis B virus DNA levels and outcomes in chronic hepatitis B. *Hepatology.* 2009;49(5 Suppl):S72–S84
84. Iloeje UH, Yang HI, Jen CL, et al. Risk and predictors of mortality associated with chronic hepatitis B infection. *Clin Gastroenterol Hepatol.* 2007;5(8);921–931
85. Iloeje UH, Yang HI, Su J, et al. Predicting cirrhosis risk based on the level of circulating hepatitis B viral load. *Gastroenterology.* 2006;130(3);678–686
86. Alfaleh F, Alshehri S, Alansari S, et al. Long-term protection of hepatitis B vaccine 18 years after vaccination. *J Infect.* 2008;57(5);404–409
87. van der Sande MA, Waight PA, Mendy M, et al. Long-term protection against HBV chronic carriage of Gambian adolescents vaccinated in infancy and immune response in HBV booster trial in adolescence. *PLoS One.* 2007;2(1):e753
88. MacKellar DA, Valleroy LA, Secura GM, et al. Two decades after vaccine license: hepatitis B immunization and infection among young men who have sex with men. *Am J Public Health.* 2001;91(6);965–971
89. Moran JS, Peterman TA, Weinstock HS, et al. Hepatitis B vaccination trials in sexually transmitted disease clinics: implications for program development. 26th National Immunization Conference; 1992 1–6 June; St. Louis, Missouri; 1992
90. Savage RB, Hussey MJ, Hurie MB. A successful approach to immunizing men who have sex with men against hepatitis B. *Public Health Nurs.* 2000;17(3);202–206

91. Gunn RA, Murray PJ, Ackers ML, et al. Screening for chronic hepatitis B and C virus infections in an urban sexually transmitted disease clinic: rationale for integrating services. *Sex Transm Dis.* 2001;28(3);166–170
92. Kato N. Molecular virology of hepatitis C virus. *Acta medica Okayama.* 2001;55(3);133–159
93. Armstrong GL, Alter MJ, McQuillan GM, et al. The past incidence of hepatitis C virus infection: implications for the future burden of chronic liver disease in the United States. *Hepatology.* 2000;31(3);777–782
94. Armstrong GL, Wasley A, Simard EP, et al. The prevalence of hepatitis C virus infection in the United States, 1999 through 2002. *Ann Intern Med.* 2006;144(10):705–714
95. Mathei C, Robaeys G, Van Ranst M, et al. The epidemiology of hepatitis C among injecting drug users in Belgium. *Acta gastro-enterologica belgica.* 2005;68(1):50–54
96. Hagan H, Thiede H, Weiss NS, et al. Sharing of drug preparation equipment as a risk factor for hepatitis C. *Am J Public Health.* 2001;91(1):42–46
97. Hagan H, Thiede H, Des Jarlais DC. Hepatitis C virus infection among injection drug users: survival analysis of time to seroconversion. *Epidemiology.* 2004;15(5):543–549
98. Hahn J, Page-Shafer K, Lum P, et al. Hepatitis C virus seroconversion among young injection drug users: relationships and risks. *J Infect Dis.* 2002;186(11):1558–1564
99. Aaron S, McMahon J, Milano D, et al. Intranasal transmission of hepatitis C virus: virological and clinical evidence. *Clin Infect Dis.* 2008;47(7):931–934
100. Koblin B, Factor S, Wu Y, et al. Hepatitis C virus infection among noninjecting drug users in New York City. *J Med Virol.* 2003;70(3):387–390
101. Thompson ND, Perz JF, Moorman AC, et al. Nonhospital health care-associated hepatitis B and C virus transmission: United States, 1998–2008. *Ann Intern Med.* 2009;150(1):33–39
102. Alter HJ, Seeff LB. Recovery, persistence, and sequelae in hepatitis C virus infection: a perspective on long-term outcome. *Sem Liver Dis.* 2000;20(1):17–35
103. Martinez-Sierra C, Arizcorreta A, Diaz F, et al. Progression of chronic hepatitis C to liver fibrosis and cirrhosis in patients coinfected with hepatitis C virus and human immunodeficiency virus. *Clin Infect Dis.* 2003;36(4):491–498
104. Merchante N, Giron-Gonzalez JA, Gonzalez-Serrano M, et al. Survival and prognostic factors of HIV-infected patients with HCV-related end-stage liver disease. *AIDS.* 2006;20(1):49–57
105. Fierer DS, Uriel AJ, Carriero DC, et al. Liver fibrosis during an outbreak of acute hepatitis C virus infection in HIV-infected men: a prospective cohort study. *J Infect Dis.* 2008;198(5):683–686
106. Poynard T, Bedossa P, Opolon P. Natural history of liver fibrosis progression in patients with chronic hepatitis C. The OBSVIRC, METAVIR, CLINIVIR, and DOSVIRC groups. *Lancet.* 1997;349(9055):825–832
107. Roffi L, Redaelli A, Colloredo G, et al. Outcome of liver disease in a large cohort of histologically proven chronic hepatitis: influence of HCV genotype. *Eur J Gastroenterol Hepatol.* 2001;13(5):501–506
108. Graham CS, Baden LR, Yu E, et al. Influence of human immunodeficiency virus infection on the course of hepatitis C virus infection: a meta-analysis. *Clin Infect Dis.* 2001;33(4):562–569
109. Seeff LB, Buskell-Bales Z, Wright EC, et al. Long-term mortality after transfusion-associated non-A, non-B hepatitis. The National Heart, Lung, and Blood Institute Study Group. *N Engl J Med.* 1992;327(27):1906–1911
110. Di Bisceglie AM, Goodman ZD, Ishak KG, et al. Long-term clinical and histopathological follow-up of chronic posttransfusion hepatitis. *Hepatology.* 1991;14(6):969–974
111. Kiyosawa K, Sodeyama T, Tanaka E, et al. Interrelationship of blood transfusion, non-A, non-B hepatitis and hepatocellular carcinoma: analysis by detection of antibody to hepatitis C virus. *Hepatology.* 1990;12(4 Pt 1):671–675
112. Centers for Disease Control and Prevention. Recommendations for prevention and control of hepatitis C virus (HCV) infection and HCV-related chronic disease. Centers for Disease Control and Prevention. *MMWR Recomm Rep.* 1998;47(RR-19):1–39

113. Aach RD, Stevens CE, Hollinger FB, et al. Hepatitis C virus infection in post-transfusion hepatitis. An analysis with first- and second-generation assays. *N Engl J Med.* 1991;325(19): 1325–1329
114. Alter JH, Jett BW, Polito AJ, et al. Analysis of the role of hepatitis C virus in transfusion-associated hepatitis. In: Hollinger FB, Lemon SM, Margolis HS, eds. *Viral Hepatitis and Liver Disease.* Baltimore: Williams and Williams, 1991:396–402
115. Koretz RL, Brezina M, Polito AJ, et al. Non-A, non-B posttransfusion hepatitis: comparing C and non-C hepatitis. *Hepatology.* 1993;17(3):361–365
116. Marranconi F, Mecenero V, Pellizzer GP, et al. HCV infection after accidental needlestick injury in health-care workers. *Infection.* 1992;20(2):111
117. Seeff LB. Hepatitis C from a needlestick injury. *Ann Intern Med.* 1991;115(5):411
118. Weinbaum C, Lyerla R, Margolis H. Prevention and control of infections with hepatitis viruses in correctional settings. Centers for Disease Control and Prevention. *MMWR Recomm Rep.* 2003;52(RR-1):1–36
119. Lanphear BP, Linnemann CC Jr, Cannon CG, et al. Hepatitis C virus infection in healthcare workers: risk of exposure and infection. *Infect Control Hosp Epidemiol.* 1994;15(12):745–750
120. Alter MJ, Kuhnert WL, Finelli L. Guidelines for laboratory testing and result reporting of antibody to hepatitis C virus. Centers for Disease Control and Prevention. *MMWR Recomm Rep.* 2003;52(RR-3):1–13
121. Ghany MG, Strader DB, Thomas DL, et al. Diagnosis, management, and treatment of hepatitis C: an update. *Hepatology.* 2009;49(4);1335–1374
122. Strader DB, Wright T, Thomas DL, et al. Diagnosis, management, and treatment of hepatitis C. *Hepatology.* 2004;39(4);1147–1171
123. Peters MG, Terrault NA. Alcohol use and hepatitis C. *Hepatology.* 2002;36(5 Suppl 1):S220–225
124. Hoofnagle JH, Wahed AS, Brown RS Jr, et al. Early changes in hepatitis C virus (HCV) levels in response to peginterferon and ribavirin treatment in patients with chronic HCV genotype 1 infection. *J Infect Dis.* 2009;199(8);1112–1120
125. Howell CD, Dowling TC, Paul M, et al. Peginterferon pharmacokinetics in African American and Caucasian American patients with hepatitis C virus genotype 1 infection. *Clin Gastroenterol Hepatol.* 2008;6(5);575–583
126. Centers for Disease Control and Prevention. A comprehensive strategy for the prevention and control of hepatitis c virus infection and its consequences. 2001. Available from: http://www.cdc.gov/hepatitis/HCV/Strategy/PDFs/NatHepCPrevStrategy.pdf. Accessed February 2, 2010

# Meningitis and Encephalitis in Adolescents

## W. Garrett Hunt, MD, FAAP*

*Section of Infectious Diseases, Department of Pediatrics, College of Medicine, The Ohio State University, Nationwide Children's Hospital, 700 Children's Drive, Columbus, OH 43205*

Meningitis is inflammation of the protective membranes that cover the brain and spinal cord, known collectively as the meninges, and encephalitis is inflammation of the brain.[1,2] Because central nervous system (CNS) infections occur within the confined space of the cranium or spinal column, they may be associated with increased intracranial and intraspinal pressure, altered blood flow, and, ultimately, neuronal injury.[3] These changes may lead to serious long-term consequences, including deafness, epilepsy, hydrocephalus, cognitive deficits, or even death, if not prevented or treated by certain emergency measures.[4,5] The objective of this review is to summarize the current epidemiology, diagnostic, and therapeutic algorithms, as well as prevention of meningitis and encephalitis in immunocompetent adolescents.

Meningitis is signaled by the clinical symptoms of fever, meningismus (neck stiffness), and headache.[6,7] When altered mental status accompanies one or more of these symptoms, encephalitis or meningoencephalitis is present.[6,8,9] Patients with encephalitis should be distinguished from those with encephalopathy, defined as cerebral dysfunction without associated inflammation. Fever, cerebrospinal fluid (CSF) pleocytosis, focal neurologic signs, and abnormalities on magnetic resonance imaging (MRI) of the brain are uncommon in patients with encephalopathy, whereas they are common in patients with encephalitis.

In general, causes of meningitis are classified as bacterial or nonbacterial, equivalent to the terms septic and aseptic, respectively (see Fig. 1). The classic definition of bacterial (septic) meningitis requires identification of pyogenic bacteria on Gram stain or growth of bacteria on a culture medium. This definition is expanded in cases of partial treatment of bacterial meningitis and by diagnostic tests such as polymerase chain reaction (PCR), which may implicate an organism not isolated by culture. If the cerebrospinal fluid culture remains sterile, by convention the meningitis is referred to as aseptic. Nonbacterial (aseptic)

---
*Corresponding author.
*E-mail address:* wgarrett.hunt@nationwidechildrens.org (W. G. Hunt).

Copyright © 2010 American Academy of Pediatrics. All rights reserved. ISSN 1934-4287

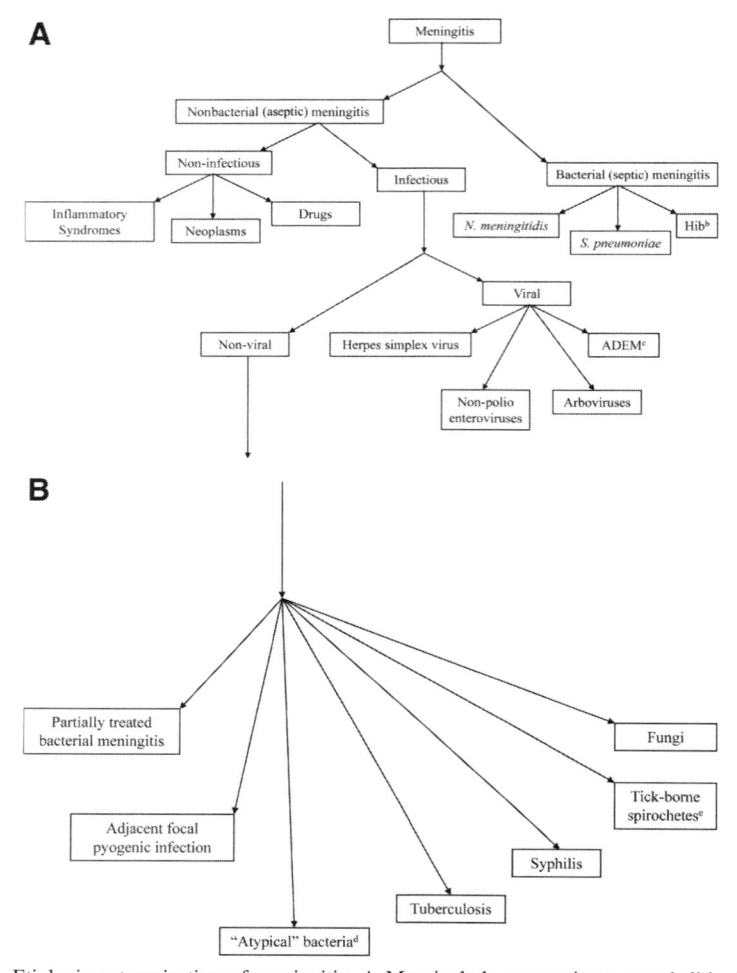

Fig 1. Etiologic categorization of meningitis. A May include concomitant encephalitis. B *Haemophilus influenzae* type B. C Acute disseminated encephalomyelitis, a postinfectious autoimmune syndrome most commonly associated with MMR vaccine, recent varicella or influenza infection, or even nonviral infections such as *Mycoplasma pneumoniae*. D Includes *M. pneumoniae* and *Bartonella henselae*. E Includes *Rickettsia rickettsii*, cause of Rocky Mountain spotted fever; *Borrelia borgdorferi*, cause of Lyme disease; *Anaplasma phagocytophilum*, the cause of human granulocytic anaplasmosis; and both *Ehrlichia chaffensis* and *E. ewingii*, causes of human monocytic ehrlichiosis.

menÜingitis refers to infectious meningitis that has a sterile cerebrospinal fluid culture, is not attributable to pyogenic bacteria or is due to noninfectious etiologies, including toxins, drugs, trauma, or systemic illness.[2,10–12] Infectious etiologies of nonbacterial meningitis include viruses, fungi, parasites, spirochetes, acid-fast bacteria, "atypical" bacteria, and adjacent focal pyogenic infections. Autoimmune inflammation following infection is referred to as acute disseminated encephalomyelitis (ADEM).[2,3,13] Recent clinical and experimental studies suggest that a subset of cases of encephalitis and nonbacterial meningitis may be mediated by antibodies to neuronal extracellular membrane antigens, specifically to the N-methyl-D-aspartate receptor (anti-N-methyl-D-aspartate receptor [NMDAR] encephalitis).[14,15] Initial distinction between bacterial and nonbacterial meningitis is important because it serves to direct history taking, diagnostic testing, antibiotic therapy, prognosis, and prevention. Meningitis may be classified further as acute (<7 days), subacute (up to 2 weeks), chronic (>1 month), or recurrent.[2,3,11] The focus of this review is to highlight the more common pathogenic agents that cause acute bacterial or nonbacterial meningitis, encephalitis, or meningoencephalitis.

**Epidemiology**

Although meningitis is a reportable disease in many countries, active national surveillance is performed for only some bacterial causes of disease. In the United States, the Centers for Disease Control and Prevention (CDC) tracks the incidence of bacterial meningitis due to *Haemophilus influenzae* type B (Hib), *Streptococcus pneumoniae*, and *Neisseria meningitidis* (see Table 1). The incidence of bacterial meningitis in countries where routine vaccination is available has decreased significantly over the past 20 years, declining 55% in the United States since the widespread introduction of the Hib conjugate vaccine in 1990.[16,17]

*N. meningitidis* and *S. pneumoniae* together cause 80% of all cases of meningitis in adults.[18,19] Both bacteria are transmitted by droplet inhalation. Meningococcal strains that most commonly cause invasive disease belong to groups A, B, C, Y, and W-135; ~75% of disease occurring in persons >11 years of age is caused by serotype C, Y, or W-135.[20] Epidemics occur in areas where many people live together for the first time, such as army barracks and college campuses.[4,16,21] The quadrivalent meningococcal vaccine became available in the United States in 2005. As of 2007, CDC has not reported any change in the incidence of meningococcal meningitis.[22]

Pneumococcal disease in general and meningitis in particular have decreased substantially since implementation of routine childhood vaccination with the heptavalent pneumococcal conjugate vaccine (PCV7). Before PCV7 was recommended and then implemented in the year 2000, serotypes 4, 6B, 9V, 14, 18C, 19F, and 23F caused most of the invasive childhood pneumococcal infections in the United States.[16] Antigens of these 7 types are contained in PCV7. The overall incidence of all serotypes of pneumococcal meningitis declined from 1.13 cases to 0.79 case per 100 000 persons between 1998–1999 and 2004–2005 (a 30.1% decline); rates of PCV7-serotype meningitis declined from 0.66 cases to 0.18 cases per 100 000 persons (a 73.3% decline) among patients of all ages.[23]

The annual number of cases of nonbacterial meningitis in the United States due to all causes is estimated to be at least 75 000.[2] In Western countries, population-

Table 1
Epidemiology, clinical features, diagnosis, and empirical therapy of selected causes of meningitis and encephalitis

|  | Epidemiology | Clinical Features | Diagnosis | Empirical Management |
|---|---|---|---|---|
| S. pneumoniae | Droplet transmission from close contact; most prevalent cause of bacterial meningitis in the United States, with single highest morbidity and mortality; splenectomized patients at increased risk of sepsis | 2 of 4 symptoms: headache, fever, stiff neck, and altered mental status | CSF Gram-stain and culture; blood culture; PCR of CSF | IV vancomycin + IV ceftriaxone ± IV rifampin[a] |
| N. meningitidis | Occurs sporadically and in epidemics, some of the latter among military recruits and US college students; droplet transmission from close contact | See above; many also with diffuse rash that can involve palms & soles, first macular, then petechial, finally purpuric | CSF Gram-stain and culture; blood culture | IV ceftriaxone prophylaxis[b] |
| H. influenzae type B | Most cases occur in children 3 months to 3 years of age; increased risk of acquiring a secondary case for household exposure to child <4 years; uncommon in developed countries | See clinical features for pneumococcus; associated with soft tissue infection, eg, buccal or preseptal cellulitis | CSF Gram-stain and culture; blood culture | IV ceftriaxone prophylaxis[b] |
| Non-Polio Enteroviruses | Echoviruses, coxsackie viruses, and enterovirus 71; peak incidence late summer and early fall | Aseptic meningitis w/o encephalitis most common; different syndromes of oral ulcers + diffuse macular and sometimes petechial exanthems | RT-PCR of throat, stool, and CSF | Supportive, IV Ig for chronic disease |

(*Continued*)

Table 1
(Continued)

|  | Epidemiology | Clinical Features | Diagnosis | Empirical Management |
|---|---|---|---|---|
| HSV 1 and 2 | 5–10% of all cases; all age groups and seasons; HSV-1 more common in adolescents and adults | Fever, HA, behavioral abnormalities, seizure, SIADH | PCR of CSF and any vesicular lesions; brain MRI (FLAIR and T2) | IV acyclovir |
| La Crosse Virus | Mosquito vector; chipmunk and squirrel reservoir; midwestern and eastern United States | Many subclinical; biphasic or fulminant onset; fever, headache, and seizure | IgM and IgG of serum and CSF | Supportive |
| Lyme Disease (*B. burgdorferi*) | Deer and lone star tick vectors; occurs in North America, Europe, and Asia | Often associated with erythema migrans; facial nerve palsy (bilateral) | IgM and IgG of serum and CSF; confirmatory Western blot of serum; brain MRI | 1) IV ceftriaxone + doxycycline[c] 2) IV cefotaxime |
| Rocky Mountain Spotted Fever (*R. rickettsii*) | American dog tick in the eastern United States. and Rocky Mountain wood tick in the west; south Atlantic, southeastern, and south central states | Fever, myalgias, and headache; rash that starts at wrists and ankles, maculopapular at first and then petechial | IgM and IgG of serum | 1) IV or oral doxycycline |
| *M. tuberculosis* | More common in developing areas of the world; risk factors include age (<4 years), alcoholism, IV drug use, HIV, and immunosuppressive therapy | Often subacute presentation; fever, night sweats, and weight loss; lethargy | TST and IGRA (false negatives possible); screen for lung disease (CXR and/or chest CT with contrast); acid-fast stain and culture | Four-drug therapy[d] |

(*Continued*)

Table 1
(Continued)

| | Epidemiology | Clinical Features | Diagnosis | Empirical Management |
|---|---|---|---|---|
| Human Immunodeficiency Virus | Sexual contact, percutaneous or mucous membrane exposure to infected blood or body fluids, mother-to-child transmission, or transfusion with contaminated blood products | Acute encephalopathy with seroconversion; most commonly presents as HIV dementia (cognitive dysfunction) | HIV EIA for HIV type 1 and type 2 followed by Western blot if +, and/or HIV cDNA PCR of blood; HIV cDNA PCR of CSF | Highly active antiretroviral therapy |
| Acute Disseminated Encephalomyelitis | More common in children | Abrupt onset of symptoms within several weeks of recent viral illness or live-virus vaccine (MMR); absence of fever | MRI: bilateral but asymmetric hyperintense lesions of white matter on T2 and FLAIR | Corticosteroids Neurology consultation |

Where treatment is listed numerically, the first is the preferred therapy.
[a] Rifampin may be used when CSF antibiotic penetration is reduced, such as when corticosteroids are given, or when an isolate is known to be ceftriaxone-intermediate or -resistant.
[b] See text.
[c] Ceftriaxone alone is effective for Lyme meningitis, but empirical doxycycline is included for cases in which RMSF and the erhlichioses are also being considered.
[d] Usually, empirical 4-drug therapy with oral isoniazid, rifampin, pyrazinamide, and ethionamide for pan-susceptible tuberculous meningitis.
CSF, cerebrospinal fluid; PCR, polymerase chain reaction; IV, intravenous; Ig, immunoglobulin; RT-PCR, reverse-transcriptase polymerase chain reaction; HA, headache; SIADH, syndrome of inappropriate antidiuretic hormone secretion; MRI, magnetic resonance imaging; FLAIR, fluid-attenuated inversion recovery; TST, tuberculin skin test; IGRA, interferon gamma release assay; CXR, chest x-ray; CT, computed tomography; HIV, human immunodeficiency virus; EIA, enzyme immunoassay; MMR, measles, mumps, rubella.

wide studies have shown that viruses are the most common etiology of meningitis, with an annual incidence of 10.9 per 100 000.[24] In studies of patients with accompanying encephalitis, a specific etiology is identified in approximately one-third or fewer of all cases.[25,26] The California Encephalitis Project investigated etiologies of encephalitis in immunocompetent hospitalized patients who met defined criteria, including alteration of consciousness for 24 hours or more and at least one of the following characteristics: fever, seizures, focal neurologic findings, CSF pleocytosis, or electroencephalogram (EEG) or neuroimaging findings consistent with meningoencephalitis.[26,27] A confirmed or probable etiology was found in only 16% of cases; these etiologies included viruses (69%), bacteria (20%), prions (7%), parasites (3%), and fungi (1%).[26]

The majority of cases of nonbacterial meningitis in immunocompetent adolescents and adults are due to non-polio enteroviruses, including enterovirus 71 (EV-71), coxsackieviruses, and echoviruses; the herpes viruses such as herpes simplex virus 1 (HSV-1) and varicella zoster virus (VZV); and the arthropod-borne viruses (arboviruses) such as Japanese encephalitis virus, West Nile virus, and La Crosse virus.[2,26] HSV is the most common cause of sporadic encephalitis in the United States, accounting for up to 2000 cases of encephalitis annually.[3] HSV-1 is responsible for at least 90% of cases of nonneonatal herpes meningoencephalitis[28]; approximately 1 of every 3 affected individuals is younger than 20 years of age.[29] The most common arthropod vectors are mosquitoes and ticks. Mosquito-borne arboviruses causing disease in North America are La Crosse virus, which is a California serogroup *Bunyavirus*; the Flaviviridae, including West Nile virus (WNV) and St. Louis encephalitis virus; and the Togaviridae, examples of which include eastern, western, and Venezuelan equine encephalitis viruses.[16] Ticks may serve as a vector for transmission of bacteria, protozoa, and viruses. *Dermacentor variabilis* (the American dog tick) in the eastern United States and *D. andersoni* (the Rocky Mountain wood tick) in the west can transmit *Rickettsia rickettsii*, the bacterial spirochete that causes Rocky Mountain spotted fever (RMSF; rarely prevalent in the Rocky Mountain states, but found in the south Atlantic, southeastern, and south central states).[16,30] *Ixodes* black-legged ticks (deer ticks) occur primarily in the northeastern and north central United States, and may transmit two causative agents of meningitis or meningoencephalitis: *Borrelia borgdorferi*, the bacterial spirochete that causes Lyme disease, and *Anaplasma phagocytophilum*, the spirochete that causes human granulocytic anaplasmosis (HGA), a syndrome similar in clinical presentation to Rocky Mountain spotted fever.[16,30] *Amblyomma americanum* (the lone star tick) is found in the southeastern and south central United States and may transmit either *Ehrlichia chaffensis* or *Ehrlichia ewingii*, causative agents of human monocytic ehrlichiosis (HME), or *B. burgdorferi*.[16,30]

Less common causes of nonbacterial meningitis in adolescents and adults include herpes viruses other than HSV-1 (HSV-2, human herpesvirus 6, Epstein-Barr virus, and cytomegalovirus), mumps virus, human immunodeficiency virus (HIV), *Mycobacterium tuberculosis* (TB), parameningeal bacterial infection, and fungi including *Cryptococcus gatti* (previously known as *Cryptococcus neoformans* var. *gatti*).[3] Rare causes of nonbacterial meningitis or meningoencephalitis include respiratory viruses (adenovirus, influenza, parainfluenza), lymphocytic choriomeningitis virus (potentially transmitted from ingestion of rodent urine), *Mycoplasma pneumoniae*, *Bartonella henselae*, leptospirosis, syphilis, rabies virus, and amebic meningoencephalitis.[3,16] In-depth discussion of these organisms and their clinical manifestations is beyond the scope of this review.

Meningitis and encephalitis may occur as the result of noninfectious causes as well, including primary or secondary (metastatic) neoplasms of the meninges (malignant meningitis)[10] and certain medications or biologics, primarily nonsteroidal anti-inflammatory drugs, antibiotics, and intravenous immune globulin.[12] Autoimmune conditions such as sarcoidosis, lupus erythematosis, anti-NMDAR encephalitis, or ADEM (postinfectious) and certain forms of vasculitis such as Kawasaki disease or Behçet's disease may cause a CSF pleocytosis.[31] Epidermoid and dermoid cysts may cause aseptic meningitis by releasing irritant matter into the subarachnoid space.[11,31] Reye's syndrome, though an encephalopathy rather than a meningoencephalitis, may present as vomiting, lethargy, and fever and can progress to hepatic dysfunction and severe encephalopathy; it is associated with aspirin ingestion and concomitant chickenpox or viral upper respiratory tract infection. Influenza encephalopathy is known to be present in a similar fashion, with rapidly progressive neurologic deterioration, seizures, and coma within 26 hours of the onset of influenza symptoms.[32]

**Pathophysiology**

Pathogenic events that result in infectious meningitis depend on the interplay between specific virulence factors of the pathogen and defense mechanisms of the host.[3] Infection is often initiated by nasopharyngeal colonization or acquisition at another skin or mucous membrane surface.[33] A recent preceding viral respiratory tract infection may promote successful bacterial colonization. If bacteria invade the intravascular space, they may travel to the blood-brain barrier. Alternatively, direct contamination of the CSF may arise from an indwelling device, skull fracture, or fistulous tract between the nasopharynx or nasal sinuses and the subarachnoid space or between the dura mater and the surface of the skin. The exact site of CNS invasion for most bacteria is unclear, but some experimental studies have identified specific bacterial surface receptors on endothelial cells of the choroid plexus and cerebral capillaries, implicating these sites as potential entry points. The exact mechanism of entry into the CNS is also unclear.

Once bacteria enter the subarachnoid space, there is an influx of leukocytes, mostly neutrophils, within the first 48 hours. This influx is typically mediated by complement components C5a, C3, and factor B.[34,35] Despite the influx of leukocytes in bacterial meningitis, host defense remains suboptimal due to lack of functional opsonic and bactericidal activity. Furthermore, data from animal models have confirmed that the marked subarachnoid space inflammation and much of the sequelae that can occur during bacterial meningitis are primarily a result of the release of inflammatory cytokines by the host.[36] Inflammatory cytokines, including IL-1, tumor necrosis factor (TNF), and prostaglandins,[37] are triggered by exposure to bacterial virulence factors that are released during the replication and lysis of bacteria in the CSF.[36,38]

Cerebral edema, increased intracranial pressure (ICP), and changes in regional blood flow contribute to the majority of sequelae of bacterial meningitis. Cerebral edema is the main factor contributing to increased intracranial pressure, which may result in life-threatening cerebral herniation or other complications. Increased ICP, coupled with narrowed or thrombosed cerebral vessels (vasculitis) and the low blood pressure often encountered in acute infection, may decrease blood flow to the brain, leading to regional hypoxia, increased lactate, CSF acidosis, apoptosis, neuronal injury, stroke, or encephalopathy.[3] Administration of antibiotics may initially worsen the process outlined above by increasing the amount of bacterial cell membrane products released through bacterial destruction, thereby potentiating the inflammatory cascade and ultimately increasing cerebral edema. It has been suggested that the administration of dexamethasone before the initiation of antibiotics may mitigate this effect.[39,40]

Viruses that cause meningitis or encephalitis use many of the same routes of pathogenesis exploited by bacteria: initiation of infection by colonization of mucosal surfaces; hematogenous dissemination (viremia); and CNS invasion across the blood-brain barrier. While the reticuloendothelial system usually clears virions within the blood, some viruses such as HSV, mumps, and measles infect and replicate in human leukocytes.[3] Subsequently, such viruses are protected from phagocytosis by macrophages, neutralization by circulating antibody, and inactivation by nonspecific serum inhibitors.[3] Respiratory viruses are acquired by the respiratory droplet route and then replicate in the upper respiratory epithelium. Alternatively, nonrespiratory viruses such as enteroviruses may initially multiply in the peritonsillar and intestinal lymphatics, lamina propria, or vascular and endothelial cells. From the primary site of replication, the virus spreads to tissues such as the liver, spleen, or muscle, from which viremia and subsequent possible CNS invasion may occur. Arboviral infections begin with subcutaneous inoculation by a vector, followed by replication in local tissue and lymph nodes. Viral invasion of the CNS, similar to that of bacteria, may occur by disruption of the blood-brain barrier. Beyond the neonatal period, HSV is believed to spread in the CNS via reactivation of latent virus from trigeminal ganglia, with transport of virus along olfactory tracts to the bitemporal areas of the brain.[41] Flaccid paralysis caused by WNV is mediated by infection and damage to anterior horn cells, pathology similar to that caused by poliomyelitis. The mechanisms of disease of *Ehrlichia* and *Anaplasma* remain poorly defined; they do not appear to cause the vasculitis and endothelial damage characteristic of other spirochetes.[2]

**Clinical Manifestations**

Initial CNS symptoms and signs of meningitis and meningoencephalitis, whether bacterial or nonbacterial, may be indistinguishable. Nevertheless, epidemiologic information, time course, and associated systemic symptoms and signs can help to differentiate specific etiologies (see Table 1). In adults, a severe headache is the most common initial symptom of meningitis, occurring in almost 90% of cases of bacterial meningitis, followed by nuchal rigidity.[7] In a review of 696 cases of community-acquired bacterial meningitis, the classic triad of diagnostic signs consisting of fever, nuchal rigidity, and altered mental status was present in only 44% of episodes.[7] However, almost all patients (95%) presented with at least 2 of 4 symptoms: headache, fever, stiff neck, or altered mental status. If neither fever, neck stiffness, nor altered mental status is reported, meningitis is extremely unlikely.[42] Other symptoms commonly associated with meningoencephalitis include photophobia, phonophobia, or difficulty with balance. Seizures occur more commonly in children (20–30%) than in adults (0–12%).[3]

Meningitis caused by *N. meningitidis* can be differentiated from most other causes by a rapidly spreading macular erythematous rash that may precede other symptoms and then quickly evolve into petechiae.[43] About one half patients with meningococcemia, with or without meningitis, presents with this rash. The rash consists of numerous small, irregular, purple or red nonblanching spots on the trunk, lower extremities, mucous membranes, conjunctiva, and occasionally the palms of the hands or soles of the feet. A group of petechiae may coalesce to form a purpuric lesion.

The initial presentation of viral meningitis may be very similar to that of bacterial meningitis. For patients with enteroviral meningitis, headache is nearly always present, nuchal rigidity is present in >50% of patients, and photophobia is common.[44–46] Fever may be biphasic. Common nonspecific symptoms include vomiting, anorexia, rash, diarrhea, cough, sore throat, congestion, and myalgia.[45,46] Particular exanthems and enanthems are associated with certain serotypes that cause meningitis and rash. Hand, foot, and mouth syndrome (vesicles on the inner portions of the gums and on the back of the hands and feet) and herpangina (vesicles and shallow ulcers on the posterior pharynx) are both associated with EV-71,[47] although both of these presentations are more common in young children than in adolescents. A diffuse petechial or morbilliform rash of the skin in combination with meningitis is associated with echovirus 9.[48] Generalized febrile seizures can complicate aseptic meningitis without implicating parenchymal brain disturbance. The clinical manifestations of mumps, including the presence of rash, are similar to enteroviruses except for several distinguishing characteristics: 1) occurrence in older children, adolescents, and young adults and 2) common association with either parotitis, which may follow or precede encephalitis, or orchitis. In a multistate outbreak of mumps reported in 2006, parotitis occurred in 66% of patients for whom there were available data; the absence of parotitis does not exclude the diagnosis of mumps or mumps meningoencephalitis.[49] The clinical presentation of HSV-1 meningoencephalitis, from most to least common, includes alteration of consciousness (confusion or behavioral abnormalities), fever, and headache.[50] Focal seizures or other focal neurologic disturbances such as dysphasia or hemiparesis may be present. HSV-1 encephalitis with coexistent orolabial herpetic lesions or ulcerative pharyngitis is more common in immunocompromised patients but has been described for immunocompetent patients.[51] VZV may be associated with meningitis or meningoencephalitis in the immunocompetent patient, typically occurring with zoster along a unilateral trigeminal nerve distribution. The diagnosis may depend on a high degree of suspicion since zoster reactivation may occur in the absence of typical skin lesions.[52] WNV infections are asymptomatic in 80% of cases. Symptomatic neuroinvasive disease occurs in <1% of those infected.[53] In addition, most recognized cases of neuroinvasive WNV present as meningoencephalitis or acute flaccid paralysis.

Meningitis due to spirochetes (RMSF and Lyme disease) has a somewhat more protracted time course than many of the viral illnesses outlined above (2–5 days). The mean incubation period for RMSF is 1 week, with presenting symptoms of fever, myalgia, severe headache, vomiting, and anorexia.[16] Skin rash may fail to develop in up to 20% of cases,[16] but when present typically appears 2–3 days after the initial symptoms and begins as a blanching, maculopapular rash of the ankles and wrists.[54] This rash often becomes petechial with time and may spread diffusely. Signs of encephalitis may develop in ~25% of cases of RMSF.[55] About 15% of patients with Lyme disease come to medical attention with early disseminated disease. This most commonly presents as multiple erythema migrans (EM) lesions (expanding annular, nonpruritic, painless rashes with erythematous borders, each up to 5 cm in diameter) and several weeks of fever, malaise, mild neck stiffness, and myalgia. Lymphocytic meningitis and cranial nerve palsies, especially facial nerve palsy, may occur with early disseminated disease. Bilateral facial nerve palsy is very suggestive of Lyme disease.

Patients with encephalopathy or ADEM typically lack fever as well as some of the other clinical characteristics of infectious meningoencephalitis or encephalitis. Factors favoring ADEM compared with infectious encephalitis include a history of recent immunization (especially measles, mumps, and rubella [MMR] or influenza) or viral illness within the preceding weeks as well as visual loss, absence of fever, and the presence of specific findings on MRI (see *Initial Management and Lumbar Puncture*). Anti-NMDAR antibody positive encephalitis may present in a similar fashion to ADEM. However, the prominence of psychiatric symptoms (including hallucinations and schizophrenia-like behavior), movement disorders (not only ataxia but also choreoathetoid movements), dysautonomia, and hyperthermia may help to distinguish this cause of encephalitis from ADEM.[14,15]

On neurologic examination, alteration in the level of consciousness is highly variable, regardless of whether meningitis is bacterial or nonbacterial.[2,56] Focal neurologic abnormalities, such as sixth cranial nerve palsies, are generally related to either increased intracranial pressure or impaired cerebral blood flow (infarction).[57] Specific pathogens, especially certain causes of nonbacterial meningitis, may result in trigeminal or facial nerve palsies. Peripheral nerve palsies have also been reported for bacterial meningitis. Nystagmus and aphasia are relatively common in adults. If papilledema is noted in a patient with meningitis, usually a complication such as venous sinus thrombosis, brain abscess, hydrocephalus, or subdural empyema has already started to develop.[57] Hemiparesis implies that cerebral vascular occlusion (stroke) has occurred. Ataxia may be noted in patients with hearing loss, reflecting injury to the inner ear. In previous reports, stiff neck was detected in 60% to 80% of children and in over 90% of adults with bacterial meningitis,[57] but in a more recent prospective study in adults, the sensitivity of this sign alone was only 30%.[58] Meningismus may be subtle or marked, in either case possibly accompanied by a positive Kernig's or Brudzinski's sign or both.[59] Although Kernig's and Brudzinski's signs are both commonly used to screen for meningitis, a recent prospective study found the sensitivity of these tests to be limited (each with a sensitivity of 5%).[58] Nevertheless, Kernig's sign, Brudzinski's sign, and meningismus do have good individual specificity for meningitis, as each sign rarely occurs with other diseases.[58]

In the early stages of illness, meningitis may present as cardiorespiratory or CNS instability that requires admission to an intensive care unit. Infection may also trigger the systemic inflammatory response syndrome. Hypotension may occur early, especially but not exclusively in meningococcal illness, and may lead to insufficient blood supply to other organs.[1] Disseminated intravascular coagulation may cause both the obstruction of blood flow to organs and a paradoxical increased risk of bleeding. In meningococcal disease, gangrene of limbs can occur.[1] Severe meningococcal or pneumococcal infections may result in adrenal gland hemorrhage and subsequent adrenocortical insufficiency, such as Waterhouse-Friderichsen syndrome, which is often lethal.[60]

## Initial Management and Lumbar Puncture

The most important test used to identify meningitis is analysis of the CSF through performance of a lumbar puncture (LP).[61] The timing of an LP in relation to other diagnostic studies, antimicrobial therapy, and adjunctive therapy (dexamethasone) is important to understand (see Fig. 2). Initial management has been based traditionally on the assumption that delay in administration of antimicrobial therapy is associated with adverse clinical outcomes. There are no prospective data to prove this association, but the practice guidelines for the management of bacterial meningitis published by the Infectious Diseases Society of America (IDSA) detail several studies that support this approach.[18]

Complications of LP range from mild local discomfort or headache to life-threatening brain herniation. The risk for herniation is increased in patients with elevated intracranial pressure. Any patient who has signs of increased intracranial pressure or who has historical risk factors, such as being immune compromised or having a history of CNS disease, should undergo a computed tomography (CT) scan of the head before lumbar puncture (see Fig. 2). If a CT is required

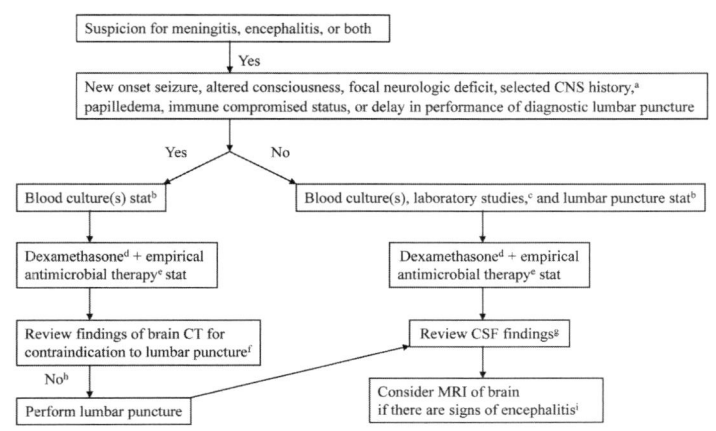

Fig 2. Management algorithm for meningitis and encephalitis. A Includes CSF shunt, hydrocephalus, or trauma; neurosurgery; or various space-occupying lesions. B "Stat" is an abbreviation of statim, meaning immediately. C May include complete blood count with differential, chem-10 (Na, K, Cl, C03, BUN, Cr, glucose, Mg, Ca, and Phos), SGOT (ALT), SGPT (AST), alkaline phosphatase, GGTP, total/direct/indirect bilirubin, lipase, amylase, lactate, blood gas, and urinalysis with microscopy and urine culture. D Administer before or at the same time as antimicrobial therapy in patients ≥17 years of age with possible pneumococcal meningitis (see text). E See Tables 2 and 3. F See text. G See text and Table 2. H Only this pathway is provided since the management of CNS mass lesions or other findings associated with increased intracranial pressure is beyond the scope of this review. I See text.

before the LP, if the LP fails (ie, CSF cannot be obtained), or if there is any other delay, then a blood culture—and in severe cases, an additional range of laboratory tests—should be obtained while intravenous access is acquired (see Fig. 2).[18] Antibiotics should be administered before the LP to prevent delay in treatment of underlying infection. In one retrospective review of 177 patients with CSF culture-proven bacterial meningitis, 39 of whom had received prior antimicrobial therapy, the combination of blood culture and CSF Gram-stain identified the causative bacterium in 92% of patients.[62]

In patients with a presentation concerning for encephalitis, MRI with gadolinium contrast should be considered after the initial evaluation is performed (see Fig. 2). MRI is more sensitive and provides more detailed diagnostic information than CT. The most common abnormalities found in encephalitis include focal areas of increased signal involving gray matter of both hemispheres, basal ganglia, brainstem, and cerebellum on T2-weighted MRI. For ADEM, there are focal areas of hyperintensity in white matter of both hemispheres, basal ganglia, brainstem, cerebellum, and spinal cord. A method complementary to T2-weighted MRI is fluid-attenuated inversion recovery, used to suppress areas of increased signal so that interfaces between sections of high and low signal intensity can be distinguished more easily. Another very sensitive technique for measuring the restriction of water diffusion due to cytotoxic edema is diffusion-weighted MRI.[63]

## Diagnosis

*Interpretation of CSF Findings*

The CSF sample is examined for presence and types of white blood cells (WBCs), red blood cells (RBCs), protein content, and glucose level. CSF is normally clear and colorless but may appear cloudy or turbid in patients with increased concentrations of WBC (>200/mm$^3$), RBC (>400/mm$^3$), protein, or bacteria (>10$^5$ colony-forming units).[3] The Gram stain of CSF is ~60% sensitive for the diagnosis of bacterial meningitis; this is reduced by another 20% if

Table 2
Typical cerebrospinal fluid (CSF) findings for children and adults at baseline and with meningitis caused by various etiologies

| CSF Parameter | Leukocytes/ mm$^3$ | PMNs (%) | Protein (mg/dL) | Glucose (mg/dL) | CSF-to-blood glucose ratio | Positive Stain[a] (%) | Positive Culture (%) | PCR |
|---|---|---|---|---|---|---|---|---|
| Normal | 0–5 | 0[b] | 5–40 | 40–80 | >0.4 | No | No | N/A |
| Viral | <1000 | 20–40[c] | <100 | N[d] | N[d] | NA | Rare | Yes[e] |
| Bacterial | >1000[f] | >70[g] | 100–500[h] | ≤40 | ≤0.4 | >60 | >70 | Yes[h] |
| Partially Treated Bacterial | >1000[f] | >70[i] | 60–100 | >40[i] | >0.4 | ~40 | <70 | Yes[h] |
| Lyme Disease | <500 | ≤10 | <100 | N | N | NA | NA | Yes[j] |
| Fungal | <500 | <20 | >100 | ≤40 | ≤0.4 | <40 | >30 | No |
| M. tuberculosis | <300 | <20[b] | >200 | ≤40 | ≤0.4 | ≤30 | ≤70 | Yes[k] |

[a] Gram or acid-fast bacillus staining for bacteria or *M. tuberculosis*, respectively.
[b] Studies in children with a non-CNS-associated illness have shown presence of PMNs in otherwise normal CSF, with up to 5% of children having as many as 3 PMNs in one study.[120]
[c] PMN predominance may be observed in early stages of meningitis.
[d] CMV, mumps, and eastern equine virus encephalitis may be associated with low serum glucose and a low CSF-to-blood glucose ratio.
[e] Commerically available PCRs include those for herpes simplex viruses 1 and 2, the non-polio enteroviruses, varicella zoster virus, and Epstein-Barr virus (see text).
[f] A small percentage of patients can present with initially normal values.
[g] Approximately 10% of patients with bacterial meningitis present with a predominance of mononuclear cells.
[h] A commercially available PCR exists for pneumococcus, and those for Hib and meningococcus look promising (see text).
[i] Both absolute neutrophil counts (and therefore percent) as well as glucose levels (and therefore CSF-to-blood glucose ratio) normalized in patients pre-treated with antibiotics within the 72 hours prior to LP.[64]
[j] PCR for *B. burgdorferi*, if obtained, should be interpreted within the context of antibody testing of the CSF and serum as well as Western blot from the serum (see text).
[k] Though not formally approved for CSF testing, the Gen-Probe Amplified *M. tuberculosis* Direct Test has shown good sensitivity and specificity in small cohorts of patients with tuberculous meningitis.
CSF, cerebrospinal fluid; PMN, polymorphonuclear cells; PCR, polymerase chain reaction; NA, not applicable; N, normal.

antibiotics are administered before CSF is obtained.[18] Microbiologic culture of the sample is 70–85% sensitive for identification of the most bacteria, but results can take up to 48 hours to become available.[18] In patients with meningitis or meningoencephalitis, the specific CSF results may vary depending on the infectious agent (see Table 2). If antimicrobial agents, particularly parenteral broad-spectrum agents, have been administered before performing the LP, distinguishing between bacterial and nonbacterial causes of meningitis may be difficult. However, in one recent study of 85 patients who received antibiotic pretreatment within 72 hours of lumbar puncture, antibiotic treatment was associated with normalizing values of glucose and protein in the cerebrospinal fluid (ie, higher glucose and lower protein) without modification of CSF WBC or absolute neutrophil counts.[64]

The normal CSF WBC count range in persons over 3 months of age is 0–5 per cubic millimeter.[65] Elevated CSF concentrations of WBCs are seen with meningitis, encephalitis, and parameningeal focus of infection. The highest median WBC counts are seen in bacterial meningitis, but these decrease gradually over the course of appropriate antibiotic therapy. The primary cell type may vary with time course of infection. Most bacterial infections cause an initial predominance of neutrophils, but the proportion of monocytes and lymphocytes increases during resolution of the infection. Viral infections usually result in a predominance of mononuclear cells, though neutrophils may be more numerous during the first 24–48 hours of symptomatic disease. A cross-sectional study that compared patients with Lyme and enteroviral meningitis found that Lyme meningitis, as opposed to enteroviral meningitis, was unlikely when cerebrospinal fluid neutrophils exceeded 10% (negative predictive value, 99%).[66]

Elevations of WBC counts may occur with traumatic LP or in patients with intracerebral or subarachnoid hemorrhage.[3] The following may be used as a correction factor to calculate the true CSF WBC in the presence of RBCs:

$$WBC_{TRUE} = WBC_{CSF} - [(WBC_{BLOOD} \times RBC_{CSF})/RBC_{BLOOD}]$$

In this equation, the amount being subtracted in brackets is the predicted WBC in the CSF that is the result of contamination from the peripheral blood stream. Several studies of meningitis and traumatic LP in children >1 month up to adulthood have examined the use of ratios of observed and predicted WBC counts in CSF. This method has been found to be helpful in predicting meningitis in these particular studies, with sensitivities varying between 80–100% and specificities of 63–97%, depending on the exact method used.[67–69] CSF RBC counts do not differ significantly between patients with biopsy-proven HSV encephalitis and nonherpetic encephalitis.[50,70]

The concentration of glucose in CSF is normally above 40% of that in blood. A ratio of simultaneous CSF glucose to blood glucose levels ≤0.4 in adolescents and adults is typically indicative of bacterial meningitis.[71] Hypoglycemia and hyperglycemia can also affect the level of glucose in the CSF. Glucose concentrations are normal in >95% of patients with encephalitis caused by HSV and the flaviviruses but may be low in some cases of cytomegalovirus, mumps, and eastern equine virus encephalitis.[50,72–74]

Several algorithms and additional laboratory tests may help to differentiate septic from aseptic meningitis. The Bacterial Meningitis Score, developed by the Pediatric Emergency Medicine Collaborative Research Committee of the American Academy of Pediatrics (AAP), classifies patients to be at very low risk of bacterial meningitis if they lack all of the following criteria: positive CSF Gram stain, CSF absolute neutrophil count of at least 1000 cells/$\mu$L, CSF protein of at least 80 mg/dL, peripheral blood absolute neutrophil count of at least 10 000 cells/$\mu$L, and a history of seizure before or at the time of presentation.[75] This algorithm may prove to be useful as a guide to clinical management of patients who present with CSF pleocytosis, but validation as part of a prospective trial is required for proof of clinical utility. C-reactive protein (CRP) may be useful in distinguishing viral from Gram-stain-negative bacterial meningitis.[76,77] A retrospective cohort study compared 55 children >3 months of age with Gram-stain-negative bacterial meningitis with 182 children with proven or suspected viral meningitis.[77] Although routine CSF tests were included in the analysis, only a normal serum CRP (cutoff <2 mg/dL) distinguished viral from Gram-stain-negative bacterial meningitis with high sensitivity (96%), specificity (93%), and negative predictive value (99%).[77] Therefore, CRP may be helpful in deciding whether to withhold antimicrobial therapy for a patient with CSF pleocytosis but negative CSF Gram stain.[18]

*Identification of Pathogens*
*Septic Meningitis* CSF bacterial culture is the standard for diagnosis of bacterial meningitis. Routine use of CSF latex agglutination testing is not recommended but may be considered in cases of pretreatment with antimicrobial therapy and when both CSF Gram stain and culture are negative.[18] PCR has been used to amplify DNA from the CSF of patients with meningitis caused by common pathogens such as *S. pneumoniae*, *N. meningitidis*, and Hib. In one study, multiplex PCR of CSF for the detection of these three organisms had sensitivities of 92.3%, 93.9%, and 88%, respectively; the overall specificity and positive predictive value of the assay was 100%.[78] Depending on regional or institutional availability, CSF PCR is rapid and may detect nonviable organisms in patients pretreated with antibiotics when both CSF Gram stain and culture are negative. False-positive results have become less common with more recent primers. It is important to evaluate patients for local or systemic disease that may have disseminated to the CNS. Cultures of blood, urine, and other appropriate sites that would be sterile in an otherwise uninfected host should be cultured, ideally before antibiotic administration. Periorbital cellulitis, arthritis, pneumonia, and

pericarditis are examples of local infections that may be caused by bacteria and disseminate to the CNS via the bloodstream.[57]

*Aseptic Meningitis, Encephalitis, and Meningoencephalitis* In general, viral culture of CSF is of limited value. Alternatively, PCR of CSF has high sensitivity and specificity for many neuroinvasive viruses, making this test the usual diagnostic study of choice for viral identification.[3,79] Enteroviral reverse-transcriptase PCR of CSF has better sensitivity than that of viral culture (65–75%) and a specificity of almost 100%. HSV DNA PCR of the CSF for the detection of both HSV-1 and HSV-2 has a sensitivity of 98% and a specificity of 94%.[80,81] Although the sensitivity of this test is high, it should be interpreted within the context of the time course of disease. In the California Encephalitis Project, 3 patients with negative CSF HSV PCR performed within 72 hours of symptom onset had positive tests 4–7 days later.[82] Furthermore, sensitivity declines as the duration of time after initiation of intravenous acyclovir increases: 98% sensitivity in patients treated ≤7 days, 47% after 8–14 days, and 21% after ≥15 days.[81] If CSF testing cannot be obtained until later in the course of disease (after 7 or more days of antiviral therapy), use of nested or quantitative HSV PCR or detection of HSV-specific intrathecal antibodies may improve sensitivity.[83,84] Furthermore, MRI with gadolinium contrast of the brain and EEG are useful in making the diagnosis of HSV encephalitis. In contrast to the detection of herpes simplex virus in CSF, VZV DNA PCR has a sensitivity of ≤30% but a specificity of >95%.[85] VZV-specific intrathecal antibody is recommended as a complementary test. For most flaviviruses, including WNV, PCR is less sensitive (<70% for WNV) than CSF anti-virus immunoglobulin (Ig) M antibody for detection of neuroinvasive disease. Intrathecal anti-WNV IgM has a sensitivity of ~10% on the first day of illness, thereafter increasing by ~10% daily and reaching 80% by the end of the first week.[86] Most arboviral infections, including La Crosse virus, are confirmed by virus-specific IgM and IgG antibodies in serum and CSF. IgM is typically detectable in serum in 3–8 days and persists for 30–90 days, but longer persistence has been documented; virus-specific IgG lasts for years.[16] In contrast to the previously discussed viruses, the diagnosis of mumps is based on CSF viral culture, although CSF and serum antibodies can also be helpful.

For most causes of nonviral, nonbacterial infectious meningitis, evaluation of acute systemic disease is important to include along with CSF analysis and testing. Of the diseases caused by spirochetes, RMSF and ehrlichiosis have the most typified laboratory abnormalities. Both are associated with elevated alanine aminotransferase and aspartate aminotransferase, thrombocytopenia, leukopenia (more common for ehrlichiosis), and hyponatremia. In addition, the erhlichioses (HME and HGA) frequently cause lymphopenia.[2] Lyme disease has nonspecific findings on routine laboratory studies. Acute infection with *R. rickettsii, E. chaffensis, E. ewingii,* or *A. phagocytophilum* induces a 4-fold increase in IgG titers from the acute period to convalescence (2–4 weeks after onset). Lyme disease requires 2-step testing, in which combined IgM and IgG serology is obtained first. Antibodies measured by enzyme-linked immunoassay should be obtained simultaneously from the serum and CSF. "If antibodies are detected from at least one of these sites," then serologic immunoblot testing (Western blot) is done next. IgM and IgG immunoblots are obtained if the patient has had symptoms for ≤1 month, versus IgG alone if the patient has had symptoms >1 month. A positive IgM immunoblot requires at least 2 of the following bands: 23/24, 39, and 41 polypeptides.[16] A positive IgG immunoblot requires 5 or more of the following bands: 18, 23/24, 28, 30, 39, 41, 45, 60, 66, and 93 kDa polypeptides.[16] PCR testing for all of the vector-borne spirochetes is available through CDC. PCRs from the blood have been validated for all of the spirochetes discussed above and from the CSF and synovial fluid for Lyme disease.

**Antimicrobial Therapy**

Meningitis has a high mortality rate if untreated,[18] and delay in treatment may be associated with worse outcomes.[87] Thus, patients for whom there is a suspicion of meningitis should receive treatment with broad-spectrum antibiotics while confirmatory tests are pending.[18,88] In the United States, empirical antimicrobial therapy for coverage of pneumococcus and meningococcus as well as other pathogens with a combination of high-dose intravenous vancomycin and either intravenous ceftriaxone or cefotaxime is used for infants and children and is "recommended by some experts for adults" according to IDSA practice guidelines.[18] In general, substitution of other antibiotics or use of additional antibiotics for initial therapy should be determined by local susceptibility patterns of pathogens, relative penetration of the antibiotic into CSF in the context of inflamed meninges, and patient-specific clinical factors (see Fig. 2). For example, focal seizures or change in mental status (encephalitis) should heighten the suspicion for HSV meningoencephalitis, which would trigger testing of the CSF and appropriate peripheral sites for HSV as well as the addition of intravenous acyclovir to the empirical antibiotic regimen. In general, antimicrobial therapy may be narrowed based on certain characteristics of the CSF, including the routine CSF parameters, and of the pathogen, including Gram stain, PCR, culture identification, and in vitro susceptibility data for an isolate from the blood or CSF, depending on the specific circumstance (see Table 3).

Intravenous aqueous penicillin G was once the empirical antibiotic of choice for meningitis due to *S. pneumoniae* and *N. meningitidis*; however, reduced susceptibility to penicillin has been detected in the United States and worldwide for both bacteria.[23,89] In the United States and abroad, resistance to third-generation cephalosporins has been reported for pneumococcus, and resistance to chloramphenicol has been reported for both Hib and pneumococcus.[23,90] Because of the concern that vancomycin penetrates poorly into the CSF, particularly in the context of steroid administration, rifampin may be added pending culture results and in vitro susceptibility testing for patients who have received steroids. More-

Table 3
Recommendations for pathogen-specific antimicrobial therapy in patients with meningitis

| Pathogen | Standard Therapy[a] | Route | Total Daily Dose in Dose/Kg (Dosing Interval in Hours) | Duration of Therapy (Days) | Alternative Agents |
|---|---|---|---|---|---|
| S. pneumoniae 1) Penicillin-susceptible (MIC <0.1) | Penicillin G or ampicillin | IV | 250\|000–400\|000 U[b] (4–6)[c] 200–400 (6)[e] | 10–14 | Ceftriaxone[d] or cefotaxime |
| Penicillin-intermediate (MIC 0.1–1.0) | Ceftriaxone or cefotaxime ± vancomycin | IV | 100 (12–24)[f] 225–300 (6)[g] 60 (6)[h] | | Cefepime or meropenem |
| Penicillin-resistant (MIC ≥1.0) | Ceftriaxone or cefotaxime plus vancomycin | IV | See above | | Cefepime or meropenem |
| Ceftriaxone-nonsusceptible (MIC >0.5) | See above + rifampin[i] | IV/PO or IV | 20 (12)[i] | | Meropenem + vancomycin |
| N. meningitidis | Penicillin G[j] or ampicillin | IV | 250\|000–300\|000 U[b](4–6)[j] 200–400 (6) | 7 | Ceftriaxone or cefotaxime |
| Haemophilus influenzae type b | Ceftriaxone[k] or cefotaxime | IV | 100 (12–24)[f] 200 (6)[f] | 7 | Meropenem ampicillin + chloramphenicol |
| HSV 1 and 2 | Acyclovir | IV | 30 (8)[l] | 14–21 | Foscarnet cidofovir |
| Lyme Disease (B. burgdorferi) | Ceftriaxone or penicillin | IV | 75–100 (24)[f] 250\|000–300\|000 U[b](4–6) | 14–28 | Doxycycline[m] |
| RMSF (R. rickettsii) | Doxycycline[m] | PO or IV | 20 (12)[m] | 7–10 | Chloramphenicol fluoroquinolone |
| Syphilis (T. pallidum) | Penicillin G, or procaine penicillin G + probenecid | IV/IM/ PO | 200\|000–300\|000 (4–6)[c] 50\|000 (24)[n] 40 (6)[o] | 10–14 | Ceftriaxone |

[a] Dexamethasone may be beneficial for meningitis due to S. pneumoniae or H. influenzae type b (Hib) if given prior to or at the same time as the first dose of antibiotics.
[b] 1 U = 0.0006 mg, so this range is = 150–240 mg/Kg per day.
[c] Penicillin G maximum daily dose for pneumococcus or syphilis is 24 million U per day.
[d] Once or twice daily alternative for convenience and cost savings.
[e] Ampicillin maximum single and daily doses for children are 2 g and 12 g, respectively, and for adults 3 g and 14 g, respectively.
[f] Ceftriaxone maximum single dose 2 g and daily dose 4 g.
[g] Cefotaxime maximum single dose 2 g and daily dose 12 g.

(Continued)

Table 3
(Continued)

[h] Vancomycin dosing is based on achievement of trough levels sustained at 15–20 μg/mL, first obtained prior to the fourth dose; when individual doses exceed 1g, the infusion period should be extended to 1.5–2 hours.[121]
[i] Consider addition of or continuation of rifampin (discontinue if isolate not susceptible) if there is no clinical improvement with empirical antibiotics in 24–48 hours, if repeat cerebrospinal fluid analysis does not show sterilization or reduction of the number of organisms, or if MIC to cefotaxime or ceftriaxone is ≥4 μg/mL; rifampin maximum single dose is 600 mg and daily dose 1.2 g.
[j] Reduced susceptibility to penicillin has been detected in the United States and worldwide. If penicillin or ampicillin is used, then another antimicrobial agent will need to be given to the index patient to eradicate colonization; maximum daily dose for meningococcus is 12 million units.
[k] Rifampin for eradication of colonization in the index patient does not need to be given if the patient receives cefotaxime or ceftriaxone.
[l] No adult maximum for intravenous dosing.
[m] Tetracyclines, including doxycycline, are generally not given to children younger than 8 years of age due to the increased risk of dental staining, although most experts consider doxycycline to be the drug of choice for children of any age for Rocky Mountain spotted fever and ehrlichiosis; doxycycline is an alternative antibiotic for Lyme disease meningitis; the maximum single dose is 100 mg and daily dose 200 mg.
[n] Maximum single and daily dose of procaine penicillin is 2.4 million U.
[o] Maximum single dose is 500 mg and daily dose 2 g.
MIC, minimum inhibitory concentration (μg/mL); IV, intravenous.

over, once susceptibility results are known, a third-generation cephalosporin should be continued, along with vancomycin, for a pneumococcal strain not susceptible to third-generation cephalosporins. Any patient who does not have expected clinical improvement or who has a pneumococcal isolate that is resistant to cefotaxime or ceftriaxone (see Table 3) should undergo a repeat lumbar puncture after 36–48 hours of therapy to document sterility of CSF.[3,18] Consideration should be given to continuing or adding rifampin, if the isolate is susceptible, for clinical or microbiologic failure or for penicillin- or cephalosporin-resistant pneumococcal strains (see Table 3).[3,16] The duration of antibiotic therapy is primarily based on expert opinion rather than well-validated clinical trials. Alternative empirical antibiotics for Hib, meningococcus, and pneumococcus include cefepime and meropenem[91]; linezolid is an additional alternative antibiotic for pneumococcus.[16]

IDSA guidelines advise that intravenous acyclovir should be initiated in all patients with suspected encephalitis pending results of diagnostic studies.[65] The dosing of intravenous acyclovir beyond the neonatal period is 10 mg/kg/dose every 8 hours (no adult maximum), continued for 2–3 weeks in patients with definitive HSV meningoencephalitis. Similarly, VZV encephalitis is typically treated with intravenous acyclovir, 15 mg/kg/dose every 8 hours for 2–3 weeks. Most of the arboviral encephalitides are treated supportively, with management of increased intracranial pressure, seizures, and behavioral disorders as needed. In general, most cases of viral meningitis other than those caused by HSV, varicella, and the arboviruses represent mild to moderate disease that requires bed rest and analgesics only. Specific antibiotics are not available for most of the viruses that cause meningitis.

A reasonable approach for patients who present with possible tick-borne meningoencephalitis is to add oral or intravenous doxycycline to the routine empirical regimen of intravenous ceftriaxone and vancomycin. Doxycycline is well-absorbed orally; thus, intravenous administration should be needed only if oral therapy cannot be tolerated.[92] Lyme meningitis is treated with intravenous penicillin or ceftriaxone for 14–28 days. For patients who are intolerant of β-lactam antibiotics, increasing evidence indicates that oral doxycycline may be adequate. For ehrlichiosis or RMSF meningoencephalitis, doxycycline should be continued until the patient has had clinical improvement, including absence of fever, for at least 3 days. The typical duration of therapy is 7–10 days.

## Adjunctive Measures

Since meningitis can cause a number of potentially severe complications, close medical surveillance is recommended, as is admission to an intensive care unit depending on hemodynamic and respiratory support required by the patient.[19] Adjunctive measures center on decreasing the likelihood of cerebral ischemia by maintaining appropriate systemic blood pressure and reducing inflammation, intracranial hypertension, and metabolic demands. Mechanical ventilation may be needed if consciousness is impaired or there is evidence of respiratory failure. Simple measures to help normalize intracranial pressure include elevation of the head of the bed to 30 degrees and, in some circumstances, hyperventilation. Intracranial pressure monitoring, a more invasive method, may allow for optimization of cerebral perfusion pressure using mannitol or other adjunctive therapies. Seizures are treated with fluid and electrolyte management, antipyretics, or anticonvulsants, as indicated.[19] Hydrocephalus due to obstructed flow of CSF may require insertion of a temporary or long-term drainage device such as a shunt.[93]

Selected patients should receive adjunctive therapy with corticosteroids, usually dexamethasone, when presenting with suspected or proven bacterial meningitis (see Fig. 2). In adolescents and adults from developed countries with low rates of HIV, corticosteroids have been shown to reduce mortality, severe hearing loss, and neurologic morbidity.[94] Experimental animal models have shown that the breakdown products of the pneumococcal cell wall following antibiotic-induced bacteriolysis may contribute to the inflammatory response in the subarachnoid space.[95] The likely mechanism for the benefit of corticosteroids is suppression of this inflammation. A meta-analysis of clinical studies in humans confirmed the benefit of adjunctive dexamethasone, 0.15 mg/kg every 6 hours for 2–4 days, for Hib meningitis.[96] In 2002, a multicenter randomized controlled trial was published that enrolled 301 adults (≥17 years of age) with meningitis who received either dexamethasone (10 mg every 6 hours for 4 days) or placebo, the first dose administered 15–20 minutes before the first dose of antibiotics.[21] At 8 weeks after enrollment, patients in the dexamethasone group had lower rates of unfavorable outcomes (15% vs. 25%; $P = .03$) and death (7% vs. 15%; $P = .04$).[18,21]

The IDSA guidelines on meningitis published in 2004 recommend the use of dexamethasone, 0.15 mg/kg every 6 hours for 2–4 days, for adolescents ≥17 years of age and adults. The first dose is administered 10–20 minutes before or concurrent with the first dose of antimicrobial therapy, but antibiotics should never be delayed to account for steroid dosing.[18] Given that most of the benefit of the treatment is confined to those with pneumococcal meningitis, IDSA Guidelines suggest that dexamethasone be discontinued if a cause of meningitis other than pneumococcus is identified.[18,97]

Adjuvant corticosteroids have a differently defined role in children and in adolescents younger than 17 years of age than in older adolescents and adults. For children, the effect of steroids appears to be greatest in cases of Hib meningitis, the incidence of which has decreased dramatically since the introduction of Hib vaccine. Thus, corticosteroids are recommended in the treatment of pediatric meningitis if the cause is *H. influenzae* type B and only if given before or simultaneously with the first dose of antibiotics. As stated in the 2009 recommendations of the AAP Committee on Infectious Diseases regarding pneumococcal meningitis, "many experts recommend the use of corticosteroids in pneumococcal meningitis; but this issue is controversial and data are not sufficient to make a recommendation for children. If used, dexamethasone should be given before or concurrently with the first dose of the antimicrobial agent."[16] The benefit of steroids for cranial nerve palsies in cases of Lyme disease is unclear, but they may be given with concomitant antimicrobial therapy.[98] There is no proven benefit of steroids for treatment of HSV encephalitis. Although not fully assessed, high-dose intravenous methylprednisolone is generally recommended for patients with ADEM.[65]

**Prognosis**

Mortality and morbidity from treated meningitis depends on a variety of factors, some of which include the infecting organism, inoculum, route of infection, time to clearance of the infecting organism from the CSF, type and timing of antimicrobial therapy, adjunctive therapy, and host characteristics such as age, immunologic status, and initial clinical presentation. With modern management, the risk of mortality from the three primary etiologies of bacterial meningitis is much lower in children, <5–10% in most studies,[2] than in adults, in whom the risk is 19–37%.[1,19] Of the bacterial meningitides, the case-fatality rate and incidence of neurologic sequelae beyond the neonatal period are greatest for pneumococcal meningitis.[2]

One of the most important factors predicting a patient's mortality or morbidity is state of consciousness at the time of admission. Patients ultimately proven to have bacterial meningitis who are comatose on admission have a significantly higher risk of mortality.[99,100] Comatose patients who survive have increased risk of deficiencies in perceptual-performance skills that last until at least school age.[101] Seizures that are focal, persistant, or late-onset are indicators of worse long-term outcome.[1,11] Sensorineural hearing loss, epilepsy, learning and behavioral difficulties, and decreased intelligence occur in ~15% of survivors.[1] Hearing loss is more likely if the CSF glucose concentration at admission is <20 mg/dL.[99] Some hearing loss may be reversible.[102] In adults, 66% of all cases emerge without disability. The most serious permanent problems are deafness in 14% and cognitive impairment in 10%.[19]

The mortality rate for treated HSV encephalitis in older children and adults is ~28% at 18 months after treatment.[70,103] Following a 10-day course of acyclovir therapy, up to 5% of patients may experience a relapse within 1 month.[104] Most cases of virologic relapse are cured with a second course of therapy. La Crosse virus encephalitis that is severe enough to require hospitalization may be associated with significant cognitive impairment in greater than one-third of patients and attention-deficit/hyperactivity disorder in 60%.[105] For Lyme disease, there is no convincing biological evidence for the existence of symptomatic chronic *B. burgdorferi* infection among patients after receipt of recommended treatment regimens.[92]

**Prevention**

*Chemoprophylaxis*

Rifampin prophylaxis continues to be recommended for eradication of colonization in all households in which there is Hib meningitis and at least one unvaccinated contact <4 years of age.[16] For exposure to an index case of meningococcal meningitis, all household and day care contacts should be given rifampin prophylaxis. Options in place of oral rifampin for meningococcal prophylaxis include a single intramuscular dose of ceftriaxone (125 mg for children <12 years of age and 250 mg for ≥12 years of age) or, in adults, one oral dose of ciprofloxacin, ofloxacin, or azithromycin. However, three cases of ciprofloxacin-resistant *N. meningitidis* were reported recently in North Dakota and Minnesota, leading the CDC to no longer recommend ciprofloxacin for meningococcal prophylaxis in selected counties of these states.[106] Topical repellants that contain N-N-diethyl-*m*-toluamide (DEET) are the most effective in preventing arthropod-borne transmission of potential pathogens. Routine administration of antimicrobial prophylaxis after a deer tick bite is not recommended, although a single dose of doxycycline, 4 mg/kg up to the adult dose of 200 mg, may be considered for children >8 years of age if an attached, engorged tick is identified in an endemic area. Expeditious removal of ticks with blunt curved forceps or tweezers, with avoidance of crushing or puncturing the body of the tick, may decrease the risk of infection.[2]

*Immunoprophylaxis*

This section will be limited to a concise review of meningococcal vaccines. A quadrivalent polysaccharide vaccine against serogroups A, C, Y, and W-135 (Menomune, Sanofi Pasteur, MPSV4) has been available in the United States since 1981.[107] The meningococcal polysaccharide vaccine elicits production of specific bactericidal, protective antibodies. The T-cell response to this vaccine, however, is less pronounced than that for two recently developed meningococcal vaccines with the same polysaccharides conjugated to diphtheria toxoid or diphtheria $CRM_{197}$ protein, respectively (Menactra, Sanofi Pasteur, MCV4, and Menveo, Novartis Vaccines and Diagnostics, MenACWY-$CRM_{197}$).[108,109] MCV4 and MenACWY-$CRM_{197}$ are associated with more robust and longer-lasting immunity than MPSV4.[107] In the United Kingdom and other countries where the conjugate vaccine against meningococcus serogroup C has been introduced, cases of meningococcal meningitis due to this serogroup have decreased substantially. There has been no serogroup replacement identified to date.[110] Group B meningococcus has proven more of a challenge for vaccine development since its capsular polysaccharide is poorly immunogenic in humans, and many of its surface proteins induce only a weak immune response or cross-react with normal human proteins.[111,112] Nevertheless, some countries (New Zealand, Cuba, Norway, and Chile) have developed vaccines effective against local strains of group B meningococcus, and some of these vaccines are used in local immunization schedules.[111]

In the United States, MCV4 was licensed for use in January 2005. The Advisory Committee on Immunization Practices (ACIP) recommends routine vaccination with a single dose of MCV4 in those 11–18 years of age.[108] On February 19, 2010, the U.S. Food and Drug Administration licensed a second quadrivalent meningococcal conjugate vaccine, MenACWY-$CRM_{197}$ (Menveo, Novartis Vaccines and Diagnostics).[109] MenACWY-CRM is licensed as a single dose for use among persons 11–55 years of age.[109] Ideally, vaccination with either conjugate vaccine occurs at the preadolescent health care visit at 11–12 years of age, as supported by the ACIP and the Society for Adolescent Medicine.[108,113,114] Persons who do not receive vaccine when they are 11–12 years of age should be offered vaccine at the first appropriate health care visit from 13–18 years of age. The ACIP recommends vaccination with MCV4 for persons 2–55 years of age who are at increased risk of disease, including college freshman living in dormitories, military recruits, microbiologists routinely exposed to *N. meningitidis*, individuals with terminal complement deficiencies, individuals with functional or anatomic asplenia, and individuals residing in or traveling to places where *N. meningitidis* is endemic.[108,115] The AAP recommends that anyone at increased risk who received MPSV4 ≥3 years previously should receive MCV4.[116] If children receive MCV4 or MPSV4 from 2–6 years of age and remain at increased risk of disease, they should be revaccinated with MCV4 in 3 years.[117] Children who were vaccinated with MCV4 at age ≥7 years and remain at increased risk should be revaccinated after 5 years.[117] The ACIP does not currently recommend that college freshmen living in dormitories who were previously vaccinated with MCV4 be revaccinated.[117] There are insufficient data on the safety of MCV4 in pregnancy to recommend its use in this situation, but MPSV4 may be used.[108] Soon after MCV4 was licensed for routine immunization in 2005, cases of Guillain-Barré Syndrome (GBS) were reported among recent recipients of MCV4.[118] Because of the ongoing risk for meningococcal disease and the limitations of the data indicating a small risk for GBS after MCV4 vaccination, the CDC has not changed its recommendations regarding MCV4, except that history of GBS before receipt of the vaccine is a relative contraindication.[119]

## CONCLUSIONS

The clinical presentation of meningoencephalitis due to distinct etiologies, including meningococcus, pneumococcus, and herpes simplex virus, may be indistinguishable. Consequently, a thorough history of present illness and physical examination are essential to achieve a complete yet focused diagnostic evaluation, which should include a lumbar puncture for cerebrospinal fluid. Patients who have seizures or focal neurologic findings by history or physical examination require CT of the brain before consideration of lumbar puncture. If lumbar puncture is to be delayed by CT or for other reasons, it is important not to delay blood culture, administration of antibiotics, and, in some circumstances, concomitant intravenous dexamethasone. The latter is a consideration if the patient is ≥17 years of age or, in a patient <17 years of age, if there is a suspicion for Hib meningitis. Empirical broad-spectrum antibiotics should include, in general, vancomycin and a third-generation cephalosporin, plus acyclovir if there are seizures or focal neurologic findings indicative of herpes simplex virus, and doxycycline if there is a particular rash or another finding suggestive of tickborne disease. Antibiotics are adjusted based on clinical progression and the results of diagnostic studies, which typically include bacterial cultures of the cerebrospinal fluid and blood and may include polymerase chain reaction amplification as well as serologic studies. Length of antibiotic therapy is primarily based on retrospective cohort data and historical precedent. Clinical care is often multidisciplinary and necessitates careful surveillance of hemodynamic, neurologic, inflammatory, and fluid and electrolyte status. Chemoprophylaxis and vaccination are important strategies for prevention of infection, disease, or both in the adolescent patient.

## REFERENCES

1. Saez-Llorens X, McCracken GH Jr. Bacterial meningitis in children. *Lancet.* 2003;361(9375): 2139–2148
2. Pickering LaP. *Principles and Practice of Pediatric Infectious Diseases.* 3rd ed. London: Churchill Livingstone; 2008

3. Mandell DaB. *Mandell, Douglas, and Bennett's Principles and Practice of Infectious Diseases.* 7th ed. London: Churchill Livingstone; 2009
4. Saez-Llorens X, McCracken GH Jr. Bacterial meningitis in children. *Lancet.* 2003;361(9375); 2139-2148
5. Schut ES, de GJ, van de BD. Community-acquired bacterial meningitis in adults. *Pract Neurol* 2008;8(1):8-23
6. Durand ML, Calderwood SB, Weber DJ, et al. Acute bacterial meningitis in adults. A review of 493 episodes. *N Engl J Med.* 1993;328(1):21-28
7. van de BD, de GJ, Spanjaard L, Weisfelt M, Reitsma JB, Vermeulen M. Clinical features and prognostic factors in adults with bacterial meningitis. *N Engl J Med.* 2004;351(18);1849-1859
8. Kilpi T, Anttila M, Kallio MJ, Peltola H. Severity of childhood bacterial meningitis and duration of illness before diagnosis. *Lancet.* 1991;338(8764):406-409
9. Whitley RJ, Gnann JW. Viral encephalitis: familiar infections and emerging pathogens. *Lancet.* 2002;359(9305):507-513
10. Chamberlain MC, Glantz M, Groves MD, Wilson WH. Diagnostic tools for neoplastic meningitis: detecting disease, identifying patient risk, and determining benefit of treatment. *Semin Oncol.* 2009;36(4 Suppl 2):S35-S45
11. Tebruegge M, Curtis N. Epidemiology, etiology, pathogenesis, and diagnosis of recurrent bacterial meningitis. *Clin Microbiol Rev.* 2008;21(3):519-537
12. Moris G, Garcia-Monco JC. The challenge of drug-induced aseptic meningitis. *Arch Intern Med.* 1999;159(11):1185-1194
13. Leake JA, Albani S, Kao AS, et al. Acute disseminated encephalomyelitis in childhood: epidemiologic, clinical and laboratory features. *Pediatr Infect Dis J.* 2004;23(8):756-764
14. Florance NR, Davis RL, Lam C, et al. Anti-N-methyl-D-aspartate receptor (NMDAR) encephalitis in children and adolescents. *Ann Neurol.* 2009;66(1):11-18
15. Gable MS, Gavali S, Radner A, et al. Anti-NMDA receptor encephalitis: report of ten cases and comparison with viral encephalitis. *Eur J Clin Microbiol Infect Dis.* 2009;28(12):1421-1429
16. American Academy of Pediatrics. *Red Book: 2009 Report of the Committee on Infectious Diseases.* 28th ed. Elk Grove Village, IL: American Academy of Pediatrics; 2009
17. Dery M, Hasbun R. Changing epidemiology of bacterial meningitis. *Curr Infect Dis Rep.* 2007;9(4):301-307
18. Tunkel AR, Hartman BJ, Kaplan SL, et al. Practice guidelines for the management of bacterial meningitis. *Clin Infect Dis.* 2004;39(9);1267-1284
19. van de Beek D, de GJ, Tunkel AR, Wijdicks EF. Community-acquired bacterial meningitis in adults. *N Engl J Med.* 2006;354(1);44-53
20. Rosenstein NE, Perkins BA, Stephens DS, et al. The changing epidemiology of meningococcal disease in the United States, 1992-1996. *J Infect Dis.* 1999;180(6):1894-1901
21. de GJ, van de BD. Dexamethasone in adults with bacterial meningitis. *N Engl J Med.* 2002;347(20):1549-1556
22. Shaw EF, Casey CG, Seale D. Summary of notifiable diseases—United States, 2007. *MMWR.* 2009;56(53):1-94
23. Hsu HE, Shutt KA, Moore MR, et al. Effect of pneumococcal conjugate vaccine on pneumococcal meningitis. *N Engl J Med.* 2009;360(3):244-256
24. Logan SA, MacMahon E. Viral meningitis. *BMJ.* 2008;336(7634):36-40
25. Kupila L, Vuorinen T, Vainionpaa R, Hukkanen V, Marttila RJ, Kotilainen P. Etiology of aseptic meningitis and encephalitis in an adult population. *Neurology.* 2006;66(1):75-80
26. Glaser CA, Honarmand S, Anderson LJ, et al. Beyond viruses: clinical profiles and etiologies associated with encephalitis. *Clin Infect Dis.* 2006;43(12):1565-1577
27. Glaser CA, Gilliam S, Schnurr D, et al. In search of encephalitis etiologies: diagnostic challenges in the California Encephalitis Project, 1998-2000. *Clin Infect Dis.* 2003;36(6);731-742
28. Fodor PA, Levin MJ, Weinberg A, Sandberg E, Sylman J, Tyler KL. Atypical herpes simplex virus encephalitis diagnosed by PCR amplification of viral DNA from CSF. *Neurology.* 1998;51(2):554-559

29. Tyler KL. Herpes simplex virus infections of the central nervous system: encephalitis and meningitis, including Mollaret's. *Herpes.* 2004;11(Suppl 2):57A–64A
30. Hunt R. *Ticks.* Columbia, SC: University of South Carolina; 2010
31. Ginsberg L, Kidd D. Chronic and recurrent meningitis. *Pract Neurol.* 2008;8(6):348–361
32. Surtees R, DeSousa C. Influenza virus associated encephalopathy. *Arch Dis Child.* 2006;91(6): 455–456
33. Stephens DS, Farley MM. Pathogenic events during infection of the human nasopharynx with Neisseria meningitidis and Haemophilus influenzae. *Rev Infect Dis.* 1991;13(1):22–33
34. Kadurugamuwa JL, Hengstler B, Bray MA, Zak O. Inhibition of complement-factor-5a-induced inflammatory reactions by prostaglandin E2 in experimental meningitis. *J Infect Dis.* 1989; 160(4):715–719
35. Stahel PF, Frei K, Fontana A, Eugster HP, Ault BH, Barnum SR. Evidence for intrathecal synthesis of alternative pathway complement activation proteins in experimental meningitis. *Am J Pathol.* 1997;151(4):897–904
36. Zwijnenburg PJ, van der Poll T, Roord JJ, van Furth AM. Chemotactic factors in cerebrospinal fluid during bacterial meningitis. *Infect Immun.* 2006;74(3):1445–1451
37. Mustafa MM, Ramilo O, Saez-Llorens X, Mertsola J, Magness RR, McCracken GH Jr. Prostaglandins E2 and I2, interleukin 1-beta, and tumor necrosis factor in cerebrospinal fluid in infants and children with bacterial meningitis. *Pediatr Infect Dis J.* 1989;8(12):921–922
38. Nolan CM, Clark RA, Beaty HN. Experimental pneumococcal meningitis: III. Chemotactic activity in cerebrospinal fluid. *Proc Soc Exp Biol Med.* 1975;150(1):134–136
39. Kadurugamuwa JL, Hengstler B, Zak O. Cerebrospinal fluid protein profile in experimental pneumococcal meningitis and its alteration by ampicillin and anti-inflammatory agents. *J Infect Dis.* 1989;159(1):26–34
40. Syrogiannopoulos GA, Olsen KD, Reisch JS, McCracken GH Jr. Dexamethasone in the treatment of experimental Haemophilus influenzae type b meningitis. *J Infect Dis.* 1987;155(2): 213–219
41. Boerman RH, Peters AC, Bloem BR, Raap AK, van der Ploeg M. Spread of herpes simplex virus to the cerebrospinal fluid and the meninges in experimental mouse encephalitis. *Acta Neuropathol.* 1992;83(3):300–307
42. Attia J, Hatala R, Cook DJ, Wong JG. The rational clinical examination. Does this adult patient have acute meningitis? *JAMA.* 1999;282(2):175–181
43. Theilen U, Wilson L, Wilson G, Beattie JO, Qureshi S, Simpson D. Management of invasive meningococcal disease in children and young people: summary of SIGN guidelines. *BMJ.* 2008;336(7657):1367–1370
44. Rotbart HA, Brennan PJ, Fife KH, et al. Enterovirus meningitis in adults. *Clin Infect Dis.* 1998;27(4):896–898
45. Singer JI, Maur PR, Riley JP, Smith PB. Management of central nervous system infections during an epidemic of enteroviral aseptic meningitis. *J Pediatr.* 1980;96(3 Pt 2):559–563
46. Wilfert CM, Lehrman SN, Katz SL. Enteroviruses and meningitis. *Pediatr Infect Dis.* 1983; 2(4):333–341
47. Tseng FC, Huang HC, Chi CY, et al. Epidemiological survey of enterovirus infections occurring in Taiwan between 2000 and 2005: analysis of sentinel physician surveillance data. *J Med Virol.* 2007;79(12):1850–1860
48. Solomon P, Weinstein L, Chang TW, Artenstein MS, Ambrose CT. Epidemiologic, clinical, and laboratory features of an epidemic of type 9 ECHO virus meningitis. *J Pediatr.* 1959;55:609–619
49. Centers for Disease Control and Prevention. Update: multistate outbreak of mumps—United States, January 1-May 2, 2006. *MMWR.* 2006;55(20):559–563
50. Whitley RJ, Soong SJ, Linneman C Jr, Liu C, Pazin G, Alford CA. Herpes simplex encephalitis. Clinical Assessment. *JAMA.* 1982;247(3):317–320
51. Kolokotronis A, Doumas S. Herpes simplex virus infection, with particular reference to the progression and complications of primary herpetic gingivostomatitis. *Clin Microbiol Infect.* 2006;12(3):202–211

52. Spiegel R, Miron D, Lumelsky D, Horovitz Y. Severe meningoencephalitis due to late reactivation of Varicella-Zoster virus in an immunocompetent child. *J Child Neurol.* 2010;25(1): 87–90
53. Hayes EB, Sejvar JJ, Zaki SR, Lanciotti RS, Bode AV, Campbell GL. Virology, pathology, and clinical manifestations of West Nile virus disease. *Emerg Infect Dis.* 2005;11(8):1174–1179
54. Thorner AR, Walker DH, Petri WA Jr. Rocky mountain spotted fever. *Clin Infect Dis.* 1998;27(6):1353–1359
55. Horney LF, Walker DH. Meningoencephalitis as a major manifestation of Rocky Mountain spotted fever. *South Med J.* 1988;81(7):915–918
56. Feigin RD, McCracken GH Jr, Klein JO. Diagnosis and management of meningitis. *Pediatr Infect Dis J.* 1992;11(9):785–814
57. Kaplan SL. Clinical presentations, diagnosis, and prognostic factors of bacterial meningitis. *Infect Dis Clin North Am* 1999;13(3):579–594
58. Thomas KE, Hasbun R, Jekel J, Quagliarello VJ. The diagnostic accuracy of Kernig's sign, Brudzinski's sign, and nuchal rigidity in adults with suspected meningitis. *Clin Infect Dis.* 2002;35(1):46–52
59. Verghese A, Gallemore G. Kernig's and Brudzinski's signs revisited. *Rev Infect Dis.* 1987; 9(6):1187–1192
60. Varon J, Chen K, Sternbach GL. Rupert Waterhouse and Carl Friderichsen: adrenal apoplexy. *J Emerg Med.* 1998;16(4):643–647
61. Marton KI, Gean AD. The spinal tap: a new look at an old test. *Ann Intern Med.* 1986;104(6): 840–848
62. Coant PN, Kornberg AE, Duffy LC, Dryja DM, Hassan SM. Blood culture results as determinants in the organism identification of bacterial meningitis. *Pediatr Emerg Care.* 1992;8(4): 200–205
63. Kiroglu Y, Calli C, Yunten N, et al. Diffusion-weighted MR imaging of viral encephalitis. *Neuroradiology.* 2006;48(12);875–880
64. Nigrovic LE, Malley R, Macias CG, et al. Effect of antibiotic pretreatment on cerebrospinal fluid profiles of children with bacterial meningitis. *Pediatrics.* 2008;122(4):726–730
65. Tunkel AR, Glaser CA, Bloch KC, et al. The management of encephalitis: clinical practice guidelines by the Infectious Diseases Society of America. *Clin Infect Dis.* 2008;47(3):303–327
66. Shah SS, Zaoutis TE, Turnquist J, Hodinka RL, Coffin SE. Early differentiation of Lyme from enteroviral meningitis. *Pediatr Infect Dis J.* 2005;24(6):542–545
67. Bonadio WA, Smith DS, Goddard S, Burroughs J, Khaja G. Distinguishing cerebrospinal fluid abnormalities in children with bacterial meningitis and traumatic lumbar puncture. *J Infect Dis.* 1990;162(1):251–254
68. Mayefsky JH, Roghmann KJ. Determination of leukocytosis in traumatic spinal tap specimens. *Am J Med.* 1987;82(6):1175–1181
69. Mazor SS, McNulty JE, Roosevelt GE. Interpretation of traumatic lumbar punctures: who can go home? *Pediatrics.* 2003;111(3):525–528
70. Whitley RJ, Alford CA, Hirsch MS, et al. Vidarabine versus acyclovir therapy in herpes simplex encephalitis. *N Engl J Med.* 1986;314(3):144–149
71. Straus SE, Thorpe KE, Holroyd-Leduc J. How do I perform a lumbar puncture and analyze the results to diagnose bacterial meningitis? *JAMA* 2006;296(16):2012–2022
72. Deresiewicz RL, Thaler SJ, Hsu L, Zamani AA. Clinical and neuroradiographic manifestations of eastern equine encephalitis. *N Engl J Med.* 1997;336(26):1867–1874
73. Kanra G, Isik P, Kara A, Cengiz AB, Secmeer G, Ceyhan M. Complementary findings in clinical and epidemiologic features of mumps and mumps meningoencephalitis in children without mumps vaccination. *Pediatr Int.* 2004;46(6):663–668
74. Miller RF, Fox JD, Thomas P, et al. Acute lumbosacral polyradiculopathy due to cytomegalovirus in advanced HIV disease: CSF findings in 17 patients. *J Neurol Neurosurg Psychiatry.* 1996;61(5):456–460

75. Nigrovic LE, Kuppermann N, Macias CG, et al. Clinical prediction rule for identifying children with cerebrospinal fluid pleocytosis at very low risk of bacterial meningitis. *JAMA*. 2007; 297(1):52–60
76. Gerdes LU, Jorgensen PE, Nexo E, Wang P. C-reactive protein and bacterial meningitis: a meta-analysis. *Scand J Clin Lab Invest*. 1998;58(5):383–393
77. Sormunen P, Kallio MJ, Kilpi T, Peltola H. C-reactive protein is useful in distinguishing Gram stain-negative bacterial meningitis from viral meningitis in children. *J Pediatr*. 1999;134(6): 725–729
78. Tzanakaki G, Tsopanomichalou M, Kesanopoulos K, et al. Simultaneous single-tube PCR assay for the detection of Neisseria meningitidis, Haemophilus influenzae type b and Streptococcus pneumoniae. *Clin Microbiol Infect*. 2005;11(5):386–390
79. DeBiasi RL, Kleinschmidt-DeMasters BK, Weinberg A, Tyler KL. Use of PCR for the diagnosis of herpesvirus infections of the central nervous system. *J Clin Virol* 2002;25 Suppl 1:S5–11
80. Tyler KL. Herpes simplex virus infections of the central nervous system: encephalitis and meningitis, including Mollaret's. *Herpes* 2004;11 Suppl 2:57A–64A
81. Lakeman FD, Whitley RJ. Diagnosis of herpes simplex encephalitis: application of polymerase chain reaction to cerebrospinal fluid from brain-biopsied patients and correlation with disease. National Institute of Allergy and Infectious Diseases Collaborative Antiviral Study Group. *J Infect Dis*. 1995;171(4):857–863
82. Weil AA, Glaser CA, Amad Z, Forghani B. Patients with suspected herpes simplex encephalitis: rethinking an initial negative polymerase chain reaction result. *Clin Infect Dis*. 2002;34(8): 1154–1157
83. Aurelius E, Johansson B, Skoldenberg B, Staland A, Forsgren M. Rapid diagnosis of herpes simplex encephalitis by nested polymerase chain reaction assay of cerebrospinal fluid. *Lancet*. 1991;337(8735):189–192
84. Schloss L, Falk KI, Skoog E, Brytting M, Linde A, Aurelius E. Monitoring of herpes simplex virus DNA types 1 and 2 viral load in cerebrospinal fluid by real-time PCR in patients with herpes simplex encephalitis. *J Med Virol*. 2009;81(8):1432–1437
85. Nagel MA, Forghani B, Mahalingam R, et al. The value of detecting anti-VZV IgG antibody in CSF to diagnose VZV vasculopathy. *Neurology*. 2007;68(13):1069–1073
86. Tardei G, Ruta S, Chitu V, Rossi C, Tsai TF, Cernescu C. Evaluation of immunoglobulin M (IgM) and IgG enzyme immunoassays in serologic diagnosis of West Nile Virus infection. *J Clin Microbiol*. 2000;38(6):2232–2239
87. Lebel MH, McCracken GH Jr. Delayed cerebrospinal fluid sterilization and adverse outcome of bacterial meningitis in infants and children. *Pediatrics*. 1989;83(2):161–167
88. Heyderman RS. Early management of suspected bacterial meningitis and meningococcal septicaemia in immunocompetent adults–second edition. *J Infect*. 2005;50(5):373–374
89. Rosenstein NE, Stocker SA, Popovic T, Tenover FC, Perkins BA. Antimicrobial resistance of Neisseria meningitidis in the United States, 1997. The Active Bacterial Core Surveillance (ABCs) Team. *Clin Infect Dis*. 2000;30(1):212–213
90. Duke T, Michael A, Mokela D, Wal T, Reeder J. Chloramphenicol or ceftriaxone, or both, as treatment for meningitis in developing countries? *Arch Dis Child*. 2003;88(6):536–539
91. Odio CM, Puig JR, Feris JM, et al. Prospective, randomized, investigator-blinded study of the efficacy and safety of meropenem vs. cefotaxime therapy in bacterial meningitis in children. Meropenem Meningitis Study Group. *Pediatr Infect Dis J*. 1999;18(7):581–590
92. Wormser GP, Dattwyler RJ, Shapiro ED, et al. The clinical assessment, treatment, and prevention of lyme disease, human granulocytic anaplasmosis, and babesiosis: clinical practice guidelines by the Infectious Diseases Society of America. *Clin Infect Dis*. 2006;43(9):1089–1134
93. Rajshekhar V. Management of hydrocephalus in patients with tuberculous meningitis. *Neurol India*. 2009;57(4):368–374

94. Assiri AM, Alasmari FA, Zimmerman VA, Baddour LM, Erwin PJ, Tleyjeh IM. Corticosteroid administration and outcome of adolescents and adults with acute bacterial meningitis: a meta-analysis. *Mayo Clin Proc.* 2009;84(5):403–409
95. Tunkel AR. *Bacterial Meningitis.* Philadelphia: Lippincott Williams & Wilkins; 2001
96. McIntyre PB, Berkey CS, King SM, et al. Dexamethasone as adjunctive therapy in bacterial meningitis. A meta-analysis of randomized clinical trials since 1988. *JAMA.* 1997;278(11):925–931
97. Chaudhuri A, Martinez-Martin P, Kennedy PG, et al. EFNS guideline on the management of community-acquired bacterial meningitis: report of an EFNS Task Force on acute bacterial meningitis in older children and adults. *Eur J Neurol.* 2008;15(7);649–659
98. Halperin JJ, Shapiro ED, Logigian E, et al. Practice parameter: treatment of nervous system Lyme disease (an evidence-based review): report of the Quality Standards Subcommittee of the American Academy of Neurology. *Neurology.* 2007;69(1):91–102
99. Arditi M, Mason EO Jr, Bradley JS, et al. Three-year multicenter surveillance of pneumococcal meningitis in children: clinical characteristics, and outcome related to penicillin susceptibility and dexamethasone use. *Pediatrics.* 1998;102(5):1087–1097
100. Kornelisse RF, Westerbeek CM, Spoor AB, et al. Pneumococcal meningitis in children: prognostic indicators and outcome. *Clin Infect Dis.* 1995;21(6):1390–1397
101. Taylor HG, Schatschneider C, Watters GV, et al. Acute-phase neurologic complications of Haemophilus influenzae type b meningitis: association with developmental problems at school age. *J Child Neurol.* 1998;13(3):113–119
102. Richardson MP, Reid A, Tarlow MJ, Rudd PT. Hearing loss during bacterial meningitis. *Arch Dis Child.* 1997;76(2):134–138
103. McGrath N, Anderson NE, Croxson MC, Powell KF. Herpes simplex encephalitis treated with acyclovir: diagnosis and long term outcome. *J Neurol Neurosurg Psychiatry.* 1997;63(3):321–326
104. Ito Y, Kimura H, Yabuta Y, et al. Exacerbation of herpes simplex encephalitis after successful treatment with acyclovir. *Clin Infect Dis.* 2000;30(1):185–187
105. McJunkin JE, de los Reyes EC, Irazuzta JE, et al. La Crosse encephalitis in children. *N Engl J Med.* 2001;344(11):801–807
106. Wu HM, Harcourt BH, Hatcher CP, et al. Emergence of ciprofloxacin-resistant Neisseria meningitidis in North America. *N Engl J Med.* 2009;360(9):886–892
107. Pace D, Pollard AJ. Meningococcal A, C, Y and W-135 polysaccharide-protein conjugate vaccines. *Arch Dis Child.* 2007;92(10):909–915
108. Centers for Disease Control and Prevention. *Prevention and control of meningococcal disease. Recommendations of the Advisory Committee on Immunization Practives (ACIP).* Atlanta, GA: Centers for Disease Control and Prevention; 2005
109. Centers for Disease Control and Prevention. *Licensure of a Meningococcal Conjugate Vaccine (Menveo) and Guidance for Use—Advisory Committee on Immunization Practices (ACIP), 2010.* Atlanta, GA: Centers for Disease Control and Prevention; 2010
110. Snape MD, Pollard AJ. Meningococcal polysaccharide-protein conjugate vaccines. *Lancet Infect Dis.* 2005;5(1):21–30
111. Harrison LH. Prospects for vaccine prevention of meningococcal infection. *Clin Microbiol Rev.* 2006;19(1):142–164
112. Segal S, Pollard AJ. Vaccines against bacterial meningitis. *Br Med Bull.* 2004;72:65–81
113. American Academy of Pediatrics, Committee on Infectious Diseases. *Prevention and control of meningococcal disease: recommendations for use of meningococcal vaccine in pediatric patients.* Chicago, IL: American Academy of Pediatrics; 2010
114. Middleman AB, Rosenthal SL, Rickert VI, Neinstein L, Fishbein DB, D'Angelo L. Adolescent immunizations: a position paper of the Society for Adolescent Medicine. *J Adolesc Health.* 2006;38(3):321–327
115. Centers for Disease Control and Prevention Advisory Committee on Immunization Practices. *Revised recommendations of the Advisory Committee on Immunization Practices to vaccinate*

all persons aged 11–18 years with meningococcal conjugate vaccine. Atlanta, GA: Centers for Disease Control and Prevention; 2007
116. McCormick JB, Gusmao HH, Nakamura S, et al. Antibody response to serogroup A and C meningococcal polysaccharide vaccines in infants born of mothers vaccinated during pregnancy. *J Clin Invest.* 1980;65(5):1141–1144
117. Centers for Disease Control and Prevention. *Updated recommendation from the Advisory Committee on Immunization Practices (ACIP) for revaccination of persons at prolonged increased risk for meningococcal disease.* Atlanta, GA: Centers for Disease Control and Prevention; 2009
118. Centers for Disease Control and Prevention. *Guillain-Barré syndrome among recipients of Menactra® meningococcal conjugate vaccine — United States, June–July 2005.* Atlanta, GA: Centers for Disease Control and Prevention; 2005
119. Centers for Disease Control and Prevention. *Update: Guillain-Barré syndrome among recipients of Menactra® meningococcal conjugate vaccine—United States, June 2005–September 2006.* Atlanta, GA: Centers for Disease Control and Prevention; 2006
120. Portnoy JM, Olson LC. Normal cerebrospinal fluid values in children: another look. *Pediatrics.* 1985;75(3):484–487
121. Rybak M, Lomaestro B, Rotschafer JC, et al. Therapeutic monitoring of vancomycin in adult patients: a consensus review of the American Society of Health-System Pharmacists, the Infectious Diseases Society of America, and the Society of Infectious Diseases Pharmacists. *Am J Health Syst Pharm.* 2009;66(1):82–98

# *Staphylococcus aureus* Infections in Adolescents

## Blanca E. Gonzalez, MD*[a], Rodrigo A. Mon, MD, FACS*[b]

[a]*Division of Pediatric Infectious Diseases and Rheumatology, Rainbow Babies and Children's Hospital, 11100 Euclid Avenue, Cleveland, OH 44106*
[b]*Department of Pediatric Surgery, The Children's Hospital of Southwest Florida, 9981 S. Health Park Drive, Lee Memorial Health Systems, Fort Myers, FL 33908*

*Staphylococcus aureus* is a major cause of morbidity and mortality in the pediatric population, causing a wide spectrum of diseases ranging from skin and soft tissue infections (SSTIs) to more severe presentations such as sepsis syndrome, necrotizing pneumonia, and necrotizing fasciitis.[1-3] Methicillin-resistant *S. aureus* (MRSA), once a pathogen of hospitals and long-term care facilities, has established itself in the community and has been associated with multiple outbreaks in schools and severe infections in adolescents.[4-7] This review will discuss the scope of *S. aureus* infections in teenagers along with treatment and prevention of the infection.

### Epidemiology

*S. aureus* are Gram-positive cocci that microscopically resemble grape clusters and form yellow colonies on agar plates. Staphylococci are commensal in the human skin, with an estimated 30% of the population colonized in the nares, axillae, and/or groin with the organism.[8] Colonization with *S. aureus*, in particular MRSA, has been shown to be a risk factor for the development of invasive infections.[9]

Although MRSA has been present since the 1960s, until recently the infection was confined mainly to hospital wards and chronically ill patients. In 1998, the death of 4 children in the Minnesota/North Dakota area marked the emergence of MRSA as a community-acquired pathogen (CA-MRSA) in the United States.[10] Over the past decade, cases of CA-MRSA have grown exponentially among children and adolescents and are now commonplace in the clinic setting.[6,7,11-14]

---

*Corresponding author.
*E-mail address*: blanca.gonzalez@uhhospitals.org (B. E. Gonzalez).

Copyright © 2010 American Academy of Pediatrics. All rights reserved. ISSN 1934-4287

The decreased affinity of MRSA to β-lactams is mediated by an altered penicillin binding protein 2A encoded by the mecA gene and carried by a mobile genetic element known as the staphylococcal chromosomal cassette (SCC). Most CA-MRSA strains carry SCC type IV, which is smaller than SCC II, commonly associated with hospital-acquired MRSA (HA-MRSA), and is why CA-MRSA does not carry resistance to as many antimicrobial agents as HA-MRSA.[15]

The predominant CA-MRSA clonal type circulating in the United States is referred to as USA300.[16,17] This clone commonly carries the pvl genes (*lukSPV* and *lukFPV*), which encode for a cytotoxin called Panton-Valentine Leukocidin (PVL) that is capable of lysing white blood cells and proposed to be the major virulence factor in certain infections, such as necrotizing pneumonia and musculoskeletal infections.[18–24]

Transmission of CA-MRSA has been summarized by the Centers for Disease Control and Prevention (CDC) to occur by the "5 Cs": crowding, contact, compromised skin, contaminated surfaces and shared items, and lack of cleanliness. Adolescent conditions and behaviors conducive to *S. aureus* transmission include acne, obesity, body modifications practices or body art, participation in contact sports, sexual activity, drug abuse, and tampon use.[4,25–33]

Tattooing and body piercing performed by nonprofessionals is a common risk factor for developing infections (Fig. 1).[28] In an outbreak of CA-MRSA among 34 people between 15 and 42 years of age who had received tattoos, the majority of the patients received their tattoos from unlicensed tattooists

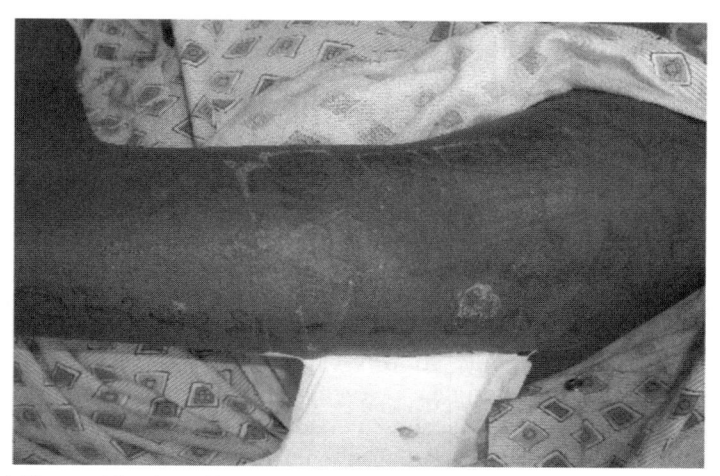

Fig 1. A 17-year-old patient with multiple *S. aureus* abscesses around site of a tattoo performed in his garage by a family member 3 weeks before admission.

who failed to abide by adequate infection control practices.[31] Most people developed SSTIs, but 4 patients developed bacteremia requiring hospitalization. Development of perichondritis is a well-recognized complication of piercing ear cartilage and may result in ear necrosis and mutilation.[28,29] Risks of acquiring CA-MRSA from sports participation include sharing of equipment, turf burns, shaving, and poor hygiene practices in the locker room.

Although toxic shock syndrome (TSS) occurs in only 1–3 per 100 000 individuals, the use of tampons increases the risk.[33] Addition of glycerol monolaurate to tampons may potentially decrease staphylococcal toxic shock toxin-1 (TSST-1) production by *S. aureus*.[34,35] Counseling adolescents on the safe use of tampons could further decrease the risk of using the product and should be part of the anticipatory guidance in premenstrual and menstrual teenagers.[36]

## Clinical Presentations

### Skin and Soft Tissue Infections

SSTIs are the most frequent manifestations of *S. aureus* and CA-MRSA in all age groups, with the spectrum of disease ranges from folliculitis, furuncles, carbuncles, and abscesses to necrotizing skin processes.[1] Patients often come to medical care complaining of spider bites because of the necrotic aspect of these wounds. However, as illustrated by a study from California, the majority of "spider bites" were in fact SSTI associated with *S. aureus*.[37] In the past years, several hospitals have reported an increase in the admissions of patients with SSTI caused by *S. aureus*, especially MRSA.[12,38]

### Musculoskeletal Infections

*S. aureus* is the most common cause of hematogenous osteomyelitis and septic arthritis in children and adolescents. CA-MRSA strains that carry the PVL genes elicit higher inflammatory responses and have been associated with more severe disease requiring aggressive surgical management.[20,21,39] Multifocal osteomyelitis has been described in patients with staphylococcal severe sepsis syndrome, many with associated venous thrombosis near the infection site.[40,41] Septic arthritis caused by PVL positive *S. aureus* strains are associated with higher C-reactive protein levels, prolonged duration of fever, and often pyomyositis/myositis.[39] The incidence of pyomyositis/myositis has also increased with the rise of CA-MRSA infections. These may be primary infections or associated to osteomyelitis and septic arthritis (Fig. 2).[14]

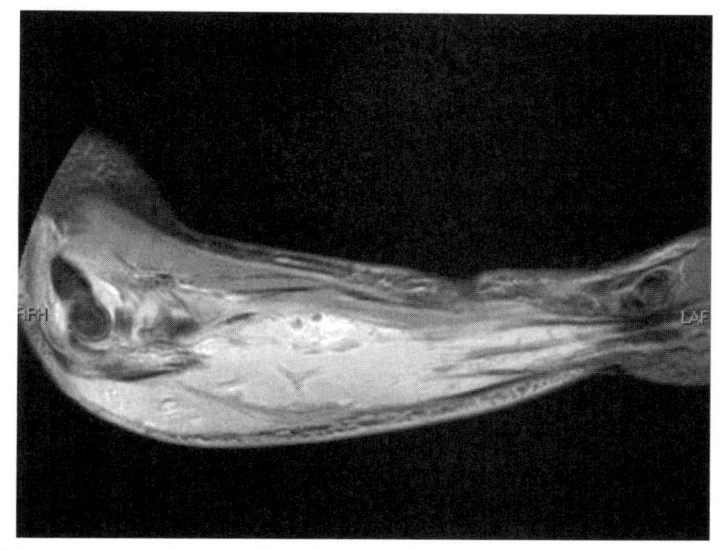

Fig 2. Magnetic resonance imaging of the right arm of a 17-year-old boy, who after a blunt trauma while playing baseball developed an osteomyelitis of the radius with a subperiosteal abscess and associated myositis.

## Pulmonary Disease

CA-MRSA involvement of the lungs in children and adolescents is widespread and span from complicated pneumonia with empyema, lung abscesses, and necrosis to septic embolisms.[22] Necrotizing pneumonia is commonly caused by PVL-containing strains and has a high associated mortality.[2]

Seasonal influenza has been associated with the development of severe staphylococcal infections. During the 2006–2007 season, influenza and *S. aureus* coinfections resulted in 22 pediatric deaths, 15 of which were CA-MRSA strains.[42] Pneumonia and acute respiratory distress syndrome (ARDS) are frequent manifestations influenza and staphylococcal superinfection.

## Endocarditis

Endocarditis (IE) associated with *S. aureus* bacteremia is less common in pediatric patients than in adults and when it does occur, it is usually associated with an underlying heart defect.[13,43] Nevertheless, IE should be investigated in adolescents who are admitted with *S. aureus* bacteremia, especially in severe sepsis syndrome and in the presence of septic pulmonary emboli (Fig. 3).

## Severe Sepsis Syndrome

In 1976, Shulman and Ayoub described a sepsis syndrome in adolescent patients caused by *S. aureus* characterized by multifocal osteomyelitis, septic arthritis,

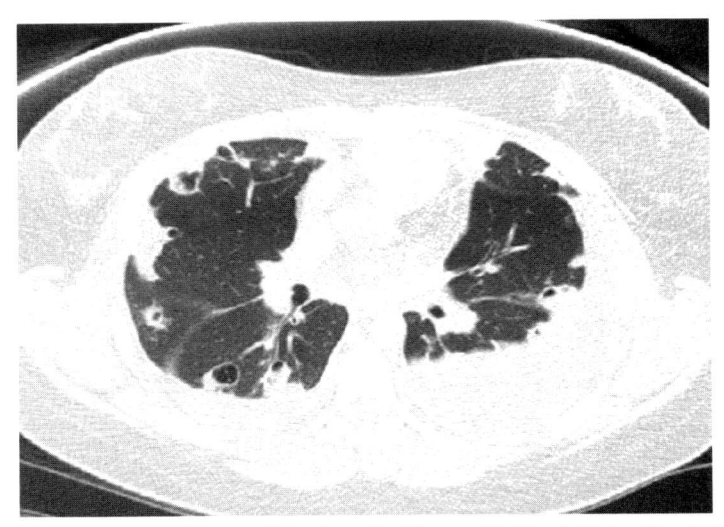

Fig 3. Computed tomography scan of the chest of a 17-year-old girl admitted with cellulitis of the left dorsum of the foot and right-side native valve endocarditis. Arrows indicate ill-defined cavitary lesions in the periphery consistent with septic pulmonary emboli.

pulmonary embolisms, and multiorgan system involvement.[44] Recently, this presentation has returned, being more commonly described, this time with CA-MRSA strains.[6,7,13,45]

Staphylococcal severe sepsis syndrome can occur in any age or gender, but teenage males seem to be affected more commonly. Many patients are athletes and a history of previous trauma frequently has been elicited.[6,7,13,45]

Patients who present with this syndrome have multiorgan system failure. Commonly osteomyelitis and septic arthritis are present with multiples sites involved. Deep venous thrombosis may be a found adjacent to the sites of bone infections and frequently account for the septic embolisms seen. Skin infections and rashes may be present and vary from abscess, pustular lesions, erythema multiforme, to subcutaneous nodules.

Less common presentations with high morbidity and mortality are necrotizing fasciitis and Watterhouse-Friderichsen syndrome/purpura fulminans and spinal epidural abscess.[3,11,30]

*Toxic Shock Syndrome*

This acute toxin mediated process is caused by strains of *S. aureus* that produce TSST-1 or other endotoxins (non menstrual TSS).[46] Patients present with fever, hypotension, and a rash that is erythrodermic or scarlatiniform and that may desquamate. Myalgias, diarrhea, emesis, mucus membrane hyperemia, changes in mental status, and hepatitis are common. Patients may develop renal failure secondary and ARDS as a consequence of the severe hypotension. Contrary to streptococcal TSS, the isolation of *S. aureus* is not required to make the diagnosis. Menstrual TSS may be associated with less mortality than nonmenstrual TSS.[46]

## Diagnosis and Treatment

### Skin and Soft Tissue Infections

SSTIs usually are easily recognized by simple inspection. In cases where the source of infection is unclear, imaging may assist with the diagnosis. Ultrasound has been shown to identify underlying purulent collections that may not be obvious on physical examination, as well as more severe complications such as pyomyositis and necrotizing fasciitis.

Incision and drainage, the mainstay of treatment of SSTI with abscess formation, can be performed in the office, in the emergency room, or at the bedside.[47,48] Regardless of the setting, adequate pain control is critical. Local anesthetic (1–2% lidocaine) is used to infiltrate the wound followed by waiting 2–3 minutes for the anesthetic to work. Once the abscess cavity is opened, a sample should be sent for cultures and Gram stain, the loculations of the cavity broken with a finger or a small instrument (mosquito clamp), and the cavity irrigated with saline followed by packing with ¼-inch packing gauze. The packing is then left in place for 24 hours, at which time it can be removed and the area reevaluated. Although the wound often will continue to drain for additional days, repacking typically is not necessary. All wounds should remain covered while actively draining to prevent transmission of infections to others.

Complications of incision and drainage are rare and include bleeding and incomplete drainage of the abscess and transient bacteremia. Follow-up should be arranged and tetanus immunization history reviewed. Parents should be advised to seek further care promptly if there is clinical worsening or fever. An excellent instructional video on performing incision and drainage is available at http://content.nejm.org/misc/videos.dtl.[48] Very large or deep abscesses are best drained in the operating room under general anesthesia as well as those in which adequate analgesia cannot be assured. Abscesses in locations that may require expert consultation, such as face or hands, should not be drained in the office.

Once the abscess has been drained, the question remains whether antimicrobial therapy offers any additional benefit. One retrospective chart review suggested that patients who had abscesses smaller than 5 cm that were drained improved regardless of the antimicrobial agent given.[49] No prospective randomized trial has been published to date addressing this issue.[50]

Knowing susceptibility patterns of the strains circulating in the community is important for the appropriate selection of empirical therapy. Clindamycin and trimethoprim-sulfamethoxazole (TMP-SMX) are largely used in the pediatric population with SSTI caused by MRSA with comparable efficacy.[51] It is important to remember that TMP-SMX is not clinically effective against group A streptococcus and may not be suitable in patients with eczema. Additionally, TMP-SMX has been associated with severe drug reactions such as Steven Johnson syndrome.[52] Limitations to use of clindamycin include pseudomembranous colitis and the frequency of CA-MRSA developing resistance to the organism.[53] Resistance to clindamycin is encoded by the erm genes and can be constitutive (resistance always present) or inducible (development of resistance after exposure to the antimicrobial agent). Detection of inducible resistance can be made using the D-test.[54] This test is performed by coating an agar plate with the bacteria to be tested and then placing an erythromycin disk at a fixed distance from a clindamycin disk on the plate. Inducible resistance is noted by a blunting of the clindamycin zone adjacent to the erythromycin into the shape of a "D" (Fig. 4).

Doxycycline has been shown to be highly active against MRSA SSTIs.[55] Requiring only 12-hour dosing and a good safety profile make it an excellent treatment option for adolescent patients. Other agents such as linezolid, daptomycin, and tigecycline have comparable outcomes to vancomycin in the treatment MRSA SSTI but less data are available.[56]

*Invasive Infections*

A multidisciplinary approach to patients with severe sepsis syndrome is essential because many organ systems may be involved. Finding the foci of

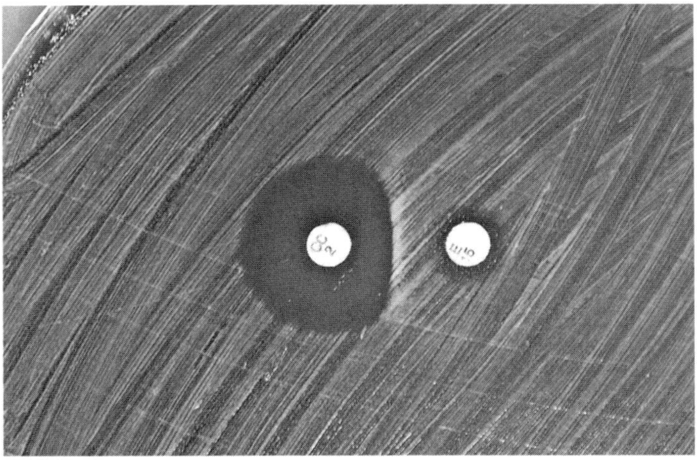

Fig 4. Inducible clindamycin resistance by disk diffusion method.

infection and prompt initiation of adequate antimicrobials is necessary because adverse outcomes have been associated with delays in initiation of therapy.[57] A complete physical evaluation may help identify the sources of infections. Bone and joints should be promptly aspirated if infection is evident. In musculoskeletal infections, initial debridement of necrotic tissue, drainage of septic arthritis and subperiosteal abscesses is critical in the treatment of these infections. In some instances, the orthopedic specialist may aspirate bone and joints at bedside to recognize those who need prompt and aggressive debridement in the operating room. Persistent bacteremia in these settings is more often related to the presence of undrained focus of infection rather than an antimicrobial failure.

Magnetic resonance imaging (MRI) is the imaging modality of choice for musculoskeletal infections, as plain films may fail to identify bone infections early in the disease process.[58] The MRI may also offer additional information regarding other comorbidities such as subperiosteal abscesses, myositis, and deep venous thrombosis. Bone scans are less useful but can be used when the foci of infection is not evident.

Patients with respiratory distress, pulmonary emboli, and severe sepsis syndrome may have an endovascular sources. Septic pulmonary emboli are commonly seen on chest radiographs or computed tomography (CT) and should alert the clinician to look for IE or deep venous thrombosis adjacent to sites of osteomyelitis.[40,41] Doppler ultrasound is the modality of choice for venous thrombosis but they may be apparent on MRI. Placement of vascular filters may be required in patients in whom anticoagulation is contraindicated or in those with persistent pulmonary embolism and respiratory compromise.[41,59]

Empirical antibiotic therapy for severely ill patients should cover resistant and nonresistant *S. aureus* and offer adequate tissue penetration. Most of the evidence supporting combination therapy is derived from endocarditis studies. Initial low-dose gentamicin is associated with nephrotoxicity in adult patients and does not improve survival.[60] Similarly, the addition of rifampin in general has not shown to improve outcomes but it may have a role in the treatment of osteomyelitis, particularly with prosthetic infections secondary to its enhanced penetration in biofilms.[61] The American Academy of Pediatrics has recommended the combined use of vancomycin plus nafcillin with or without gentamicin as initial empirical therapy in critically ill patients with staphylococcal infections.[62]

For MSSA, the drug of choice remains nafcillin or oxacillin as it has been shown to be superior to vancomycin for MSSA pneumonia and endocarditis.[63] For MRSA bacteremia, vancomycin is still the standard of care. Vancomycin is slowly bactericidal; therefore, some clinicians would combine this drug with other antibiotics initially.[64]

Over the last decade, there has been a vancomycin "creep," with an increase of minimum inhibitory concentration (MIC) to values closer to 1 µg/ml.[63,65,66] In addition, there are S. aureus strains that are susceptible to vancomycin but have subpopulations that are intermediate or resistant to vancomycin. These heteroresistant vancomycin intermediate S. aureus (hVISA) strains are not detected by automated laboratory methods and have resulted in vancomycin treatment failures.[66] To reflect this rising resistance, the U.S. Food and Drug Administration (FDA) has lowered the vancomycin breakpoints from MIC of $\leq$4, 8–16 and $\geq$32 µg/ml (susceptible, intermediate, and resistant, respectively) to $\leq$2, 4–8 and $\geq$16 µg/ml.[67] Vancomycin dosing should be optimized in the hospital setting, especially for strains that have higher MICs to vancomycin to avoid treatment failures. Some authors propose dosing vancomycin at 60 mg/kg/d (rather than the typical 40 mg/kg/d) to achieve an $AUC_{24}$/MIC >400, a value that has been associated with improved outcomes in adults.[68,69] Once the MIC are 2 µg/ml or above, it seems prudent to use an alternative antibiotic.

Linezolid has excellent tissue penetration, especially in the pulmonary lining, and has the added benefit of decreasing PVL production.[70] It has been shown to be equivalent and possibly superior to vancomycin for the treatment of ventilator-associated pneumonia and has been used successfully in individual patients in the treatment of MRSA endocarditis.[71,72] However, there is scant literature on the use of linezolid monotherapy in patients with MRSA bacteremia. The drug is also myelosuppressive; therefore, close monitoring is required.

Daptomycin has been shown to be effective in the treatment of S. aureus bacteremia and bone and joint infections.[73] It has FDA approval for the treatment of right-sided endocarditis. Conversely, it is inhibited by surfactant precluding its use in treatment of pneumonia. There have been reports of patients developing resistance to daptomycin while receiving the drug.[74,75] The only failure reported in pediatrics to date has been in a 15-year-old boy with MRSA bacteremia. The organism became nonsusceptible to daptomycin after 5 days of therapy. Suboptimal serum concentrations of the drug were thought to have played a role in the development of resistance.[74] Current trials are ongoing to study the pharmacokinetics of this drug in patients younger than 18 years of age.

Clindamycin is an excellent drug for MRSA-invasive infections. Martinez et al showed that monotherapy was effective in pediatric patients with MRSA bacteremia, bone and joint infections, and pneumonia.[76] It also has the advantage of suppressing PVL and other toxins. Its use for MRSA infections has been hindered by the development of resistance in many areas in the United States.[77]

Other antimicrobials with activity against MRSA include ceftobripole, telvavancin, tigecycline, and quinupristin/dalfopristin. The latter has shown a favorable response in pediatric patients with invasive Gram-positive infections who were intolerant to alternative therapy as well as in patients with invasive infections.[78]

However, much is still to be learned about the use of quinupristin/dalfopristin and other newer drugs to treat staphylococcal infections in the pediatric population.

The use of intravenous immunoglobulin is recommended in patients with TSS that is unresponsive to several hours of aggressive therapy as it may neutralize antibodies.[62] Intravenous immunoglobulin may also be useful in severe sepsis syndrome or severe necrotizing pneumonia as in vitro studies have shown that it may reduce the cytotoxic effect of PVL.[79]

**Prevention**

Hygiene is possibly the most important measure to prevent staphylococcal infections. From outbreaks, we have learned that simple interventions such as frequent handwashing, covering wounds, not sharing clothes or personal items, and showering after physical activities are enough to stop the spread of bacteria.[4,80]

Many patients with recurrent infections seek the help of an infectious disease specialist for eradication of the *S. aureus*. A study that surveyed 100 pediatric infectious disease physicians from various parts of the United States found that there was no consensus in decolonization practices.[81] The lack of randomized pediatric studies makes it difficult to decide if, when, and how to decolonize patients with recurrent SSTI. Mupirocin is frequently used intranasally to eliminate the carrier state. Resistance does not seem to arise commonly with short treatment courses, but eradication may fail when patients are colonized with strains with high level mupirocin resistance (MIC ≥152 μg/ml).[82]

Use of antibacterial soaps including chlorhexidine baths is often tried as a means to reduce recurrence of staphylococcal-associated SSTIs. As an alternative, bleach baths have been used in pediatric patients to prevent recurrent MRSA infections.[83] Although no trials have been done to show their efficacy, a recent in vitro study which measured the optimal amount of bleach needed to kill MRSA found that a dilution of 2.5 μL/ml of bleach (or what is equivalent to one-half cup in 13 gallons of water, approximately a quarter-filled standard 50-gallon bathtub) was sufficient to decrease the amount of bacteria by 3 logs when incubated for 5 minutes.[84] Without data to support the effectiveness of these protocols, it should be emphasized that hygiene is still the most successful preventative measure.

**CONCLUSIONS**

Staphylococcal infections cause a high burden of disease in the teenage population. The development of a vaccine to help prevent these infections has become a necessity. In the meantime, efforts should be made to prevent and control the spread of *S. aureus* in the community.

## ACKNOWLEDGMENTS

We thank Dr. Edward O. Mason for kindly supplying us the D-test image.

## REFERENCES

1. Daum RS. Clinical practice. Skin and soft-tissue infections caused by methicillin-resistant staphylococcus aureus. *N Engl J Med.* 2007;357:380–390
2. Gillet Y, Issartel B, Vanhems P, et al. Association between staphylococcus aureus strains carrying gene for panton-valentine leukocidin and highly lethal necrotising pneumonia in young immunocompetent patients. *Lancet.* 2002;359:753–759
3. Miller LG, Perdreau-Remington F, Rieg G, et al. Necrotizing fasciitis caused by community-associated methicillin-resistant staphylococcus aureus in los angeles. *N Engl J Med.* 2005;352:1445–1453
4. Methicillin-resistant Staphylococcus aureus among players on a high school football team–New York City, 2007. *MMWR Morb Mortal Wkly Rep.* 2009;58:52–55
5. Rihn JA, Posfay-Barbe K, Harner CD, et al. Community-acquired methicillin-resistant staphylococcus aureus outbreak in a local high school football team unsuccessful interventions. *Pediatr Infect Dis J.* 2005;24:841–843
6. Gonzalez BE, Martinez-Aguilar G, Hulten KG, et al. Severe staphylococcal sepsis in adolescents in the era of community-acquired methicillin-resistant staphylococcus aureus. *Pediatrics.* 2005;115:642–648
7. Castaldo ET, Yang EY. Severe sepsis attributable to community-associated methicillin-resistant staphylococcus aureus: An emerging fatal problem. *Am Surg.* 2007;73:684–687
8. Gorwitz RJ, Kruszon-Moran D, McAllister SK, et al. Changes in the prevalence of nasal colonization with staphylococcus aureus in the united states, 2001–2004. *J Infect Dis.* 2008;197:1226–1234
9. Safdar N, Bradley EA. The risk of infection after nasal colonization with staphylococcus aureus. *Am J Med.* 2008;121:310–315
10. Centers for Disease Control and Prevention. Four pediatric deaths from community-acquired methicillin-resistant Staphylococcus aureus–Minnesota and North Dakota, 1997–1999. *JAMA* 1999;282:1123–1125
11. Adem PV, Montgomery CP, Husain AN, et al. Staphylococcus aureus sepsis and the waterhouse-friderichsen syndrome in children. *N Engl J Med.* 2005;353:1245–1251
12. Kaplan SL, Hulten KG, Gonzalez BE, et al. Three-year surveillance of community-acquired staphylococcus aureus infections in children. *Clin Infect Dis.* 2005;40:1785–1791
13. Miles F, Voss L, Segedin E, Anderson BJ. Review of Staphylococcus aureus infections requiring admission to a paediatric intensive care unit. *Arch Dis Child.* 2005;90:1274–1278
14. Pannaraj PS, Hulten KG, Gonzalez BE, Mason EO Jr, Kaplan SL. Infective pyomyositis and myositis in children in the era of community-acquired, methicillin-resistant Staphylococcus aureus infections. *Clin Infect Dis.* 2006;43:953–960
15. Daum RS, Ito T, Hiramatsu K, et al. A novel methicillin-resistance cassette in community-acquired methicillin-resistant Staphylococcus aureus isolates of diverse genetic backgrounds. *J Infect Dis.* 2002;186:1344–1347
16. McCaskill ML, Mason EO Jr, Kaplan SL, et al. Increase of the USA300 clone among community-acquired methicillin-susceptible staphylococcus aureus causing invasive infections. *Pediatr Infect Dis J.* 2007;26:1122–1127
17. Mishaan AM, Mason EO Jr, Martinez-Aguilar G, et al. Emergence of a predominant clone of community-acquired Staphylococcus aureus among children in Houston, Texas. *Pediatr Infect Dis J.* 2005;24:201–206
18. Boyle-Vavra S, Daum RS. Community-acquired methicillin-resistant Staphylococcus aureus: The role of Panton-Valentine leukocidin. *Lab Invest.* 2007;87:3–9

19. Badiou C, Dumitrescu O, Croze M, et al. Panton-Valentine leukocidin is expressed at toxic levels in human skin abscesses. *Clin Microbiol Infect.* 2008;14:1180–1183
20. Bocchini CE, Hulten KG, Mason EO Jr, et al. Panton-Valentine leukocidin genes are associated with enhanced inflammatory response and local disease in acute hematogenous Staphylococcus aureus osteomyelitis in children. *Pediatrics.* 2006;117:433–440
21. Dohin B, Gillet Y, Kohler R, et al. Pediatric bone and joint infections caused by panton-valentine leukocidin-positive staphylococcus aureus. *Pediatr Infect Dis J.* 2007;26:1042–1048
22. Gonzalez BE, Hulten KG, Dishop MK, et al. Pulmonary manifestations in children with invasive community-acquired staphylococcus aureus infection. *Clin Infect Dis.* 2005;41:583–590
23. Labandeira-Rey M, Couzon F, Boisset S, et al. Staphylococcus aureus Panton-Valentine leukocidin causes necrotizing pneumonia. *Science.* 2007;315:1130–1133
24. Loffler B, Hussain M, Grundmeier M, et al. Staphylococcus aureus Panton-Valentine leukocidin is a very potent cytotoxic factor for human neutrophils. *PLoS Pathog.* 2010;6:e1000715
25. Cohen PR. Cutaneous community-acquired methicillin-resistant Staphylococcus aureus infection in participants of athletic activities. *South Med J.* 2005;98:596–602
26. Craven DE, Rixinger AI, Goularte TA, McCabe WR. Methicillin-resistant Staphylococcus aureus bacteremia linked to intravenous drug abusers using a "shooting gallery." *Am J Med.* 1986;80:770–776
27. Jones TF, Creech CB, Erwin P, et al. Family outbreaks of invasive community-associated methicillin-resistant staphylococcus aureus infection. *Clin Infect Dis.* 2006;42:e76–e78
28. Braverman PK. Body art: Piercing, tattooing, and scarification. *Adolesc Med Clin.* 2006;17:505–519
29. Staley R, Fitzgibbon JJ, Anderson C. Auricular infections caused by high ear piercing in adolescents. *Pediatrics.* 1997;99:610–611
30. Bruns AS, Sood N. Community-acquired methicillin-resistant Staphylococcus aureus epidural abscess with bacteremia and multiple lung abscesses: Case report. *Am J Crit Care.* 2009;18:88, 86–87
31. Methicillin-resistant staphylococcus aureus skin infections among tattoo recipients–Ohio, Kentucky, and Vermont, 2004–2005. *MMWR Morb Mortal Wkly Rep.* 2006;55:677–679
32. Cook HA, Furuya EY, Larson E, Vasquez G, Lowy FD. Heterosexual transmission of community-associated methicillin-resistant Staphylococcus aureus. *Clin Infect Dis.* 2007;44:410–413
33. Hajjeh RA, Reingold A, Weil A, et al. Toxic shock syndrome in the United States: Surveillance update, 1979 1996. *Emerg Infect Dis.* 1999;5:807–810
34. Projan SJ, Brown-Skrobot S, Schlievert PM, Vandenesch F, Novick RP. Glycerol monolaurate inhibits the production of beta-lactamase, toxic shock toxin-1, and other staphylococcal exoproteins by interfering with signal transduction. *J Bacteriol.* 1994;176:4204–4209
35. Strandberg KL, Peterson ML, Schaefers MM, et al. Reduction in staphylococcus aureus growth and exotoxin production and in vaginal interleukin 8 levels due to glycerol monolaurate in tampons. *Clin Infect Dis.* 2009;49:1711–1717
36. Omar HA, Aggarwal S, Perkins KC. Tampon use in young women. *J Pediatr Adolesc Gynecol.* 1998;11:143–146
37. Suchard JR. "Spider bite" lesions are usually diagnosed as skin and soft-tissue infections. *J Emerg Med.* 2009 Nov 23; Epub ahead of print
38. Sircar KD, Bancroft E, Nguyen DM, Mascola L. Hospitalization of paediatric patients for methicillin-resistant Staphylococcus aureus skin and soft-tissue infection, 1998–2006. *Epidemiol Infect.* 2009:1–6
39. Carrillo-Marquez MA, Hulten KG, Hammerman W, Mason EO, Kaplan SL. USA300 is the predominant genotype causing Staphylococcus aureus septic arthritis in children. *Pediatr Infect Dis J.* 2009;28:1076–1080
40. Crary SE, Buchanan GR, Drake CE, Journeycake JM. Venous thrombosis and thromboembolism in children with osteomyelitis. *J Pediatr.* 2006;149:537–541
41. Gonzalez BE, Teruya J, Mahoney DH Jr, et al. Venous thrombosis associated with staphylococcal osteomyelitis in children. *Pediatrics.* 2006;117:1673–1679

42. Finelli L, Fiore A, Dhara R, et al. Influenza-associated pediatric mortality in the United States: Increase of Staphylococcus aureus coinfection. *Pediatrics.* 2008;122:805–811
43. Day MD, Gauvreau K, Shulman S, Newburger JW. Characteristics of children hospitalized with infective endocarditis. *Circulation.* 2009;119:865–870
44. Shulman ST, Ayoub EM. Severe staphylococcal sepsis in adolescents. *Pediatrics.* 1976;58:59–66
45. Cunnington A, Brick T, Cooper M, et al. Severe invasive panton-valentine leucocidin positive staphylococcus aureus infections in children in London, UK. *J Infect.* 2009;59:28–36
46. Descloux E, Perpoint T, Ferry T, et al. One in five mortality in non-menstrual toxic shock syndrome versus no mortality in menstrual cases in a balanced French series of 55 cases. *Eur J Clin Microbiol Infect Dis.* 2008;27:37–43
47. Tsuei B. Principles of abscess drainage. In: Berry S, ed. Mont Reid surgical handbook. 4th ed. Orlando: Mosby; 1997:732–733
48. Fitch MT, Manthey DE, McGinnis HD, Nicks BA, Pariyadath M. Videos in clinical medicine. Abscess incision and drainage. *N Engl J Med.* 2007;357:e20
49. Lee MC, Rios AM, Aten MF, et al. Management and outcome of children with skin and soft tissue abscesses caused by community-acquired methicillin-resistant staphylococcus aureus. *Pediatr Infect Dis J.* 2004;23:123–127
50. Hankin A, Everett WW. Are antibiotics necessary after incision and drainage of a cutaneous abscess? *Ann Emerg Med.* 2007;50:49–51
51. Hyun DY, Mason EO, Forbes A, Kaplan SL. Trimethoprim-sulfamethoxazole or clindamycin for treatment of community-acquired methicillin-resistant Staphylococcus aureus skin and soft tissue infections. *Pediatr Infect Dis J.* 2009;28:57–59
52. Mistry RD, Schwab SH, Treat JR. Stevens-Johnson syndrome and toxic epidermal necrolysis: Consequence of treatment of an emerging pathogen. *Pediatr Emerg Care.* 2009;25:519–522
53. Baxter R, Ray GT, Fireman BH. Case-control study of antibiotic use and subsequent clostridium difficile-associated diarrhea in hospitalized patients. *Infect Control Hosp Epidemiol.* 2008;29:44–50
54. Siberry GK, Tekle T, Carroll K, Dick J. Failure of clindamycin treatment of methicillin-resistant Staphylococcus aureus expressing inducible clindamycin resistance in vitro. *Clin Infect Dis.* 2003;37:1257–1260
55. Ruhe JJ, Menon A. Tetracyclines as an oral treatment option for patients with community onset skin and soft tissue infections caused by methicillin-resistant Staphylococcus aureus. *Antimicrob Agents Chemother.* 2007;51:3298–3303
56. Stryjewski ME, Chambers HF. Skin and soft-tissue infections caused by community-acquired methicillin-resistant staphylococcus aureus. *Clin Infect Dis* 2008;46 Suppl 5:S368–S377
57. Kim SH, Park WB, Lee KD, et al. Outcome of Staphylococcus aureus bacteremia in patients with eradicable foci versus noneradicable foci. *Clin Infect Dis.* 2003;37:794–799
58. Browne LP, Mason EO, Kaplan SL, et al. Optimal imaging strategy for community-acquired Staphylococcus aureus musculoskeletal infections in children. *Pediatr Radiol.* 2008;38:841–847
59. Greenfield LJ, Proctor MC. Vena caval filter use in patients with sepsis: Results in 175 patients. *Arch Surg.* 2003;138:1245–1248
60. Cosgrove SE, Vigliani GA, Fowler VG Jr, et al. Initial low-dose gentamicin for Staphylococcus aureus bacteremia and endocarditis is nephrotoxic. *Clin Infect Dis.* 2009;48:713–721
61. Perlroth J, Kuo M, Tan J, Bayer AS, Miller LG. Adjunctive use of rifampin for the treatment of staphylococcus aureus infections: A systematic review of the literature. *Arch Intern Med.* 2008;168:805–819
62. Staphylococcal infections. In: Pickering LK BC, Kimberlin DW, Long SS, eds. *Red Book: 2009 Report of the Committee on Infectious Diseases.* 28th ed. Elk Grove Village, IL: American Academy of Pediatrics; 2009;601–615
63. Baddour LM, Wilson WR, Bayer AS, et al. Infective endocarditis: diagnosis, antimicrobial therapy, and management of complications. *Circulation.* 2005;111:e394–e434
64. Fergie J, Purcell K. The treatment of community-acquired methicillin-resistant staphylococcus aureus infections. *Pediatr Infect Dis J.* 2008;27:67–68

65. Wang G, Hindler JF, Ward KW, Bruckner DA. Increased vancomycin MICs for Staphylococcus aureus clinical isolates from a university hospital during a 5-year period. *J Clin Microbiol.* 2006;44:3883–3886
66. Deresinski S. Counterpoint: Vancomycin and staphylococcus aureus–an antibiotic enters obsolescence. *Clin Infect Dis.* 2007;44:1543–1548
67. Infectious Disease Society of America. FDA lowers vancomycin breakpoints for Staphylococcus aureus. *Clin Infect Dis.* 2008; 47:iii–iv 2009
68. Frymoyer A, Hersh AL, Benet LZ, Guglielmo BJ. Current recommended dosing of vancomycin for children with invasive methicillin-resistant Staphylococcus aureus infections is inadequate. *Pediatr Infect Dis J.* 2009;28:398–402
69. Moise-Broder PA, Forrest A, Birmingham MC, Schentag JJ. Pharmacodynamics of vancomycin and other antimicrobials in patients with Staphylococcus aureus lower respiratory tract infections. *Clin Pharmacokinet.* 2004;43:925–942
70. Dumitrescu O, Boisset S, Badiou C, et al. Effect of antibiotics on Staphylococcus aureus producing Panton-Valentine leukocidin. *Antimicrob Agents Chemother.* 2007;51:1515–1519
71. Drees M, Boucher H. New agents for Staphylococcus aureus endocarditis. *Curr Opin Infect Dis.* 2006;19:544–550
72. Wunderink RG, Rello J, Cammarata SK, Croos-Dabrera RV, Kollef MH. Linezolid vs vancomycin: Analysis of two double-blind studies of patients with methicillin-resistant Staphylococcus aureus nosocomial pneumonia. *Chest.* 2003;124:1789–1797
73. Lalani T, Boucher HW, Cosgrove SE, et al. Outcomes with daptomycin versus standard therapy for osteoarticular infections associated with Staphylococcus aureus bacteraemia. *J Antimicrob Chemother.* 2008;61:177–182
74. Jacobson LM, Milstone AM, Zenilman J, Carroll KC, Arav-Boger R. Daptomycin therapy failure in an adolescent with methicillin-resistant Staphylococcus aureus bacteremia. *Pediatr Infect Dis J.* 2009;28:445–447
75. Marty FM, Yeh WW, Wennersten CB, et al. Emergence of a clinical daptomycin-resistant staphylococcus aureus isolate during treatment of methicillin-resistant Staphylococcus aureus bacteremia and osteomyelitis. *J Clin Microbiol.* 2006;44:595–597
76. Martinez-Aguilar G, Hammerman WA, Mason EO Jr, Kaplan SL. Clindamycin treatment of invasive infections caused by community-acquired, methicillin-resistant and methicillin-susceptible Staphylococcus aureus in children. *Pediatr Infect Dis J.* 2003;22:593–598
77. Mongkolrattanothai K, Aldag JC, Mankin P, Gray BM. Epidemiology of community-onset Staphylococcus aureus infections in pediatric patients: An experience at a children's hospital in Central Illinois. *BMC Infect Dis.* 2009;9:112
78. Drew RH, Perfect JR, Srinath L, Kurkimilis E, Dowzicky M, Talbot GH. Treatment of methicillin-resistant Staphylococcus aureus infections with quinupristin-dalfopristin in patients intolerant of or failing prior therapy. *J Antimicrob Chemother.* 2000;46:775–784
79. Gauduchon V, Cozon G, Vandenesch F, et al. Neutralization of Staphylococcus aureus Panton Valentine leukocidin by intravenous immunoglobulin in vitro. *J Infect Dis.* 2004;189:346–353
80. Kazakova SV, Hageman JC, Matava M, et al. A clone of methicillin-resistant Staphylococcus aureus among professional football players. *N Engl J Med.* 2005;352:468–475
81. Creech CB, Beekmann SE, Chen Y, Polgreen PM. Variability among pediatric infectious diseases specialists in the treatment and prevention of methicillin-resistant Staphylococcus aureus skin and soft tissue infections. *Pediatr Infect Dis J.* 2008;27:270–272
82. Patel JB, Gorwitz RJ, Jernigan JA. Mupirocin resistance. *Clin Infect Dis.* 2009;49:935–941
83. Kaplan SL. Commentary: Prevention of recurrent staphylococcal infections. *Pediatr Infect Dis J.* 2008;27:935–937
84. Fisher RG, Chain RL, Hair PS, Cunnion KM. Hypochlorite killing of community-associated methicillin-resistant Staphylococcus aureus. *Pediatr Infect Dis J.* 2008;27:934–935

# Sexually Transmitted Infections in Adolescents: Advances in Epidemiology, Screening, and Diagnosis

Elise D. Berlan, MD, MPH[*,a],
Cynthia Holland-Hall, MD, MPH[a]

[a]Section of Adolescent Medicine, Nationwide Children's Hospital and Department of Pediatrics, The Ohio State University College of Medicine, 700 Children's Drive, Columbus, OH 43205

Clinicians who care for young people strive to keep adolescents healthy and help them make decisions that promote wellness as they mature into young adults. Caring for adolescent patients requires an understanding of sexually transmitted infections (STI). Many adolescents are sexually active and STIs disproportionately affect this age group.[1,2] This article provides an in-depth review of the epidemiology of STIs that commonly affect American adolescents and reviews advances in understanding racial/ethnic disparities in STIs among adolescents. Up-to-date diagnostic and screening approaches that minimize invasive experiences for adolescents and expedite clinical decision-making are presented. Advances in human papillomavirus (HPV) vaccination are discussed, including the vaccination of boys.

## Advances in Epidemiology

Adolescents in the United States are disproportionately affected by STIs.[1,2] Traditionally, the implicated reasons have included behavioral risk factors, biological susceptibility in adolescent girls, and challenges accessing health care.[3] Efforts to understand individual risks are increasingly being placed into understanding sexual networks and population-level factors such as poverty, segregation, and incarceration. Information about the prevalence of STIs comes from various sources, including national surveillance data, national population-level surveys, and studies of special populations, such as youth entering the National Job Training Program (Job Corps), juvenile detention facilities, military recruits, and young women seen in family planning clinics.

*Corresponding author.
*E-mail address*: elise.berlan@nationwidechildrens.org (E. D. Berlan).

Copyright © 2010 American Academy of Pediatrics. All rights reserved. ISSN 1934-4287

National surveillance data from the Centers for Disease Control and Prevention (CDC) demonstrate disparate rates of STIs by age, gender, and race/ethnicity.[2] CDC estimates there are >15 million new cases of STIs annually, with almost half occurring in adolescents and young adults, despite this age group comprising only approximately one-quarter of the sexually active population. Caution must be used when interpreting national surveillance data, because such data represent reported cases only. Because many infections are asymptomatic and undiagnosed, reported rates underrepresent the true prevalence of infection in the entire population.

*Chlamydia trachomatis* is an obligate intracellular organism that causes uncomplicated lower genitourinary (GU) tract infections in males and females (urethritis, proctitis, epididymitis, cervicitis) as well as upper tract disease. Most chlamydia infections are asymptomatic.[4] Untreated chlamydia infection can lead to pelvic inflammatory disease (PID) and subsequent infertility, chronic pelvic pain, and ectopic pregnancy. Infection in pregnant women may lead to neonatal pneumonia and ophthalmia. Chlamydia infections are the most common reportable infection in the United States. In 2008, >1.3 million chlamydia infections were reported, and estimates are that the true disease burden is closer to 2.8 million cases annually. Chlamydia reports have increased since the late 1980s, due largely to enhanced screening efforts and the availability of more sensitive testing modalities. Girls ages 15–19 have the highest age-specific rate of infection and number of cases (3275.8 per 100 000 population), followed by women ages 20–24 (3179.9 per 100 000 population). Boys and young men also have very high rates of infection (701.6 per 100 000 population and 1056.1 per 100 000 population, respectively; Fig. 1).[2]

*Neisseria gonorrhea* is a Gram-negative bacterium that causes lower GU tract disease in males and females (urethritis, proctitis, epididymitis, cervicitis) and also PID and its sequelae, neonatal ophthalmia, and disseminated gonococcal infection. The epidemiology of gonococcal infection is similar to that of chlamydia, with girls and young women having the highest rates of infections (636.8

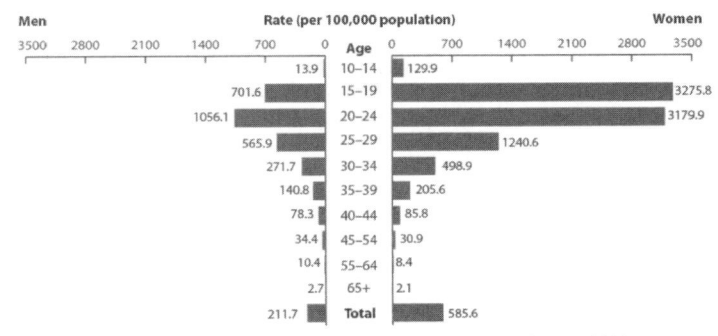

| Men | Age | Women |
|---|---|---|
| 13.9 | 10–14 | 129.9 |
| 701.6 | 15–19 | 3275.8 |
| 1056.1 | 20–24 | 3179.9 |
| 565.9 | 25–29 | 1240.6 |
| 271.7 | 30–34 | 498.9 |
| 140.8 | 35–39 | 205.6 |
| 78.3 | 40–44 | 85.8 |
| 34.4 | 45–54 | 30.9 |
| 10.4 | 55–64 | 8.4 |
| 2.7 | 65+ | 2.1 |
| 211.7 | Total | 585.6 |

Fig 1. *Chlamydia trachomatis* age- and sex-specific rates: United States, 2008.

per 100 000 population for girls ages 15–19 and 608.6 per 100 000 population for young women ages 20–24). Adolescent boys and young men also have, relative to other age groups, high rates of infection (278.3 per 100 000 population and 433.6 per 100 000 population, respectively). Gonorrhea rates declined in 2008 for the first time in 4 years. Thirteen percent of isolates in the CDC Gonococcal Isolate Surveillance Program are quinolone resistant. Cases of chlamydia and gonorrhea are strikingly more common among blacks (discussed later) and in the Southern states.[2]

Two large population-based studies contribute to our understanding of the prevalence of STIs in adolescents and young adults in the United States. Studies that screen a representative sample of the US population allow more accurate estimates of STI prevalence in the general population. The National Longitudinal Study of Adolescent Health (Add Health) follows a large nationally representative cohort of adolescents and young adults. Biological samples were obtained from participants during wave 3 (2001–2002) of this study, allowing for highly accurate prevalence estimates of STIs at that time. The prevalence of chlamydia among female and male Add Health participants ages 18–26 was 4.7% and 3.7%, respectively. Among females who tested positive for chlamydia, fewer than 5% reported vaginal or urinary symptoms. Similarly, most participants with gonorrhea infection were asymptomatic. Among persons with gonorrhea infection, 70% were coinfected with chlamydia. However, among persons with chlamydia, far fewer had gonococcal co-infection (6.2% females, 8.6% males).[4,5]

*Trichomonas vaginalis* is a motile, flagellated parasite that causes asymptomatic and symptomatic lower GU infection in males and females. Trichomoniasis may increase transmission of human immunodeficiency virus (HIV),[6] commonly is concurrent with other STIs,[7] is associated with preterm delivery and low birth weight,[8] and possibly PID.[9] Because trichomoniasis is not a reportable infection, national surveillance data from CDC are not available. However, the prevalence as assessed by polymerase chain reaction (PCR) among Add Health participants at wave 3 was 2.8% among females and 1.7% among males, and more prevalent in the South. Most of these infections were asymptomatic.[10]

The most recent population-based data indicate particularly high rates of STIs in adolescent females. National Health and Nutrition Examination Survey (NHANES) 2003–2004 data include interview and biological specimens from over 800 girls ages 14–19. This survey found that the prevalence of chlamydia was 3.9%, gonorrhea was 1.3%, herpes simplex virus type 2 (HSV-2) was 1.9%, and HPV (including 23 oncogenic serotypes and types 6 and 11) was 18.3% among this sample of female adolescents in the United States. The prevalence of any STI was 24.1%. Among sexually experienced girls, the prevalence of any STI increased to nearly 40%, including 20.4% positivity among girls reporting only a single sexual partner. The prevalence of chlamydia among sexually active girls in the survey was 7%. Within one year after coitarche, 25.6% of participants had acquired at least one infection, with HPV being the most common.[11]

Studies within special populations also further our knowledge about the distribution of the STI burden in the United States. The median state-specific rates of test positivity for chlamydia and gonorrhea among women ages 15–24 seeking care in federally funded family planning clinics in 2008 were 7.4% and 0.9%, respectively.[2] Female military recruits represent a high-risk population, with recent studies estimating the chlamydia prevalence at 12% in this population.[12,13] Gonorrhea and chlamydia prevalence are high among young people entering the National Job Training Program (Job Corps). Participants in Job Corps are generally economically disadvantaged and racial/ethnic minorities. In 2008, the mean state-specific prevalence of chlamydia infection among youth entering Job Corps was 12.8% in females and 7% in males. The prevalence of gonorrhea was 2.7% in females and 0.8% in males.[2] Youth entering juvenile detention are also highly vulnerable to STIs. The median facility-specific prevalence of chlamydia among girls and boys entering detention in 2008 was 13.8% and 6.1%. For gonorrhea infection, the median facility-specific prevalence was 3.6% in girls and 0.9% in boys.[2]

**Advances in Understanding Racial/Ethnic Disparities**

*Individual Risk Factors*

STI rates and prevalence differ dramatically by race/ethnicity in the United States. The most striking disparities exist between black and white Americans. According to the 2008 CDC surveillance data, the rate of chlamydia in black Americans is eight times that of white Americans and almost half (49%) of all the reported chlamydia cases occurred in blacks. About 71% of all gonorrhea cases occurred in blacks, and the rate for gonorrhea infection overall is 20 times higher for black Americans compared with white Americans. The rate was highest for female black adolescents. The primary and secondary syphilis rates for blacks are almost 8 times higher than for whites. Syphilis rates for black adolescents have been increasing strikingly since the mid-2000s.[2] Black Americans bear a disproportionate burden of HIV infection; almost half of new HIV infections occur in blacks, although blacks comprise only 12% of the general population.[14] Black females are 15 times more likely than white females to be infected with HIV, with heterosexual sexual contact being the most common mode of transmission (80%) to women.[15]

In Add Health wave 3, the prevalence of chlamydia infection in black adolescents was 6 times higher than in white adolescents. The prevalence of gonorrhea in black males was 36 times higher than in white males; the prevalence in black females was 14 times higher than in white females.[5] Blacks were much more likely to have Trichomonas infection, with black females nearly 10 times more likely to be infected than white females.[10] In NHANES 2003–2004, black females were 3 times more likely to have any STI compared with white females.[11]

Behavioral risk factors are known to increase personal risk for acquiring an STI. Young people acquire STIs very quickly after sexual debut. Two independent studies found that the risk of any STI was 25% within 1 year after first sex.[11,16] The risk of having an STI increases with time since sexual debut.[11] Early sexual debut is associated with having an STI. Add Health Wave 3 participants who had earlier coitarche were more likely to have a current STI.[17] Similarly, participants in the 1992 National Health Interview Survey who had a later sexual debut had reduced odds for self-reported STI.[18] Individuals with earlier sexual debut are also more likely to report other behavioral risk factors for STI acquisition.[18,19] Looking at racial/ethnic differences in sexual behaviors, the 2007 Youth Risk Behavior Survey (YRBS), a nationally representative sample of American youth in high school, found that 66.5% of black respondents compared with 43.7% of white respondents reported ever having sexual intercourse.[20] Analysis of data from the 1997–2007 YRBS found that black males had earlier sexual debut than any other racial/ethnic group.[21] In the 2007 YRBS, 16.3% of black respondents reported sex before age 13, compared with 4.4% of whites.[20]

The risk of having an STI increases with number of sexual partners.[11,18,22] Research exploring the association between race/ethnicity and number of sexual partners has been inconclusive. In the 2007 YRBS, 27.6% of black respondents reported 4 or more lifetime sexual partners, compared with 11.5% of white respondents.[20] In Add Health waves 1 and 2, a slightly higher proportion of blacks than whites reported multiple partners.[23] However, when the Add Health wave 3 data were analyzed using advanced modeling techniques, black youth were much more likely than white youth to belong to the behavior cluster characterized by, among other behaviors, few sexual partners (median = 1). More than a third of blacks were in this group, compared with 12.7% of whites.[24]

Having partners overlapping in time (concurrency) is a major risk factor for having an STI and accelerates the transmission of STIs in a population.[25] Overall, adolescents' assessments of sex partner concurrency (ie, whether their sex partner has additional sex partners) are highly inaccurate.[26] In a study of patients seen in an urban STI clinic, almost two-thirds reported having both a steady and at least one nonsteady partner in the last 3 months.[27] Reports of concurrency do not differ by race/ethnicity in Add Health waves 1 and 2.[23] In the 1995 National Survey of Family Growth (NSFG), black young women were more likely than white women to report a male partner with concurrency.[28]

Age of partner and condom use are also associated with having a STI. In Add Health waves 1 and 2, age discordance >2 years and condom nonuse increased the risk of self-reported STI.[22] However, in this sample, age discordance did not differ by race/ethnicity.[23] Condom use among adolescents has increased significantly since the early 1990s.[20] Analyses of current national level data comparing condom use by race/ethnicity are lacking. The results of older studies suggest that black adolescents may be more likely to use condoms than white adolescents.[29,30]

*Contextual Risk Factors*

Undisputedly, the individual risk factors described above affect individual-level risk for acquiring and transmitting infections. However, individual risk factors may not entirely explain racial/ethnic disparities in STIs. Accordingly, it is necessary to test the strength of the relationship between behavioral risk factors and STIs and assess whether other more powerful factors may be present. In a landmark 1998 study by Ellen et al, after controlling for age, gender, sociodemographic factors, and sexual behaviors in a national sample, African American youth were still at almost 4 times the risk of having an STI compared with white youth. The introduction of sexual behaviors into their model attenuated the odds for an STI only minimally. Findings were similar in several other large studies, including NHANES and NSFG.[11,28] In the analyses of wave 3 Add Health conducted by Hallfor et al, black adolescents were more likely to cluster in lower risk behavior categories, with the largest cluster being "few partners, low alcohol and tobacco, and other drug use." White youth were more broadly distributed in behavior clusters, with a much higher proportion in "higher substance use" and "multiple sexual partners" clusters. The likelihood of blacks engaging in very low risk behavior having an STI were remarkable; compared with white youth with similar low risk behavior, blacks were 29 times more likely to have an STI.[24] These striking findings suggest that factors other than personal behavior are largely responsible for the racial/ethnic disparities in STIs.

The most salient population-level factors include mating patterns, concurrency, and sexual network dynamics. Data about such factors are quite limited for adolescents. Network dynamics in the adult black population likely impact the STI risk for younger blacks. Analysis of a nationally representative probability sample (The National Health and Life Study) found that black adults were more likely than whites and Hispanics to have sexual partnerships within their own race (*assortive mating*). As well, black adults with low-risk sexual behavior (reporting only one sexual partner in the last year) were much more likely to have sexual partnerships with higher risk adults (reporting >4 sexual partners in the last year) than whites and Hispanics (*dissortive mating*).[31] Such mating patterns allow for relative containment of infections within the black population and promote the distribution of STIs to persons whose individual sexual behaviors are not particularly high risk.

Initial investigations into network dynamics in adolescents have been fruitful. Urban black adolescents whose recent sex partners identified other sex partners were more likely to have a partner with an STI and to have significant age discordance than those whose recent partners did not identify other partners.[25] Additional studies in this cohort, The Bayview Networks Study, suggest that females may have fewer direct partners than males, but the highly connected sexual partnerships of their male partners put them at increased STI risk.[32] Position in sexual network is important in determining STI risk. Adolescents in confirmed dyadic partnerships were less likely to have an STI compared with adolescents whose partners reported having other partners in the last 3 months. Those adolescents who were at the center of nondyadic components (had reported multiple partners who all reported other partners) were at highest risk for having chlamydia or gonorrhea, followed by adolescents at the periphery of nondyadic components (had reported only one partner, but the partner reported other partners).[33]

Excellent and detailed reviews of the impact of social contexts (poverty, racism, sex ratio, segregation, incarceration) on sexual partnerships and transmission of sexually transmitted infections are available and should be required reading for clinicians interested in better understanding racial/ethnic disparities in STIs.[34–36] In addition, 2 recent manuscripts are noteworthy and permit a deeper, more contextually sensitive understanding of adolescent sexual networks. Both are qualitative studies of mate selection among black inner city youth in Baltimore. Analysis of 50 semistructured interviews found that female participants desire monogamous romantic partners, but often accept nonmonogamous partners to fulfill their desire for emotional intimacy. Males desire casual sex and romantic partners and gain social status when they have multiple partners.[37] In another study of adolescent girls, participants identified pervasive life concerns such as family disruption, partner safety, and bleak vocational and educational opportunities, which psychologically trump concerns about partner concurrency.[38]

## Advances in Diagnostics

### Vaginal Swab Specimens

Perhaps the most important advance in recent years in STI diagnostics is the use of vaginal swabs for screening for gonorrhea and chlamydia. Numerous studies demonstrate that when tested using nucleic acid amplification tests (NAAT), vaginal swab samples, either patient- or clinician-collected, are as accurate as endocervical samples, and superior to first-catch urine samples for the diagnosis of gonorrhea and chlamydia.[13,39–43] Many studies have found the vaginal swab sample to be equivalent to endocervical samples, and several have found it superior. In a 2008 study of self-obtained vaginal swabs in adolescents, using the BDProbeTec ET assay, the self-obtained vaginal swab sample was more sensitive for chlamydia than first-catch urine and endocervical samples (97.3% vs. 89.2% and 90.1%, respectively) using any 2 positive tests as the "gold standard." Results were similar for gonorrhea. The specificities of the vaginal swab specimens for chlamydia and gonorrhea were 94.7% and 94.8%, respectively.[42] The

FDA has approved the Gen-Probe APTIMA Combo 2 assay and the BDProbeTec ET assay for vaginal swab specimens using appropriate collection kits.

Women find the self-collection technique to be easy and acceptable. Most women surveyed after self-vaginal swab report it was easy or very easy to collect, and both adolescent and adult women report first-catch urine and vaginal swab samples acceptable.[12,41,44,45] Vaginal swabs offer significant advantages over cervical and urine specimens for screening. Compared with cervical specimens, vaginal swabs are less invasive and cost-saving since they do not require a pelvic examination. In addition, the quality of urine specimens may deteriorate in transport and more processing of these specimens is required in the laboratory. A recent study of women attending STI clinics demonstrated self-obtained vaginal swabs to be the least expensive and most cost-effective modality for preventing PID, compared with cervical and urine samples.[41] The ease of use and the stability of self-obtained vaginal swab specimens may be particularly beneficial in promoting screening in nontraditional, nonclinical settings, such as field settings for military personnel, community venues, and Internet-based home screening.[12,13,43] Not surprisingly, vaginal swabs are now considered the preferred sample type for screening.[40,46,47]

*Extragenital Screening with Nucleic Acid Amplification Tests*

Nationally representative prevalence data for gonorrhea and chlamydia infections among adolescent males who have sex with males (MSM) are not available. These infections, however, are believed to be common in this population.[48] CDC recommends *at least* annual screening of MSM for urethral and rectal gonorrhea and chlamydia (the latter for those who engage in receptive anal intercourse), and for pharyngeal gonorrhea (for those who engage in receptive oral intercourse).[49] Classically, rectal and pharyngeal testing have been done with culture. The availability of the more sensitive NAAT, although not FDA approved for nongenital specimens, has prompted many to consider NAATs for this purpose. Use of NAATs for extragenital screening has been demonstrated to be clinically superior to culture.[48,50] Consequently, testing with NAAT is currently recommended for extragenital gonorrhea and chlamydia after internal validation of the method by the individual laboratory to satisfy Centers for Medicare and Medicaid Services (CMS) regulations for Clinical Laboratory Improvement Amendments (CLIA) compliance, according to an expert panel convened by the CDC and the Association of Public Health Laboratories.[46] Use of NAATs may facilitate testing adolescent MSM in both clinical and nontraditional venues, and improve diagnosis of gonorrhea and chlamydia in this population.

*Rapid Diagnostic Tests*

Rapid diagnostic tests, often referred to as point-of-care tests, allow a patient to receive test results and any necessary treatment before completion of the clinic visit. They should be easily performed by clinic personnel with a modest amount of training, and should generate results within a 30- to 60-minute timeframe or less. Although they may be convenient to use across clinical settings, they are particularly well-suited for use in populations who are unable or unlikely to return for follow-up visits, or who may be difficult to locate to communicate abnormal test results. The current standard of care for the diagnosis of trichomoniasis is the visualization of motile trichomonads in a sample of vaginal fluid, using light microscopy. It is widely acknowledged, however, that the sensitivity of this diagnostic test is limited to only 36% to 75%, depending on the experience of the user.[51] Culture is considered the gold standard, but is not performed in most settings. Xenostrip-Tv (Xenotope Diagnostics Inc., San Antonio, TX) and the second generation OSOM Trichomonas Rapid Test (Genzyme Diagnostics, Cambridge, MA) are qualitative assays that detect *T. vaginalis* antigen using color immunochromatographic (dipstick) technology. The OSOM Trichomonas Rapid Test is performed on a vaginal swab specimen, or the saline solution used for making wet mounts from vaginal swabs. It is CLIA waived and can be completed in <30 minutes. Huppert et al have studied this test in high-prevalence settings and have reported sensitivities of 83–90% compared with a composite reference standard (CRS) that included positive culture, wet mount, and/or rapid testing; one study included NAAT in the CRS as well.[52,53] The sensitivity of wet mount in these studies was clearly inferior, at 56–71%. Specificity of the OSOM test was 99–100%. Campbell et al studied this test in a low-prevalence setting and reported a sensitivity of 95% and specificity of 100%, compared with a CRS defined as a positive NAAT plus either a positive OSOM test or wet mount.[54]

Although bacterial vaginosis (BV) is not considered a sexually transmissible infection, it is the most common cause of vaginal discharge among sexually active women. The BVBlue Test (Gryphus Diagnostics, LLC, Knoxville, TN) measures the activity of sialidase, an enzyme produced by bacterial pathogens such as *Gardnerella vaginalis*, *Bacteroides spp.*, and *Prevotella spp*, in vaginal fluid specimens. It is also a CLIA-waived test; results are read after 10 minutes. Sensitivity for diagnosis of BV is 88–92% compared with Nugent criteria applied to Gram stain, and 88% compared with Amsel criteria applied to wet mount. Specificity is 91–98%.[55,56] BVBlue performed significantly better than individual tests that do not require a microscope (ie, vaginal pH and the amine release test).

The development of highly sensitive rapid diagnostic tests for gonococcal and chlamydial infections has proven more challenging, and published research in this area is surprisingly limited. Rapid tests for these organisms use various antigen detection techniques such as enzyme immunoassay (EIA). Reported sensitivities for the various rapid tests for chlamydia range from 25–73%, with specificities of 98–100%.[57-59] Rapid tests for gonococcal infections have similarly low sensitivities of 60-to 70%.[60,61] The Chlamydia Rapid Test (Diagnostics Development Unit, University of Cambridge), a newer assay, seems to have better performance and utilizes vaginal swabs rather than endocervical samples, but more research on this test is needed.[62] At this time, rapid tests for gonococcal and chlamydial infections should only be considered for use in high-prevalence settings with concerns about poor follow-up, such as some developing countries. If testing is to be performed in a laboratory after the patient's visit is complete, more accurate tests should be used. They are therefore not appropriate for use in most private office settings at this time.

**Advances in Screening**

Because chlamydia and, to a lesser degree, gonorrhea are usually asymptomatic infections, routine screening is necessary to decrease morbidity related to long-term sequelae.[63] The CDC recommends *at least* annual chlamydia screening in adolescent females,[49] with many experts recommending more frequent screening for higher risk individuals, including males.[64-67] Experts argue for more frequent screening, such as every 6 months, because adolescents who are positive for chlamydia quickly reacquire infections. In one study, Burstein et al found the mean time to chlamydia reinfection was 6.3 months among urban adolescent girls.[67] Similarly, Orr et al demonstrated that 40–73% of urban adolescents and young adults in their study were reinfected with chlamydia, gonorrhea, or *Trichomonas vaginalis* within 7 months of an initial STI diagnosis.[64]

Health care providers in the United States often fail to perform routine chlamydia screening of sexually active adolescents and young women.[68-70] Shafer and colleagues demonstrated the effectiveness of an innovative quality improvement intervention on chlamydia screening practices for girls and boys at pediatric clinics in a large health maintenance organization (HMO). The intervention involved engagement of clinical leadership, providing a toolkit, using Plan-Do-Study-Act rapid cycles,[71] and planning to sustain the changes. Their intervention dramatically increased screening.[68,72] A technically similar intervention was also effective in increasing screening rates among adolescents seen for urgent care in the same HMO.[73]

Alternatively, testing in nontraditional settings may also expand chlamydia screening among young people and is endorsed by the CDC. Several recent studies have demonstrated the feasibility of screening adolescents in alternative settings. Given the many hours adolescents spend online, and their concerns about confidentiality in a clinical setting, the Internet may prove to be a useful way to reach young people for chlamydia screening. Researchers have demonstrated the feasibility of this approach, using a self-administered vaginal swab collection kit, obtained via a website called www.iwantthekit.org.[43] Auerswald and colleagues demonstrated the feasibility, acceptability, and effectiveness of street-based urine screening for gonorrhea and chlamydia in urban homeless youth.[74] NAAT-based chlamydia screening in school-based health centers offers the ability to screen large numbers of asymptomatic youth.[75] Persistent quality improvement efforts on the part of health care providers as well as use of nontraditional screening approaches are necessary to diminish the burden of STIs in adolescents.

**Advances in Human Papillomavirus Prevention and Screening**

HPV infection is considered the most common sexually transmitted infection in the United States and occurs quickly after sexual debut.[1,11,76] HPV infection is known to cause a range of clinical problems, including genital warts, anogenital cancers, and cervical cancer. In 2006, a quadrivalent vaccine protecting against HPV types 6, 11, 16, and 18 (Gardasil; Merck and Co, Inc.) was FDA approved for girls and young women ages 9–26 for prevention of cervical cancer and genital warts. A bivalent vaccine against oncogenic HPV types 16 and 18 (Cervarix; GlaxoSmithKline) was FDA approved for use in girls and young women ages 10–25 in October 2009. Currently the CDC Advisory Committee on Immunization Practices (ACIP) recommends the routine immunization of girls with either the bivalent or the quadrivalent vaccine at age 11–12, with catch-up immunization of females up to 25 years old. In October 2009, the FDA also approved the use of Gardasil in boys and young men to prevent genital warts. Initial cost-benefit analyses of the use of Gardasil in males do not support routine vaccination of males.[77] Accordingly, the ACIP has issued a permissive recommendation to allow the use of Gardasil in boys and young men for the prevention of genital warts.

The American Congress of Obstetricians and Gynecologists (ACOG) recently updated guidelines for cervical cancer screening in adolescents.[78] The current ACOG recommendation is to begin cervical cancer screening of all immunocompetent women at age 21, using a Papanicolaou smear, regardless of reported sexual activity. The data that informed this recommendation include the very low rate of cervical cancer in the American adolescent population (1–2 per million) as well as the high morbidity and cost associated with screening adolescents and the aggressive follow-up of abnormal screening tests. Health care providers are encouraged to change their clinical practice. Although HPV testing using PCR is available, currently there is no recommended use for this test in adolescents. It is critical to note that the changes in cervical cancer screening guidelines do not imply that pediatricians ought not to do routine gynecologic care for their adolescent patients, including chlamydia screening. Instead, implementation of these recommendations will minimize the invasiveness of medical procedures being done to adolescent girls and hopefully improve their experiences and the care they receive.

**CONCLUSIONS**

STIs continue to be a major public health concern affecting adolescents and young adults. Advances in understanding the epidemiology of disease may help providers better assess their patients' personal risks, as well as the contribution of communities and sexual networks. Advances in screening and the availability of a wide variety of testing modalities allow more health care providers, and potentially those who have contact with adolescents in other areas as well, to identify and address this need.

## REFERENCES

1. Weinstock H, Berman S, Cates W Jr. Sexually transmitted diseases among american youth: Incidence and prevalence estimates, 2000. *Perspect Sex Reprod Health.* 2004;36:6–10
2. Centers for Disease Control and Prevention. Sexually transmitted diseases surveillance, 2008. Atlanta, GA: US Department of Health and Human Services; 2009
3. Shrier LA. Bacterial sexually transmitted infections: Gonorrhea, chlamydia, pelvic inflammatory disease, and syphilis. In: Emans SJ, Laufer MR, Goldstein DP, eds. *Pediatric and Adolescent Gynecology.* 5th ed. Philadelphia: Lippincott Williams & Wilkins; 2005:525
4. Miller WC, Ford CA, Morris M, et al. Prevalence of Chlamydial and gonococcal infections among young adults in the united states. *JAMA.* 2004;291:2229–2236
5. Miller WC, Zenilman JM. Epidemiology of Chlamydial infection, gonorrhea, and trichomoniasis in the united states–2005. *Infect Dis Clin North Am.* 2005;19:281–296
6. Laga M, Manoka A, Kivuvu M, et al. Non-ulcerative sexually transmitted diseases as risk factors for HIV-1 transmission in women: Results from a cohort study. *AIDS.* 1993;7:95–102
7. Allsworth JE, Ratner JA, Peipert JF. Trichomoniasis and other sexually transmitted infections: Results from the 2001–2004 National Health and Nutrition Examination Surveys. *Sex Transm Dis.* 2009;36:738–744
8. Cotch MF, Pastorek JG 2nd, Nugent RP, et al. Trichomonas vaginalis associated with low birth weight and preterm delivery. The vaginal infections and prematurity study group. *Sex Transm Dis.* 1997;24:353–360
9. Cherpes TL, Wiesenfeld HC, Melan MA, et al. The associations between pelvic inflammatory disease, Trichomonas vaginalis infection, and positive herpes simplex virus type 2 serology. *Sex Transm Dis.* 2006;33:747–752
10. Miller WC, Swygard H, Hobbs MM, et al. The prevalence of trichomoniasis in young adults in the United States. *Sex Transm Dis.* 2005;32:593–598
11. Forhan SE, Gottlieb SL, Sternberg MR, et al. Prevalence of sexually transmitted infections among female adolescents aged 14 to 19 in the United States. *Pediatrics.* 2009;124:1505–1512
12. Hsieh YH, Howell MR, Gaydos JC, et al. Preference among female army recruits for use of self-administered vaginal swabs or urine to screen for Chlamydia trachomatis genital infections. *Sex Transm Dis.* 2003;30:769–773
13. Shafer MA, Moncada J, Boyer CB, et al. Comparing first-void urine specimens, self-collected vaginal swabs, and endocervical specimens to detect Chlamydia trachomatis and Neisseria gonorrhoeae by a nucleic acid amplification test. *J Clin Microbiol.* 2003;41:4395–4399
14. Hall HI, Song R, Rhodes P, et al. Estimation of HIV incidence in the United States. *JAMA.* 2008;300:520–529
15. Centers for Disease Control and Prevention (CDC). Subpopulation estimates from the HIV incidence surveillance system–United States, 2006. *MMWR Morb Mortal Wkly Rep.* 2008;57: 985–989
16. Tu W, Batteiger BE, Wiehe S, et al. Time from first intercourse to first sexually transmitted infection diagnosis among adolescent women. *Arch Pediatr Adolesc Med.* 2009;163:1106–1111
17. Kaestle CE, Halpern CT, Miller WC, Ford CA. Young age at first sexual intercourse and sexually transmitted infections in adolescents and young adults. *Am J Epidemiol.* 2005;161:774–780
18. Ellen JM, Aral SO, Madger LS. Do differences in sexual behaviors account for the racial/ethnic differences in adolescents' self-reported history of a sexually transmitted disease? *Sex Transm Dis.* 1998;25:125–129

19. Sandfort TG, Orr M, Hirsch JS, Santelli J. Long-term health correlates of timing of sexual debut: Results from a national US study. *Am J Public Health*. 2008;98:155–161
20. Centers for Disease Control and Prevention. YRBSS: Youth Risk Behavior Surveillance System. Available at: http://www.cdc.gov/HealthyYouth/yrbs/index.htm. Accessed January 30, 2010
21. Cavazos-Rehg PA, Krauss MJ, Spitznagel EL, et al. Age of sexual debut among US adolescents. *Contraception*. 2009;80:158–162
22. Ford K, Lepkowski JM. Characteristics of sexual partners and STD infection among American adolescents. *Int J STD AIDS*. 2004;15:260–265
23. Ford K, Sohn W, Lepkowski J. American adolescents: Sexual mixing patterns, bridge partners, and concurrency. *Sex Transm Dis*. 2002;29:13–19
24. Hallfors DD, Iritani BJ, Miller WC, Bauer DJ. Sexual and drug behavior patterns and HIV and STD racial disparities: The need for new directions. *Am J Public Health*. 2007;97:125–132
25. Ellen JM, Brown BA, Chung SE, et al. Impact of sexual networks on risk for gonorrhea and Chlamydia among low-income urban African American adolescents. *J Pediatr*. 2005;146:518–522
26. Lenoir CD, Adler NE, Borzekowski DL, Tschann JM, Ellen JM. What you don't know can hurt you: Perceptions of sex-partner concurrency and partner-reported behavior. *J Adolesc Health*. 2006;38:179–185
27. Senn TE, Carey MP, Vanable PA, Coury-Doniger P, Urban M. Sexual partner concurrency among STI clinic patients with a steady partner: Correlates and associations with condom use. *Sex Transm Infect*. 2009;85:343–347
28. Harawa NT, Greenland S, Cochran SD, Cunningham WE, Visscher B. Do differences in relationship and partner attributes explain disparities in sexually transmitted disease among young white and black women? *J Adolesc Health*. 2003;32:187–191
29. Warren CW, Santelli JS, Everett SA, et al. Sexual behavior among U.S. high school students, 1990–1995. *Fam Plann Perspect*. 1998;30:170–200
30. Shafii T, Stovel K, Davis R, Holmes K. Is condom use habit forming? Condom use at sexual debut and subsequent condom use. *Sex Transm Dis*. 2004;31:366–372
31. Laumann EO, Youm Y. Racial/ethnic group differences in the prevalence of sexually transmitted diseases in the United States: A network explanation. *Sex Transm Dis*. 1999;26:250–261
32. Fichtenberg CM, Muth SQ, Brown B, Padian NS, Glass TA, Ellen JM. Sexual network structure among a household sample of urban African American adolescents in an endemic sexually transmitted infection setting. *Sex Transm Dis*. 2009;36:41–48
33. Fichtenberg CM, Muth SQ, Brown B, et al. Sexual network position and risk of sexually transmitted infections. *Sex Transm Infect*. 2009;85:493–498
34. Aral SO. Sexual network patterns as determinants of STD rates: Paradigm shift in the behavioral epidemiology of STDs made visible. *Sex Transm Dis*. 1999;26:262–264
35. Adimora AA, Schoenbach VJ. Social context, sexual networks, and racial disparities in rates of sexually transmitted infections. *J Infect Dis*. 2005;191 Suppl 1:S115–S122
36. Aral SO, Lipshutz J, Blanchard J. Drivers of STD/HIV epidemiology and the timing and targets of STD/HIV prevention. *Sex Transm Infect*. 2007;83 Suppl 1:i1–i4
37. Andrinopoulos K, Kerrigan D, Ellen JM. Understanding sex partner selection from the perspective of inner-city black adolescents. *Perspect Sex Reprod Health*. 2006;38:132–138
38. Tsui EK, Leonard L, Lenoir C, Ellen JM. Poverty and sexual concurrency: A case study of STI risk. *J Health Care Poor Underserved*. 2008;19:758–777
39. Schachter J, McCormack WM, Chernesky MA, et al. Vaginal swabs are appropriate specimens for diagnosis of genital tract infection with Chlamydia trachomatis. *J Clin Microbiol*. 2003;41:3784–3789
40. Schachter J, Chernesky MA, Willis DE, et al. Vaginal swabs are the specimens of choice when screening for Chlamydia trachomatis and Neisseria gonorrhoeae: Results from a multicenter evaluation of the APTIMA assays for both infections. *Sex Transm Dis*. 2005;32:725–728
41. Blake DR, Maldeis N, Barnes MR, et al. Cost-effectiveness of screening strategies for Chlamydia trachomatis using cervical swabs, urine, and self-obtained vaginal swabs in a sexually transmitted disease clinic setting. *Sex Transm Dis*. 2008;35:649–655

42. Fang J, Husman C, DeSilva L, Chang R, Peralta L. Evaluation of self-collected vaginal swab, first void urine, and endocervical swab specimens for the detection of Chlamydia trachomatis and Neisseria gonorrhoeae in adolescent females. *J Pediatr Adolesc Gynecol.* 2008;21:355–360
43. Masek BJ, Arora N, Quinn N, et al. Performance of three nucleic acid amplification tests for detection of Chlamydia trachomatis and Neisseria gonorrhoeae by use of self-collected vaginal swabs obtained via an internet-based screening program. *J Clin Microbiol.* 2009;47:1663–1667
44. Chernesky MA, Hook EW 3rd, Martin DH, et al. Women find it easy and prefer to collect their own vaginal swabs to diagnose Chlamydia trachomatis or Neisseria gonorrhoeae infections. *Sex Transm Dis.* 2005;32:729–733
45. Serlin M, Shafer MA, Tebb K, et al. What sexually transmitted disease screening method does the adolescent prefer? Adolescents' attitudes toward first-void urine, self-collected vaginal swab, and pelvic examination. *Arch Pediatr Adolesc Med.* 2002;156:588–591
46. Association of Public Health Laboratories. Expert consultation meeting summary report; January 13–15, 2009. Available from: http://www.aphl.org/aphlprograms/infectious/std/documents/ctgclabguidelinesmeetingreport.pdf. Accessed January 10, 2010
47. Hobbs MM, van der Pol B, Totten P, et al. From the NIH: Proceedings of a workshop on the importance of self-obtained vaginal specimens for detection of sexually transmitted infections. *Sex Transm Dis.* 2008;35:8–13
48. Schachter J, Moncada J, Liska S, Shayevich C, Klausner JD. Nucleic acid amplification tests in the diagnosis of Chlamydial and gonococcal infections of the oropharynx and rectum in men who have sex with men. *Sex Transm Dis.* 2008;35:637–642
49. Centers for Disease Control and Prevention, Workowski KA, Berman SM. Sexually transmitted diseases treatment guidelines, 2006. *MMWR Recomm Rep.* 2006;55:1–94
50. Centers for Disease Control and Prevention (CDC). Clinic-based testing for rectal and pharyngeal Neisseria gonorrhoeae and Chlamydia trachomatis infections by community-based organizations–five cities, United States, 2007. *MMWR Morb Mortal Wkly Rep.* 2009;58:716–719
51. Wiese W, Patel SR, Patel SC, Ohl CA, Estrada CA. A meta-analysis of the papanicolaou smear and wet mount for the diagnosis of vaginal trichomoniasis. *Am J Med.* 2000;108:301–308
52. Huppert JS, Batteiger BE, Braslins P, et al. Use of an immunochromatographic assay for rapid detection of Trichomonas vaginalis in vaginal specimens. *J Clin Microbiol.* 2005;43:684–687
53. Huppert JS, Mortensen JE, Reed JL, et al. Rapid antigen testing compares favorably with transcription-mediated amplification assay for the detection of Trichomonas vaginalis in young women. *Clin Infect Dis.* 2007;45:194–198
54. Campbell L, Woods V, Lloyd T, Elsayed S, Church DL. Evaluation of the OSOM trichomonas rapid test versus wet preparation examination for detection of Trichomonas vaginalis vaginitis in specimens from women with a low prevalence of infection. *J Clin Microbiol.* 2008;46:3467–3469
55. Myziuk L, Romanowski B, Johnson SC. BVBlue test for diagnosis of bacterial vaginosis. *J Clin Microbiol.* 2003;41:1925–1928
56. Bradshaw CS, Morton AN, Garland SM, Horvath LB, Kuzevska I, Fairley CK. Evaluation of a point-of-care test, BVBlue, and clinical and laboratory criteria for diagnosis of bacterial vaginosis. *J Clin Microbiol.* 2005;43:1304–1308
57. Rani R, Corbitt G, Killough R, Curless E. Is there any role for rapid tests for Chlamydia trachomatis? *Int J STD AIDS.* 2002;13:22–24
58. Yin YP, Peeling RW, Chen XS, et al. Clinic-based evaluation of Clearview Chlamydia MF for detection of Chlamydia trachomatis in vaginal and cervical specimens from women at high risk in China. *Sex Transm Infect.* 2006;82 Suppl 5:v33–7
59. Blanding J, Hirsch L, Stranton N, et al. Comparison of the Clearview Chlamydia, the PACE 2 assay, and culture for detection of Chlamydia trachomatis from cervical specimens in a low-prevalence population. *J Clin Microbiol.* 1993;31:1622–1625
60. Alary M, Gbenafa-Agossa C, Aina G, et al. Evaluation of a rapid point-of-care test for the detection of gonococcal infection among female sex workers in Benin. *Sex Transm Infect.* 2006;82 Suppl 5:v29–v32

61. Benzaken AS, Galban EG, Antunes W, et al. Diagnosis of gonococcal infection in high risk women using a rapid test. *Sex Transm Infect.* 2006;82 Suppl 5:v26–v28
62. Mahilum-Tapay L, Laitila V, Wawrzyniak JJ, et al. New point of care chlamydia rapid test–bridging the gap between diagnosis and treatment: Performance evaluation study. *BMJ.* 2007; 335:1190–1194
63. Scholes D, Stergachis A, Heidrich FE, Andrilla H, Holmes KK, Stamm WE. Prevention of pelvic inflammatory disease by screening for cervical chlamydial infection. *N Engl J Med.* 1996;334: 1362–1366
64. Orr DP, Johnston K, Brizendine E, Katz B, Fortenberry JD. Subsequent sexually transmitted infection in urban adolescents and young adults. *Arch Pediatr Adolesc Med.* 2001;155:947–953
65. Batteiger BE, Tu W, Ofner S, et al. Repeated chlamydia trachomatis genital infections in adolescent women. *J Infect Dis.* 2010;201:42–51
66. Peterman TA, Tian LH, Metcalf CA, et al. High incidence of new sexually transmitted infections in the year following a sexually transmitted infection: A case for rescreening. *Ann Intern Med.* 2006;145:564–572
67. Burstein GR, Gaydos CA, Diener-West M, Howell MR, Zenilman JM, Quinn TC. Incident Chlamydia trachomatis infections among inner-city adolescent females. *JAMA.* 1998;280:521–526
68. Shafer MA, Tebb KP, Pantell RH, et al. Effect of a clinical practice improvement intervention on Chlamydial screening among adolescent girls. *JAMA.* 2002;288:2846–2852
69. Hoover K, Tao G. Missed opportunities for Chlamydia screening of young women in the United States. *Obstet Gynecol.* 2008;111:1097–1102
70. Hoover K, Tao G, Kent C. Low rates of both asymptomatic Chlamydia screening and diagnostic testing of women in US outpatient clinics. *Obstet Gynecol.* 2008;112:891–898
71. Langley G, Nolan K, Provost L, Norman C. *The Improvement Guide: A Practical Approach to Enhancing Organizational Performance.* San Francisco, CA: Josey-Bass; 1996
72. Tebb KP, Pantell RH, Wibbelsman CJ, et al. Screening sexually active adolescents for Chlamydia trachomatis: What about the boys? *Am J Public Health.* 2005;95:1806–1810
73. Tebb KP, Wibbelsman C, Neuhaus JM, Shafer MA. Screening for asymptomatic Chlamydia infections among sexually active adolescent girls during pediatric urgent care. *Arch Pediatr Adolesc Med.* 2009;163:559–564
74. Auerswald CL, Sugano E, Ellen JM, Klausner JD. Street-based STD testing and treatment of homeless youth are feasible, acceptable and effective. *J Adolesc Health.* 2006;38:208–212
75. Joffe A, Rietmeijer CA, Chung SE, et al. Screening asymptomatic adolescent men for Chlamydia trachomatis in school-based health centers using urine-based nucleic acid amplification tests. *Sex Transm Dis.* 2008;35:S19–S23
76. Dunne EF, Unger ER, Sternberg M, et al. Prevalence of HPV infection among females in the United States. *JAMA.* 2007;297:813–819
77. Kim JJ, Goldie SJ. Cost effectiveness analysis of including boys in a human papillomavirus vaccination programme in the United States. *BMJ.* 2009;339:b3884
78. ACOG Committee on Practice Bulletins–Gynecology. ACOG practice bulletin no. 109: Cervical cytology screening. *Obstet Gynecol.* 2009;114:1409–1420

# Human Papillomavirus Disease and Vaccines in Adolescents

## Anna-Barbara Moscicki, MD*

*Division of Adolescent Medicine, University of California San Francisco, 3333 California Street, San Francisco, CA 94118*

The road to discovery of human papillomavirus (HPV) as the cause of cervical cancer has likely affected adolescents more than any group, both positively and negatively. With the development of sensitive assays for HPV, it became clear that adolescents were infected with HPV more often than any other age group. This led to increased cervical cancer screening in this age group, which unfortunately led to the discovery that HPV-associated disease was also epidemic in this group. The medical intervention spiral began with increased colposcopy, biopsy, and treatment. Meanwhile, cervical cancer rates never changed in this age group. In reflection, the decision to initiate screening cervical cancer in this age group was not evidence-based. Recently, we have also broadened our understanding about HPV-associated disease in men. In this chapter, we cover the advances in science that have led to new screening recommendation for cervical cancer and the advances in prevention: vaccines for both adolescent women and men.

## Biology of HPV

Understanding the viral replication cycle is essential to understanding the clinical implications of HPV DNA and disease detection in adolescents. The target cell for HPV infection is the epithelial basal cell. The virus life cycle is dependent on the ability of these cells to divide, differentiate, and move toward the epithelial surface.[1] In the basal layer, the early proteins (termed E6 and E7) facilitate replication and maintenance of the viral genome and cause cellular proliferation as well. As the cell matures, different HPV proteins are expressed that continue to maintain viral genomic replication. Expression of the late proteins, which create the essential outer capsid, occurs in the upper layer of the epithelium. This is followed by packaging of the DNA into the capsid and eventual release of infectious virions from the normally desquamated epithelial cell.

---

*Corresponding author.
*E-mail address*: moscickia@peds.ucsf.edu (A. B. Moscicki).

Copyright © 2010 American Academy of Pediatrics. All rights reserved. ISSN 1934-4287

Without cell differentiation, the virus cannot replicate. The period between basal cell infection and release of virus is thought to be somewhere between 3 weeks and 3 months.

Viral replication and its associated protein expression induce the development of the low-grade squamous intraepithelial lesion (LSIL), which is characterized by mild basal cell proliferation and nuclear enlargement. These changes are in part due to the expression of the oncogenes E6 and E7 and perinuclear halos secondary to E4 expression, which interferes with cytoskeletal structure. As the intraepithelial lesions advance in grade, expression of products important in cell transformation, such as E6 and E7, predominate resulting in chromosomal abnormalities and the aneuploidy characteristic of the higher-grade squamous intraepithelial lesions (HSIL). Hallmarks of cancer development include viral integration and interference with telomerase activity.[2] As a point of clarification, the cytological diagnoses of LSIL and HSIL correspond to the histologic diagnoses of cervical intraepithelial neoplasia (CIN) 1 and CIN 2 or 3, respectively.[3]

Because the virus is nonlytic, the inflammatory response to HPV is much more subtle than other infections such as *C. trachomatis*. During early HPV infection, the host remains somewhat immunologically unaware of the virus because the virions are released in the outer epithelial layer, away from the submucosa, the primary site of immune surveillance. It appears that an initial HPV infection triggers an innate immune response[4] through activation of Toll-like receptors (TLRs), which recognize genetically imprinted pathogen-associated membrane proteins or through activation of natural killer cells.[5] Innate immune responses are thought to be responsible for rapid clearance—those seen within weeks to a few months.

Chronic HPV infections are likely cleared by the development of adaptive immune responses,[6,7] dependent on presentation of viral antigens to antigen-presenting cells (APCs), such as Langerhans and dendritic cells.[8] Successful adaptive immune responses may take months to years to develop and oncogenic HPV types, specifically HPV 16, are able to downregulate both the innate and the adaptive immune response through numerous mechanisms.[4] Because HPV infections are localized to the epithelium, it is believe that the majority of both innate and adaptive immune responses are mucosal. These immune parameters are important to remember when we review the efficacy of preventive vaccines.

**Epidemiology and the Natural History of HPV and SIL in Adolescents**

Anogenital HPV infections are extremely common in the sexually active adolescent, with over 50% having a positive HPV DNA test over a 3-year period.[9-12] Numerous studies have shown that a recent new sex partner is the strongest risk for acquiring HPV.[10,12-14] Other risks include having a sexually transmitted infection, which may reflect partner risk or inflammation resulting in a break in the epithelial barrier. Fortunately, in adolescents 50% of HPV infections are cleared within 6 months and 90% within 2–3 years.[15–18] Since LSIL is a reflection of viral replication and HPV is most common in the adolescent age group, it is not surprising that LSIL is also most common in adolescents with a prevalence ranging from 2–14%.[19] In parallel with HPV DNA clearance rates, over 90% of LSIL diagnosed in adolescents or young women also resolve spontaneously.

HSIL is far less common than LSIL, but adolescents and young women have a prevalence equivalent to older women with rates around 0.7%. The greatest single risk for HSIL development is HPV persistence. However, in one study, 7% of adolescents developed a HSIL shortly after HPV acquisition, suggesting some women develop HSIL without lengthy persistence.[20] Other risk factors include smoking cigarettes[21] and prolonged oral contraceptive use.[22] Since nicotine can be measured directly in cervical mucous, proposed mechanism for cigarette use includes local immune suppression and/or local carcinogenic affect. The role for oral contraceptives is more elusive, but estrogen has been shown to induce cellular proliferation as well as enhance HPV oncogene transcription.[23,24]

Reinfection with numerous HPV types is common in adolescents contributing to the high prevalence rate observed in young women. This vulnerability is thought to be due in part to a naïve immune response since the rate of HPV declines with age, even when controlling for sexual activity.[9,11,25–27] Clearance of infection appears to protect women from repeat infections with that genotype. This was well illustrated in the HPV vaccine trials where women seropositive for HPV 16 but HPV DNA 16 negative at baseline (ie, evidence of previously cleared infection) had low rates of HPV 16 infection during the trial although they were in the placebo arm.[28–30]

## Adolescents and Biological Vulnerabilities to HPV, SIL and Cancer

Several studies, including a recent collaborative study of over 45 000 women have shown age of first intercourse to be an important risk factor for the future development of cervical cancer.[31–34] In that study, an increase in the risk for the development of cervical cancer was noted in women initiating intercourse before 24 years of age, with risk increasing with each declining year until age 17.[34] Some speculate that the risk of cancer increases because there is a longer time allowed for HPV persistence. Biologically, adolescence reflects a period of dramatic changes in an area of the cervix referred to as the transformation (T) zone where squamous cell cancers develop.[35]

Most neonates are born with an abrupt squamo-columnar junction visible on the ectocervix. This junction remains quiescent until puberty when estrogen and increased acidity of the vagina induces uncommitted basal cells of the columnar epithelium to become squamous cells through a process referred to squamous metaplasia. Consequently, the cervix in the adolescent is predominantly made up of columnar and metaplastic cells, whereas adults are predominantly squamous epithelium. Theoretically, the former epithelium may be more vulnerable to wounds induced by intercourse, douching or tampons leading to breeches in the epithelium and easy access for HPV. No study to date has shown that ectopy (eg, the presence of the columnar and metaplastic epithelium on the exocervix) is a risk for HPV acquisition. However, Castle et al[36] found that infections with HPV types including 16, 31, 33, 35, 52, 58, and 67 were more common in women with large areas of ectopy, but not common in women with mature cervixes. This observation might be related to age and immunologic memory which goes hand in hand with cervical maturation.

More important than the presence of columnar epithelium is likely the presence of active metaplastic epithelium. Cells that are rapidly undergoing differentiation and replication are "fuel for the fire" for SIL development.[37] A recent study showed that both oral contraceptive and smoking enhance metaplasia in young women.[38] This is quite interesting in light of both of these being risks for cervical cancer.

**Cervical Cancer Rates and Screening**

Despite the age of sexual debut decreasing and cervical cancer screening increasing in adolescents, cervical cancer rates have basically remained unchanged in the 15- 19-year-old group. From 1990–2006, Surveillance Epidemiology and End Results statistics show that an average of 14 cervical cancers occurred annually in girls age 15–19 years, reflecting an incidence rate of 0.1 per 100 000.[39] This rate is unchanged from that reported in 1973–1977 when screening was initiated.[40] In a recent study in England where there are active screening programs, Sasieni et al[41] found that screening women aged 20–24 years had no detectable impact on reducing cervical cancer rates in women under the age of 30 years. In comparison, there was a dramatic reduction noted for women 30 years and above. In another study, Gustoffson et al[42] compared rates of cervical cancer before and after screening programs were in place using data from several different countries including the United States. They showed that cervical cancer was significantly reduced among women between the ages of 35 and 55 years. No differences were found for women 25–35 years of age and those older than 70 years. Barnholtz-Sloan et al[43] reported that U.S. incidence cervical cancer rates showed significant decreases in incidence between 1995–1999 and 2000–2004 for all age groups and race/ethnicities except for Hispanic/all races women aged 15–24 years and non-Hispanic/other women aged 15–24 years. Changes in white and black women aged 15–24 years decreased but only marginally. These data support the notion that cervical cancer screening by cytology does not effectively prevent the rare cervical cancer case in the adolescent.

## Risk Factors that Influence Clearance of HPV and SIL and Progression to CIN3

It has been shown that the longer HPV persists, the more likely it will not be cleared.[44] HPV persistence is key in the development of cervical cancers. However, how long persistence is required remains unknown. Persistence is likely necessary but not sufficient and other important carcinogenic events are needed before cancer develops.

Currently, CIN3 is considered a true precancer since regression is unlikely and progression to cervical cancer is estimated to be around 15% if left untreated. CIN1 is considered benign because of high rates of regression and rare progression. The diagnosis of CIN2 is clinically challenging and reproducibility being quite poor. Histologic readings are often either downgraded or upgraded on repeat analysis.[45] Recent studies also show that CIN2 appears to regress in ~60% of young women.[46,47] In the ASCUS/LSIL triage study trial, depending on their study arm, some women with CIN2 were treated with excisional therapy at the end of the study.[48] Many of these women no longer had evidence of CIN2. One of the protective factors associated with progression to CIN3 included young age at biopsy. Women aged 18–21 years of age had a 52% reduced risk of having CIN3 on follow-up compared with women aged 22–23 years.[48] Another reason that CIN2 may commonly appear to regress is the low reproducibility of CIN2 lesions.[49] Castle et al[48] demonstrated that when CIN2 lesions were downgraded to CIN 1 by another review, the lesion was less likely to progress to CIN3 than those lesions that remained a CIN2 by the second review.

Although CIN3 does occur in adolescents, it is uncommon and the risk for CIN3 in this age group has not been well studied. Although there have been rare cases of spontaneous CIN3 shortly after HPV acquisition, the risk factors are likely similar to those in older women.[50] The lower progression rates from HPV or LSIL to CIN3 seen in adolescents is probably due to the fact that adolescents have not had enough time for progression to occur. However, better elucidation of the natural history of CIN3 among adolescents is unlikely to be garnered since it is considered unethical to leave potentially cancerous lesions untreated.

## Cervical Cancer Screening

As discussed above, since cervical cancer screening has not changed cervical cancer rates over the last 3 decades in 15- to 19-year-olds or 20- to 24-year-olds and screening young women does not influence rates of cancer diagnosed under the 30 years of age,[41] screening recommendations have been revised. A recent statement from a conference headed by the American Society for Colposcopy and Cervical Pathology and Centers for Disease Control and Prevention with 22 other organizations attending recommended that in the United States, cervical screening should start at the age of 21 years with no caveats related to the age of onset of sexual activity.[51] This recommendation has been made an official guideline of the American College of Obstetrics and Gynecology and several other groups are moving to adopt this recommendation. The previous guideline recommending that screening begin at 21 years old or by 3 years after sexual debut (whichever comes first) has been difficult to follow, had poor adherence, and raised concern about causing more harm than good.[52]

## Management

Although screening for cervical cancer in adolescent populations is now not recommended, the uptake of guidelines often take years. Consequently, guidelines have been developed to minimize harm to adolescents with abnormal cytology.[53,54] First, these guidelines underscore the lack of utility in using HPV DNA testing in screening, triage, or follow-up of abnormal cytology. There is no place for HPV testing in the adolescents because of its high prevalence. For abnormal cytology, the guidelines recommend observation. In the case of atypical squamous cells of undetermined significance and LSIL, only repeat cytology screening at 12-month intervals is recommended. If the abnormality persists after 2 years, only then is it recommended to refer the women to colposcopy. In the case of HSIL, referral of all to colposcopy is recommended. If CIN1 is diagnosed, follow-up with cytology is recommended at 12-month intervals. If CIN2 is diagnosed, observation is also recommended with 6-month intervals using cytology and colposcopy for up to 2 years. If CIN2 is persistent at 2 years, then treatment is recommended.

One of the reasons that the new recommendations embrace observation (or no screening) is that treatment for CIN can be harmful with risks for preterm delivery and low birth rate.[55–58] The decision to treat should be the exception not the norm in adolescent populations and histologic criteria, not cytologic are required for treatment. Often, the histologic report does not distinguish CIN2 from CIN3 resulting in a CIN2/3 diagnosis. In this case, it is recommended to treat the lesion as a CIN2 since these lesions are more common than CIN3.

## Prevention

The mainstay of prevention is vaccination. Two vaccines, a quadrivalent (HPV-4) containing serotypes HPV 6, 11, 16, and 18 (Gardasil' Merck & Co; Whitehouse Station, NJ) and a bivalent vaccine (HPV-2) containing serotypes 16 and 18 (Cervarix GlaxoSmithKline Biologicals; Rixensart, Belgium) have been approved by the U.S. Food and Drug Administration (FDA). Both of these vaccines are composed of noninfectious, recombinant HPV viral-like particles (VLP), comprising the major capsid protein, L1. Both vaccines are also adjuvanted with HPV-4 using aluminum hydroxyphosphate sulfate while HPV-2 utilizes a proprietary adjuvant, aluminum hydroxide with 3-deacylated monophosphoryl lipid A. The VLP with or without adjuvant elicits a strong systemic immune response measurable by neutralizing antibodies and cell-mediated immunity.[59–62] Although specific antibodies are present in cervical secretions of women who have received the vaccine,[63] it is thought that these HPV specific antibodies are present in cervical secretions secondary to transudation or exudation from blood into the cervical mucous at the site rather than local synthesis.

**Vaccine Efficacy Against Cervical Cancer**

Both the HPV-4 and HPV-2 vaccines are highly efficacious in preventing HPV vaccine-associated CIN—the predetermined efficacy correlate for the development of cervical cancer.[30,64–71] In the Per Protocol studies (where all subjects were HPV vaccine type naïve at entry, received all 3 doses on schedule, and cases start counting after the last vaccination), both vaccines had efficacies close to 100% (Tables 1 and 2). A subanalysis comprising women who were also HPV vaccine type naïve at entry but only received one or two doses of vaccine demonstrated efficacy almost equivalent to the per protocol analysis for both the HPV-4 and HPV-2 vaccines.[69,30] Per protocol efficacy for HPV-4 has been demonstrated for up to 42 months[70] and for up to 6.4 years for HPV-2.[30] Antibody levels (both anti IgG antibodies and neutralizing antibodies) for HPV 16 and 18 after HPV-2 have remained 5- to 13-fold higher than levels found in natural infections for up to 75 months after vaccination with no evidence of decline.[30] In contrast, women immunized with HPV-4 showed declines in antibodies for HPV-11 and -18 with final titers comparable to levels after natural infection.[28] Due to this finding, a study evaluating a booster dose of HPV-4

Table 1
Vaccine efficacy of gardasil against high-grade cervical disease and genital lesions

|  | Vaccine n | Vaccine Cases | Placebo n | Placebo Cases | Observed Efficacy, % (95% CI) |
|---|---|---|---|---|---|
| Per Protocol[a] |  |  |  |  |  |
| CIN 2 or worse[b] | 7864 | 2 | 7865 | 110 | 98.2 (93.3–99.8) |
| VIN/VaIN 2/3 or worse[b] | 7900 | 0 | 7902 | 23 | 100.0 (82.6–100.0) |
| Condyloma[c] | 2261 | 0 | 2279 | 48 | 100.0 (92.0–100.0) |
| Intention to treat[d] |  |  |  |  |  |
| CIN 2 or worse[b] | 8823 | 142 | 8860 | 293 | 51.5 (40.6–60.6) |
| VIN/VaIN 2/3 or worse[b] | 8956 | 9 | 8969 | 43 | 79.0 (56.4–91.0) |
| Condyloma[c] | 2723 | 21 | 2732 | 86 | 76.0 (61.0–86.0) |

[a] Per protocol must have met all inclusion criteria, naïve to HPV vaccine types, completed 3 doses on schedule and starting counting cases after month 7.
[b] Pooled analysis from 3 clinical trials.[70]
[c] Data from Future I only.[68]
[d] Intention-to-treat group included women who received at least one dose of the vaccine and could have been HPV infected or had disease at enrollment or day 1, respectively.

Table 2
Vaccine efficacy of cervarix against HPV 16/18-associated high-grade cervical disease

|  | Vaccine n | Vaccine Cases | Placebo n | Placebo Cases | Observed Efficacy, % (96.1% CI) |
| --- | --- | --- | --- | --- | --- |
| Per Protocol[a] |  |  |  |  |  |
| CIN 2 or worse | 7344 | 4 | 7312 | 56 | 92.9 (79.9–98.3) |
| CIN 2 or worse, corrected for lesion HPV type[b] | 7344 | 1 | 7312 | 53 | 98.1 (88.4–100.0) |
| Intention to treat[c] |  |  |  |  |  |
| CIN 2 or worse | 8667 | 82 | 8682 | 174 | 52.8 (37.5–64.7) |

[a] Per protocol must have met all inclusion criteria naïve to HPV vaccine types completed 3 doses and started counting case day after third vaccination.
[b] HPV 16/18 in lesion and in preceding sample if multiple types found in lesion.
[c] Referred to as total vaccinated cohort.[30] Included women who were given at least one does, case counting occurred day after first vaccination and included women regardless of serostatus or DNA status at visit 0.

vaccine was performed.[28] A total of 114 women were given a fourth dose of HPV-4 vaccine 60 months after completing the primary 3-dose series. About 75% of the women who had undetectable antibody levels of HPV 11 prebooster and 96.7% of the women with undetectable levels of HPV 18 prebooster had significant rises in titers postbooster suggesting that the vaccine induces long-term boostable memory. Antibody response after a natural HPV exposure post-vaccination remains unknown. Using antibody decay models, it is estimated that the protection against HPV-16 from either vaccine will last decades, with 99% of people having lifelong detectable levels of antibody.[72]

Vaccine efficacy based on an intention to treat analysis which included women who before vaccination were not HPV naïve to the vaccine containing serotypes was greatly reduced for both the HPV-4 and HPV-2 vaccines (Tables 1 and 2). As vaccine trials are often designed to test maximal vaccine efficacy, many exclusionary criteria are present making it difficult to extrapolate study results to the general population. The initial studies of the HPV-4 vaccine excluded women who had a history of either 1) >4 lifetime sexual partners, 2) abnormal cytology or genital warts, or 3) were pregnant. Subsequent HPV-4 studies allowed women with a history of abnormal Pap smears or genital warts, but excluded women with either of the other two previously listed criteria. Participants in trials of the HPV-2 vaccine had more liberal criteria with exclusion occurring if women had a history of 7 or more lifetime partners. Since U.S. data shows that, on average, sexually active women aged 19–21 years have had 4 or more sexual partners, concern could be raised about the applicability of data from the HPV-4 trials to the general population.[73]

To address some of these concerns, Kjaer et al[70] performed a pooled analysis of 3 clinical trials of HPV-4 vaccine to determine the efficacy of preventing CIN2+ related to the serotypes in the vaccine among subgroups. Not surprisingly, vaccine efficacy in the intention to treat group (inclusive of non-HPV-naïve women) was significantly reduced among women with a greater number of sexual partners. Among women with no sexual partners, the percent reduction of CIN2+ histology was 86.5% as compared with 54.5% in those with 1–2 partners and 48.1% in women with 3 or more partners. Vaccine efficacy was inversely related to the age of the subject. Those age 17 or less had a 69% reduction in CIN-2+ histology, whereas those 21 years or older had a reduction of only 31.1%. Vaccine efficacy was also adversely affected by a history of having an abnormal Pap. None of these differences were found when limiting analysis to the per protocol (HPV naïve only) group. Similar subgroup analysis for the HPV-2 vaccine is not available.

While both the HPV-4 and HPV-2 vaccine are highly efficacious in preventing HPV disease from serotypes in the vaccine, neither vaccine has demonstrated therapeutic efficacy. In the HPV-2 trials, women who were serologically positive and DNA positive[30] had an efficacy of −13.8. Efficacy rose to 35.2% in women who were serologically negative and DNA positive, and climbed to 68.8% among women who were serologically positive but DNA negative (past history but cleared) prevaccination. A similar pattern of results was shown with the HPV-4 vaccine. Olsson et al[29] recently reported more data on women who were seropositive but DNA negative and found a similar efficacy for CIN2/3 of 100%; 0 cases (of 1243 women) occurred in the vaccine group compared with 4 (of 1283) women in the placebo group. Although this data may show some vaccine efficacy, it also demonstrates that the majority of women appear protected after natural clearance. These data support the notion that this is not a therapeutic vaccine. It also underscores the importance of vaccinating naïve women.

Obviously the largest population without evidence of previous HPV exposure is sexually naïve individuals. Markowitz et al[74] examined vaccine HPV type seropositivity in blood among 4303 persons aged 14–59 years of age who participated in the 2003–2004 National Health and Nutrition Examination Survey. The seroprevalence of HPV 6, 11, 16, and 18 among female subjects was 17%, 7.1%, 15.6%, and 6.5%, respectively. The prevalence of infection with at least one HPV vaccine type was 32.5% among females. Broken down by age, 9.3% of those 14–19 years were exposed to at least one of the vaccine types— extremely few were exposed to all 4 types. When the data for the entire group was broken down by sexual behavior, women reporting >10 sexual partners had a prevalence of almost 60% for any one of the vaccine-containing types. Interestingly, the rates were also higher among women if they reported having their first intercourse under the age of 16 years (41%). The vaccine efficacy studies combined with the seroprevalence data from the epidemiologic studies continue to support the decision to target younger girls to maximize the benefits from this vaccine. Although there is evidence to show that women will continue to benefit from the vaccine at an individual level after 19 years of age, vaccination in this older age group is far less beneficial from a public health perspective.

In the United States, the Advisory Committee for Immunization Practices (ACIP) recommends vaccination to be targeted to 11- to 12-year-olds along with the adolescent platform which includes tetanus, diphtheria and acellular pertussis, meningococcal, and varicella if needed (www.cdc.gov). ACIP also recommends immunization as early as 9 years of age since immunobridging studies showed adequate immune response in this age group. Catchup vaccination is also recommended for women up to the age of 26 years. The American Cancer Society has been more conservative with its recommendation suggesting that the evidence does not support large public health vaccination efforts for women older than age 19.[75] Certainly, individual based data show that many women will continue to derive benefit from the vaccine and that number of sexual partners and past history of abnormal cytology play a role in probability of benefit from the vaccine. Although these types of risk factors remain difficult to screen for in clinical settings,[76] health care providers should be able to counsel women regarding expectations from the vaccine if the individual has already begun sexual activity.

## Vaccine Indications for Noncervical Genital Disease in Females

HPV-4 also has indications for the prevention of condyloma, which is caused by predominantly HPV-6 and -11 and noncervical genital disease including vulvar intraepithelial neoplastic (VIN) lesions and vaginal intraepithelial neoplastic (VAIN) lesions.[66,68,70] Although HPV-16 and -18 cause a large proportion of VIN and VAIN, the HPV-2 clinical trials did not include these as measured outcomes.[71]

## HPV-Related Penile, Anal, and Oropharyngeal Cancers

### Anal Cancer

Approximately 90% of anal cancers are associated with HPV and of those HPV-associated cancers, 90% are due to HPV-16 and -18.[77] Rates of anal cancers are highest in HIV-infected men who have sex with men (MSM).[78,79] Anal HPV infections are also common in adolescent and adult women with rates ranging from 13% to 50%.[80,81] Overall statistics for anal cancers demonstrate that women actually have higher rates than men.[82] In addition, the incidence of anal cancer is rising in both men and women[83] with the annual average incidence of anal cancer in women being 1935 while in men it is 1083. The higher incidence of anal cancer in women than men seems counterintuitive, but may be due to anal intercourse occurring more commonly than realized in heterosexual women and that the majority of men engage in heterosexual practices. As in men, the highest rates of anal HPV in women are found in those who are HIV infected.[79] A study of HIV-infected adolescent girls found that almost 60% had anal HPV infections.[81] Risks for anal cancer in women include a history of cervical, vaginal, and vulvar cancer and CIN3.[84-86] The association of anal cancer with HIV and other HPV-associated cancers underscore the importance of the immune response (or lack thereof) in controlling HPV infection.

*Penile Cancer*

As found in the vulvar cancers, HPV is associated with specific histologic types of penile cancers. Almost 100% of basaloid and warty penile cancers are associated with high risk HPV types (ie, HPV types associated with cancer), whereas only 30–40% of keratinizing squamous cell cancers are associated with HPV.[87]

*Oropharyngeal Cancer*

HPV is also associated with oropharyngeal cancers in both men and women.[88] Overall, ~25% of head and neck cancers are linked to HPV. The tonsil and the base of the tongue appear the most vulnerable with ~50% being associated with HPV. The sexual behaviors related to an increased risk of these cancers include multiple sexual partners, reporting oral sex, and for men, having sex with other men.[89] HPV DNA detection of the oropharynx is much lower than anogenital infections in both men and women. Most studies have published rates of oral HPV around 4–5%.[90] These figures are likely underestimations since most studies sampled the buccal mucosa or tongue, whereas HPV likely sits deep in tonsillar crypts or at the base of the tongue. Currently, there are no screening recommendations for oropharyngeal cancers.

**Epidemiology and Natural History of Anogenital HPV in Males**

As in the cervix, HPV is frequently found in samples obtained from the anus and male genital area. With better sampling techniques and extremely sensitive DNA detection kits, rates of HPV in the male anogenital area are similar to women. Approximately 20% of men (range 1.3–72.9%) will have HPV DNA detected in the anogenital area.[91] However, in MSM, the rates of anal HPV are much higher, with a prevalence of more than 90% being reported.[92,93] Like women, risks for HPV in the anogenital area in men is associated with a greater number of lifetime sexual partners.[92,94] However, unlike women, young men are as likely as older men to be HPV positive.[87,92] This is true whether the men are heterosexual or MSM.

Natural history studies of HPV in men show that HPV clears faster in heterosexual men than in women. One study found that over a 1-year period, 94% of men cleared penile/scrotal HPV compared with a clearance rate of only 80% in women with anogenital infection.[95] HPV infections of the anus in both men and women also appear to clear faster than cervical infections in women.[92,96] On the other hand, similar to cervical infection in HIV-infected women, HIV-infected men and women are unlikely to clear their anal infections.[81,93]

Few studies have examined the rate of intraepithelial lesions in men. Most importantly, there are no natural history studies of intraepithelial lesions in males demonstrating that they result in cancer. However, in studies examining HPV in penile (PIN) or anal (AIN) intraepithelial neoplastic lesions (which are histologically equivalent to CIN), HPV is found in a similar proportions as CIN.[97] About 80–90% of AIN and PIN are associated with high-risk HPV.

## Screening for Anal and Penile Cancer

Since no study has proven that intraepithelial neoplastic (IN) lesions in males progress to invasive cancer, screening for IN in males remains controversial. Because penile cancers in the United States are rare, there are no screening recommendations. In contrast, the rate of anal cancer in HIV-infected MSM is estimated to be equal to that of cervical cancer before cytology screening was initiated in the United States.[92] Studies have shown that it is cost-effective to screen MSM.[98] If abnormal, high-resolution anoscopy by a trained provider is recommended. Treatment is recommended if AIN is found on histology.[92] Although anal cancers are also more prevalent in HIV-infected women, HIV-uninfected MSM, and in women with cervical cancer, there are no screening recommendations for these groups. Clearly, studies are needed to better assess the utility of screening in groups other than HIV-infected MSM.[99]

## HPV Vaccine in Males

Clearly, if anogenital and oropharyngeal cancers can be prevented with HPV vaccination, there is a direct benefit to men in HPV vaccination. As noted, most of the HPV-associated anogenital and oropharyngeal cancers are HPV 16/18 associated and as in women nearly all external genital warts are associated with HPV 6/11. Recent data were released on the quadrivalent HPV vaccine trial in men. The trial examined 3463 men aged 16–23 years. Men were excluded if they had a history of external genital warts, genital lesions thought to be associated with HPV, and >5 lifetime sexual partners. The data showed similar results as seen in the women with an efficacy rate of 89% in preventing external genital warts in the per protocol group (received all 3 vaccines and were naïve to HPV 6, 11, 16, and 18 at baseline). In the full cohort who received at least one vaccination and included all subjects regardless of baseline HPV status, the efficacy was 67%. The FDA approved the quadrivalent vaccine in men based on this data and ACIP gave permissive recommendations for boys aged 11–12 years with a recommendation for catchup of males 13–26 years of age. There was also a substudy within the men's trial examining young MSM. The study enrolled 602 MSM aged 16–26 years of age and found an efficacy rate of 77.5% in preventing HPV 6/11/16/18 AIN in the per protocol group.

## CONCLUSIONS

HPV is extremely common in adolescents and likely related to numerous factors including sexual behavior, immunologic, and biological vulnerability. In addition to cervical cancer in women, HPV in both men and women has been associated with other anogenital cancers and cancers in nongenital areas, specifically the oropharynx. The data now show that the majority of adolescents will clear HPV including HPV-associated lesions such as CIN1 and CIN2 and that progression to cancer is extremely rare. Most disappointingly, the current cervical cancer screening technique of cytology does not appear to prevent the few cases of invasive cervical cancer that occurs in these young women. These data support the postponement of cervical cancer screening until 21 years of age. In those adolescents diagnosed with HPV-associated diseases, observation is preferred. Prevention of cervical cancer and genital warts in adolescents should focus on the successful administration of the HPV vaccine. The data clearly show that the group most likely to benefit are persons that have not experienced sexual intercourse. There is also benefit on a personal level for those who have initiated sexual intercourse but the benefit declines quickly with age and number of sexual partners.

## REFERENCES

1. Doorbar J. Molecular biology of human papillomavirus infection and cervical cancer. *Clin Sci (Lond)*. 2006;110(5);525–541
2. Durst M, Kleinheinz A, Hotz M, Gissman L. The physical state of human papillomavirus type 16 DNA in benign and malignant genital tumours. *J Gen Virol*. 1985;66(7):1515–1522
3. Solomon D, Davey D, Kurman R, et al. The 2001 Bethesda System: terminology for reporting results of cervical cytology. *JAMA*. 2002;287(16);2114–2119
4. Stanley M. Immune responses to human papillomavirus. *Vaccine*. 2006;24 Suppl 1:S16–S22
5. Woodworth CD. HPV Innate Immunity. *Front Biosci*. 2002;7(7);d2058–d2071
6. Farhat S, Nakagawa M, Moscicki AB. Cell-mediated immune responses to human papillomavirus 16 E6 and E7 antigens as measured by interferon gamma enzyme-linked immunospot in women with cleared or persistent human papillomavirus infection. *Int J Gynecol Cancer*. 2009;19(4):508–512
7. Molling JW, de Gruijl TD, Glim J, et al. CD4(+)CD25hi regulatory T-cell frequency correlates with persistence of human papillomavirus type 16 and T helper cell responses in patients with cervical intraepithelial neoplasia. *Int J Cancer*. 2007;121(8):1749–1755
8. Frazer IH. Interaction of human papillomaviruses with the host immune system: a well evolved relationship. *Virology*. 2009;384(2):410–414
9. Moscicki AB, Ellenberg JH, Vermund SH, et al. Prevalence of and risks for cervical human papillomavirus infection and squamous intraepithelial lesions in adolescent girls: impact of infection with human immunodeficiency virus. *Arch Ped Adolesc Med*. 2000;154:127–134
10. Moscicki AB, Hills N, Shiboski S, et al. Risks for incident human papillomavirus infection and low-grade squamous intraepithelial lesion development in young females. *JAMA*. 2001;285(23); 2995–3002
11. Moscicki AB, Palefsky J, Gonzales J, Schoolnik G. Human papillomavirus infection in sexually active adolescent females: Prevalence and risk factors. *Pediatr Res*. 1990;28:507–513
12. Winer RL, Lee SK, Hughes JP, Adam DE, Kiviat NB, Koutsky LA. Genital human papillomavirus infection: incidence and risk factors in a cohort of female university students. *Am J Epidemiol*. 2003;157(3);218–226
13. Brown DR, Shew ML, Qadadri B, et al. A longitudinal study of genital human papillomavirus infection in a cohort of closely followed adolescent women. *J Infect Dis*. 2005;191(2):182–192
14. Munoz N, Mendez F, Posso H, et al. Incidence, duration, and determinants of cervical human papillomavirus infection in a cohort of Colombian women with normal cytological results. *J Infect Dis*. 2004;190(12):2077–2087
15. Evander M, Edlund K, Gustaffson A, et al. Human papillomavirus infection is transient in young women: a population-based cohort study. *J Infect Dis*. 1995;171:1026–1030

16. Ho GY, Bierman R, Beardsley L, Chang CJ, Burk RD. Natural history of cervicovaginal papillomavirus infection in young women. *N Engl J Med*. 1998;338(7):423–428
17. Moscicki AB, Ellenberg JH, Fahrat S, Xu J. HPV persistence in HIV infected and uninfected adolescent girls: risk factors and differences by phylogenetic types. *J Infect Dis*. 2004;190(1):37–45
18. Moscicki AB, Shiboski S, Broering J, et al. The natural history of human papillomavirus infection as measured by repeated DNA testing in adolescent and young women. *J Pediatr*. 1998;132:277–284
19. Mount SL, Papillo JL. A Study of 10,296 pediatric and adolescent Papanicolaou smear diagnoses in northern New England. *Pediatrics*. 1999;103(3):539–546
20. Woodman CB, Collins S, Winter H, et al. Natural history of cervical human papillomavirus infection in young women: a longitudinal cohort study. *Lancet*. 2001;357(9271);1831–1836
21. International Collaboration. Comparison of risk factors for invasive squamous cell carcinoma and adenocarcinoma of the cervix: collaborative reanalysis of individual data on 8,097 women with squamous cell carcinoma and 1,374 women with adenocarcinoma from 12 epidemiological studies. *Int J Cancer*. 2007;120(4):885–891
22. Appleby P, Beral V, Berrington de Gonzalez A, et al. Cervical cancer and hormonal contraceptives: collaborative reanalysis of individual data for 16,573 women with cervical cancer and 35,509 women without cervical cancer from 24 epidemiological studies. *Lancet*. 2007;370(9599):1609–1621
23. Modiano JF, Kokai Y, Weiner DB, Pykett MJ, Nowell PC, Lyttle CR. Progesterone augments proliferation induced by epidermal growth factor in a feline mammary adenocarcinoma cell line. *J Cell Biochem*. 1991;45(2):196–206
24. Ruutu M, Wahlroos N, Syrjanen K, Johansson B, Syrjanen S. Effects of 17beta-estradiol and progesterone on transcription of human papillomavirus 16 E6/E7 oncogenes in CaSki and SiHa cell lines. *Int J Gynecol Cancer*. 2006;16(3);1261–1268
25. Burchell A, Winer R, de Sanjose S, Franco E. Epidemiolgy and transmission dynamics of genital human papillomavirus infection. *Vaccine Monographs*. 2006;24(Suppl 3):52–62
26. De Sanjose S. La investigacion sobre la infeccion por virus del papiloma human y el cancer de cuello uterino en Espana. In: de Sanjose S, Garcia A, eds. *El Virus del papiloma human y cancer: Epidemiologia y Prevencion*. Madrid: EMISA; 2006
27. Franceschi S, Herrero R, Clifford GM, et al. Variations in the age-specific curves of human papillomavirus prevalence in women worldwide. *Int J Cancer*. 2006;119(11):2677–2684
28. Olsson SE, Villa LL, Costa RL, et al. Induction of immune memory following administration of a prophylactic quadrivalent human papillomavirus (HPV) types 6/11/16/18 L1 virus-like particle (VLP) vaccine. *Vaccine*. 2007;25(26):4931–4939
29. Olsson SE, Kjaer SK, Sigurdsson K, et al. Evaluation of quadrivalent HPV 6/11/16/18 vaccine efficacy against cervical and anogenital disease in subjects with serological evidence of prior vaccine type HPV infection. *Hum Vaccin*. 2009;5(10)
30. Paavonen J, Naud P, Salmeron J, et al. Efficacy of human papillomavirus (HPV)-16/18 AS04-adjuvanted vaccine against cervical infection and precancer caused by oncogenic HPV types (PATRICIA): final analysis of a double-blind, randomised study in young women. *Lancet*. 2009;374(9686):301–314
31. Green J, Berrington de Gonzalez A, Sweetland S, et al. Risk factors for adenocarcinoma and squamous cell carcinoma of the cervix in women aged 20–44 years: the UK National Case-Control Study of Cervical Cancer. *Br J Cancer*. 2003;89(11);2078–2086
32. Herrero R, Brinton LA, Reeves WC, et al. Sexual behavior, venereal diseases, hygiene practices, and invasive cervical cancer in a high-risk population. *Cancer*. 1990;65(2):380–386
33. Sierra-Torres CH, Tyring SK, Au WW. Risk contribution of sexual behavior and cigarette smoking to cervical neoplasia. *Int J Gynecol Cancer*. 2003;13(5):617–625
34. Cervical carcinoma and sexual behavior: collaborative reanalysis of individual data on 15,461 women with cervical carcinoma and 29,164 women without cervical carcinoma from 21 epidemiological studies. *Cancer Epidemiol Biomarkers Prev*. 2009;18(4):1060–1069
35. Moscicki AB, Singer A. The cervical epithelium during puberty and adolescence. In: Jordan JA, Singer A, eds. *The Cervix: 2nd ed*. Malden: Blackwell; 2006:81–101

36. Castle PE, Jeronimo J, Schiffman M, et al. Age-related changes of the cervix influence human papillomavirus type distribution. *Cancer Res.* 2006;66(2);1218–1224
37. Moscicki AB, Grubbs-Burt V, Kanowitz S, Darragh T, Shiboski S. The significance of squamous metaplasia in the development of low grade squamous intra-epithelial lesions in young women. *Cancer.* 1999;85:1139–1144
38. Hwang LY, Ma Y, Benningfield SM, et al. Factors that influence the rate of epithelial maturation in the cervix in healthy young women. *J Adolesc Health.* 2009;44(2):103–110
39. Watson M, Saraiya M, Ahmed F, et al. Using population-based cancer registry data to assess the burden of human papillomavirus-associated cancers in the United States: overview of methods. *Cancer.* 2008;113(10 Suppl):2841–2854
40. Chan PG, Sung HY, Sawaya GF. Changes in cervical cancer incidence after three decades of screening US women less than 30 years old. *Obstet Gynecol.* 2003;102(4);765–773
41. Sasieni P, Castanon A, Cuzick J. Effectiveness of cervical screening with age: population based case-control study of prospectively recorded data. *BMJ.* 2009;339:b2968
42. Gustafsson L, Ponten J, Zack M, Adami HO. International incidence rates of invasive cervical cancer after introduction of cytological screening. *Cancer Causes Control.* 1997;8(5):755–763
43. Barnholtz-Sloan J, Patel N, Rollison D, Kortepeter K, Mackinnon J, Giuliano A. Incidence trends of invasive cervical cancer in the United States by combined race and ethnicity. *Cancer Causes Control.* 2009;20(7):1129–1138
44. Plummer M, Schiffman M, Castle PE, Maucort-Boulch D, Wheeler CM. A 2-year prospective study of human papillomavirus persistence among women with a cytological diagnosis of atypical squamous cells of undetermined significance or low-grade squamous intraepithelial lesion. *J Infect Dis.* 2007;195(11):1582–1589
45. Heatley MK. How should we grade CIN? *Histopathology.* 2002;40(4):377–390
46. Moore K, Cofer A, Elliot L, Lanneau G, Walker J, Gold MA. Adolescent cervical dysplasia: histologic evaluation, treatment, and outcomes. *Am J Obstet Gynecol.* 2007;197(2):e141–e146
47. Castle PE, Schiffman M, Wheeler CM, Solomon D. Evidence for frequent regression of cervical intraepithelial neoplasia-grade 2. *Obstet Gynecol.* 2009;113(1):18–25
48. Castle PE, Stoler MH, Solomon D, Schiffman M. The relationship of community biopsy-diagnosed cervical intraepithelial neoplasia grade 2 to the quality control pathology-reviewed diagnoses: an ALTS report. *Am J Clin Pathol.* 2007;127(5):805–815
49. Moscicki AB, Ma Y, Wibbelsman C, et al. Risks for cervical intraepithelial neoplasia 3 among adolescents and young women with abnormal cytology. *Obstet Gynecol.* 2008;112(6):1335–1342
50. Winer RL, Kiviat NB, Hughes JP, et al. Development and duration of human papillomavirus lesions, after initial infection. *J Infect Dis.* 2005;191(5);731–738
51. Moscicki AB, Cox JT. Practice improvement in cervical screening and management (PICSM): symposium on management of cervical abnormalities in adolescents and young women. *J Low Genit Tract Dis.* 2010;14(1):73–80
52. Saslow D, Runowicz CD, Solomon D, et al. American Cancer Society guideline for the early detection of cervical neoplasia and cancer. *CA Cancer J Clin.* 2002;52(6);342–362
53. American College of Obstetricians and Gynecologists. *ACOG Guidelines for Women's Health Care.* Washington, DC: The American College of Obstetricians and Gynecologists; 2007.
54. American Society for Colposcopy and Cervical Pathology. Available at: www.asccp.org. Accessed June 26, 2010
55. Kyrgiou M, Koliopoulos G, Martin-Hirsch P, Arbyn M, Prendiville W, Paraskevaidis E. Obstetric outcomes after conservative treatment for intraepithelial or early invasive cervical lesions: systematic review and meta-analysis. *Lancet.* 2006;367(9509);489–498
56. Norman JE. Preterm labour. Cervical function and prematurity. *Best Pract Res Clin Obstet Gynaecol.* 2007;21(5):791–806
57. Sadler L, Saftlas A, Wang W, Exeter M, Whittaker J, McCowan L. Treatment for cervical intraepithelial neoplasia and risk of preterm delivery. *JAMA.* 2004;291:2100–2106
58. Samson S-L, Bentley JR, Fahey TJ, McKay DJ, Gil GH. The effect of loop electrosurgical excision. *Obstet Gynecol.* 2005;105:325–332

59. Coeshott CM, Smithson SL, Verderber E, et al. Pluronic F127-based systemic vaccine delivery systems. *Vaccine.* 2004;22(19):2396–2405
60. Pinto LA, Castle PE, Roden RB, et al. HPV-16 L1 VLP vaccine elicits a broad-spectrum of cytokine responses in whole blood. *Vaccine.* 2005;23(27):3555–3564
61. Pinto LA, Edwards J, Castle PE, et al. Cellular immune responses to human papillomavirus (HPV)-16 L1 in healthy volunteers immunized with recombinant HPV-16 L1 virus-like particles. *J Infect Dis.* 2003;188(2):327–338
62. Schreckenberger C, Kaufmann AM. Vaccination strategies for the treatment and prevention of cervical cancer. *Curr Opin Oncol.* 2004;16(5):485–491
63. Schiller JT, Nardelli-Haefliger D. Chapter 17: Second generation HPV vaccines to prevent cervical cancer. *Vaccine.* 2006;24 Suppl 3:S147–S153
64. Koutsky LA, Ault KA, Wheeler CM, et al. A controlled trial of a human papillomavirus type 16 vaccine. *N Engl J Med.* 2002;347(21);1645–1651
65. Mao C, Koutsky LA, Ault KA, et al. Efficacy of human papillomavirus-16 vaccine to prevent cervical intraepithelial neoplasia: a randomized controlled trial. *Obstet Gynecol.* 2006;107(1):18–27
66. Villa LL, Costa RL, Petta CA, et al. Prophylactic quadrivalent human papillomavirus (types 6, 11, 16, and 18) L1 virus-like particle vaccine in young women: a randomised double-blind placebo-controlled multicentre phase II efficacy trial. *Lancet Oncol.* 2005;6(5):271–278
67. Emeny RT, Wheeler CM, Jansen KU, et al. Priming of human papillomavirus type 11-specific humoral and cellular immune responses in college-aged women with a virus-like particle vaccine. *J Virol.* 2002;76(15):7832–7842
68. Garland SM, Hernandez-Avila M, Wheeler CM, et al. Quadrivalent vaccine against human papillomavirus to prevent anogenital diseases. *N Engl J Med.* 2007;356(19):1928–1943
69. The FUTURE II Study Group. Quadrivalent vaccine against human papillomavirus to prevent high-grade cervical lesions. *N Engl J Med* 2007;356(19):1915–1927
70. Kjaer SK, Sigurdsson K, Iversen OE, et al. A pooled analysis of continued prophylactic efficacy of quadrivalent human papillomavirus (Types 6/11/16/18) vaccine against high-grade cervical and external genital lesions. *Cancer Prev Res (Phila Pa).* 2009;2(10):868–878
71. Paavonen J, Jenkins D, Bosch FX, et al. Efficacy of a prophylactic adjuvanted bivalent L1 virus-like-particle vaccine against infection with human papillomavirus types 16 and 18 in young women: an interim analysis of a phase III double-blind, randomised controlled trial. *Lancet.* 2007;369(9580):2161–2170
72. Fraser C, Tomassini JE, Xi L, et al. Modeling the long-term antibody response of a human papillomavirus (HPV) virus-like particle (VLP) type 16 prophylactic vaccine. *Vaccine.* 2007;25(21):4324–4333
73. Mosher WD, Chandra A, Jones J. Sexual behavior and selected health measures: men and women 15–44 years of age, United States, 2002. *Adv Data.* 2005;362:1–55
74. Markowitz LE, Sternberg M, Dunne EF, McQuillan G, Unger ER. Seroprevalence of human papillomavirus types 6, 11, 16, and 18 in the United States: National Health and Nutrition Examination Survey 2003-2004. *J Infect Dis.* 2009;200(7):1059–1067
75. Saslow D, Castle PE, Cox JT, et al. American Cancer Society Guideline for human papillomavirus (HPV) vaccine use to prevent cervical cancer and its precursors. *CA Cancer J Clin.* 2007;57(1):7–28
76. Dempsey AF, Gebremariam A, Koutsky LA, Manhart L. Using risk factors to predict human papillomavirus infection: implications for targeted vaccination strategies in young adult women. *Vaccine.* 2008;26(8):1111–1117
77. Daling JR, Sherman KJ. Relationship between human papillomavirus infection and tumours of anogenital sites other than the cervix. *IARC Sci Publ.* 1992(119):223–241
78. Frisch M, Biggar RJ, Goedert JJ. Human papillomavirus-associated cancers in patients with human immunodeficiency virus infection and acquired immunodeficiency syndrome. *J Natl Cancer Inst.* 2000;92(18):1500–1510
79. Palefsky JM, Gillison ML, Strickler HD. Chapter 16: HPV vaccines in immunocompromised women and men. *Vaccine.* 2006;24 Suppl 3:S140–S146

80. Goodman MT, Shvetsov YB, McDuffie K, et al. Acquisition of anal human papillomavirus (HPV) infection in women: the Hawaii HPV Cohort study. *J Infect Dis.* 2008;197(7):957–966
81. Moscicki AB, Durako SJ, Houser J, et al. Human papillomavirus infection and abnormal cytology of the anus in HIV-infected and uninfected adolescents. *AIDS.* 2003;17(3);311–320
82. American Cancer Society. *Cancer facts and figures, 2008.* Atlanta, GA: American Cancer Society; 2008
83. Partridge JM, Koutsky LA. Genital human papillomavirus infection in men. *Lancet Infect Dis.* 2006;6(1):21–31
84. Melbye M, Smith E, Wohlfahrt J, et al. Anal and cervical abnormality in women–prediction by human papillomavirus. *Int J Cancer.* 1996;68:559–564
85. Ogunbiyi OA, Scholefield JH, Robertson G, Smith JH, Sharp F, Rogers K. Anal human papillomavirus infection and squamous neoplasia in patients with invasive vulvar cancer. *Obstet Gynecol.* 1994;83(2):212–216
86. Park IU, Ogilvie JW Jr, Anderson KE, et al. Anal human papillomavirus infection and abnormal anal cytology in women with genital neoplasia. *Gynecol Oncol.* 2009;114(3):399–403
87. Giuliano AR, Tortolero-Luna G, Ferrer E, et al. Epidemiology of human papillomavirus infection in men, cancers other than cervical and benign conditions. *Vaccine.* 2008;26 Suppl 10:K17–K28
88. Kreimer AR, Clifford GM, Boyle P, Franceschi S. Human papillomavirus types in head and neck squamous cell carcinomas worldwide: a systematic review. *Cancer Epidemiol Biomarkers Prev.* 2005;14(2):467–475
89. Heck JE, Berthiller J, Vaccarella S, et al. Sexual behaviours and the risk of head and neck cancers: a pooled analysis in the International Head and Neck Cancer Epidemiology (INHANCE) consortium. *Int J Epidemiol.* 2010;39(1):166–181
90. Kreimer AR, Bhatia RK, Messeguer AL, Gonzalez P, Herrero R, Giuliano AR. Oral human papillomavirus in healthy individuals: a systematic review of the literature. *Sex Transm Dis.* 2010;37(6):386–391
91. Dunne EF, Nielson CM, Stone KM, Markowitz LE, Giuliano AR. Prevalence of HPV infection among men: A systematic review of the literature. *J Infect Dis.* 2006;194(8):1044–1057
92. Palefsky JM, Rubin M. The epidemiology of anal human papillomavirus and related neoplasia. *Obstet Gynecol Clin North Am.* 2009;36(1):187–200
93. de Pokomandy A, Rouleau D, Ghattas G, et al. Prevalence, clearance, and incidence of anal human papillomavirus infection in HIV-infected men: the HIPVIRG cohort study. *J Infect Dis.* 2009;199(7):965–973
94. Nyitray A, Nielson CM, Harris RB, et al. Prevalence of and risk factors for anal human papillomavirus infection in heterosexual men. *J Infect Dis.* 2008;197(12):1676–1684
95. van Doornum GJ, Prins M, Juffermans LH, et al. Regional distribution and incidence of human papillomavirus infections among heterosexual men and women with multiple sexual partners: a prospective study. *Genitourinary Med.* 1994;70(4):240–246
96. Shvetsov YB, Hernandez BY, McDuffie K, et al. Duration and clearance of anal human papillomavirus (HPV) infection among women: the Hawaii HPV cohort study. *Clin Infect Dis.* 2009;48(5):536–546
97. Aynaud O, Ionesco M, Barrasso R. Penile intraepithelial neoplasia. Specific clinical features correlate with histologic and virologic findings. *Cancer.* 1994;74(6):1762–1767
98. Goldie SJ, Kuntz KM, Weinstein MC, Freedberg KA, Palefsky JM. Cost-effectiveness of screening for anal squamous intraepithelial lesions and anal cancer in human immunodeficiency virus-negative homosexual and bisexual men. *Am J Med.* 2000;108(8):634–641
99. Chiao EY, Giordano TP, Palefsky JM, Tyring S, El Serag H. Screening HIV-infected individuals for anal cancer precursor lesions: a systematic review. *Clin Infect Dis.* 2006;43(2):223–233

# Human Immunodeficiency Virus Infection in Adolescents

Corinne Lehmann, MD, MEd*[a], Lawrence J. D'Angelo, MD, MPH[b]

[a]Departments of Pediatrics and Internal Medicine, Division of Adolescent Medicine, Cincinnati Children's Hospital Medical Center/University of Cincinnati College of Medicine, 3333 Burnet Avenue, Cincinnati, OH 45229
[b]Department of Pediatrics, Medicine, Prevention, and Community Health & Epidemiology, Division of Adolescent and Young Adult Medicine, Children's National Medical Center/George Washington University, 111 Michigan Avenue NW, Washington, DC 20010

It is currently estimated that over 1 million people are infected with the human immunodeficiency virus (HIV) in the United States.[1] While significant declines have been seen in the number of children perinatally infected with HIV, adolescents and young adults (15–29 years) have seen either stable or steadily increasing rates of HIV infection over the years 2003–2007. In 2006, persons aged 13–29 years accounted for 34% of all new infections, the largest number of new HIV infections in any age group. In the overall population, new HIV infections increased 15% in the time period 2003–2007.[2] Some of the increase in the number of infections may be attributed to improved laboratory-based tracking technology, which can improve detection of more recent infections, as well as additional information that states are now reporting to the Centers for Disease Control and Prevention (CDC). However, many providers are concerned that the reported rates of HIV infection in youth reflect a true increase in HIV incidence unrelated to the new ways of tracking recent HIV infections.[3]

Specific populations of adolescents are disproportionately affected by HIV. In an analysis of CDC data from the previous time period of 1999–2003, Rangel and colleagues noted the increase in HIV diagnoses were driven by increased cases in young men who have sex with men (MSM).[4] For HIV-infected males, MSM is the transmission mode in 83–87% of cases. Young men made up 69% of youth diagnosed with HIV infection in the age range of 13–19 years in 2007, increasing to 77% in the 20–24 year range. Overall in the years 2003–2007, MSMs had a 26% increase in annual HIV diagnoses.[2] African-American youth have been

*Corresponding author.
E-mail address: corinne.lehmann@cchmc.org (C. Lehmann).

hardest hit by the HIV epidemic, making up 72% of teens 13–19 years diagnosed in 2007.[2] Hispanics and youth living in the South are also disproportionately affected by HIV.[4] While the rates of HIV infection in young women have remained stable for several years, HIV and acquired immune deficiency syndrome (AIDS) is the number one killer of African-American women ages 24–34 years. At the current time, MSM and racial minorities are the patients most severely impacted by the rise in new HIV infections.

**Defining Which Adolescents Are Infected: HIV Testing in Teens**

To initiate treatment and prevention for HIV-infected individuals, we need to assure that as many HIV-infected people as possible know their diagnosis. In 2003, an estimated 25% of the then nearly 1 million HIV infected Americans were unaware of their HIV status. This led the CDC to expand its recommendations in 2006 to endorse HIV screening for all Americans aged 13–64 years.[5] Earlier guidance only called to regularly test people with a higher risk of acquiring HIV infection and all pregnant women. The new recommendations were clearly intended to shift providers from only doing risk-based screening to routinely screening all patients. For the adolescent and young adult age group, this was particularly relevant. Although data from 2006 showed that the overall percentage of individuals unaware of their infected status decreased to 21%, for those 13–29 years old, 47.8% remained unaware that they were HIV infected.[6] It is fair to point out that not all recommendations support this comprehensive screening approach. While the US Preventative Services Task Force gave an "A" recommendation to screening all adolescents and adults at increased risk for HIV infection and all pregnant women, the recommendation to routinely screen all adolescents and adults who are not at increased risk for HIV infection was given a "C" recommendation (no recommendation for or against the routine screen).[7]

The 2006 CDC recommendations further endorsed discontinuing all written consent and mandatory prevention counseling before HIV testing. This "opt-out" approach would allow providers to verbally notify patients that HIV testing will be performed and then allow time for the patient either to ask questions about the testing or to decline. Nonetheless, these consent recommendations have yet to be fully implemented since most states still have their own laws regarding testing that may require written or at least direct verbal consent, as well as pre- and posttest counseling. While some states have amended their laws to make testing easier, others have not done so or have developed legal revisions that are not consistent with current CDC guidelines.[8] In addition, although all states allow minors to consent to testing, the minimum age of consent varies. Other differences in state laws impact how the risk information obtained from an adolescent may be handled. Eighteen states allow providers to inform parents when their teen requests or receives sexually transmitted infection (STI) testing or treatment if the provider feels that this would be in the best interest of the patient. Only one state, Iowa, requires providers to inform parents of a positive HIV test. Thirty-one states explicitly state that HIV testing and treatment are part of the STI services to which teens can consent.[9] The Alan Guttmacher Institute (www.guttmacher.org) maintains up-to-date information on each state's laws regarding minors' rights to consent to reproductive health care. Many providers who care for adolescents are still "catching up" with implementation of the changes in the CDC guidelines and state laws. A study in 2008 evaluating the implementation of routine adolescent HIV testing in a US urban emergency department revealed that 78% of providers were still unaware of the revised testing guidelines. Although 58% of the providers stated that the patient or guardian would refuse testing, of the those patients routinely offered screening (37% of eligible patients), only 13% opted out.[10]

Besides provider-based behaviors, many other patient-related issues create additional barriers to adolescent HIV testing. These include stigma/fear of diagnosis, payment concerns, inadvertent insurance or billing disclosure, testing type (blood versus oral), time, access to testing, and perceived lack of risk. In a study of youth seeking HIV testing in Maryland, teens cited having a free test, rapid test results, a convenient location, and the ability to speak with someone about testing as factors that would make testing easier.[11] In a community-based survey in Pittsburgh of youth ages 14–24 years, the most common reasons for not being tested were fear of testing positive, not knowing anyone living with HIV, and fear of needles.[12] Another study conducted by Kowalczyk Mullins et al in an urban teen clinic found that 70% of teens preferred rapid testing, which was also associated with improved receipt of HIV test results.[13] Among youth with sexually acquired HIV infection in an urban Georgia clinic, the most common reason given for getting an HIV test was routine health care; few adolescents initiated the HIV testing themselves.[14] To increase the rates of HIV testing in teens, providers need to offer testing as part of routine care; be knowledgeable about state laws around STI testing, consent, and disclosure; and have rapid, low-cost testing available in their offices.

Many behaviors put youth at risk for acquiring HIV and some youth are at greater risk of becoming infected than others. In a recent survey of 352 HIV-infected youth from 5 US cities, 60% had problem-level substance use and 42% had higher risk sexual behavior.[15] Youth who are homeless, runaway, in foster care, victims of abuse, incarcerated, substance using, or mentally ill are all at increased risk for HIV infection.[16] For males, being gay, bisexual, or transgender is associated with increased rates infection. Identifying males in this high-risk group can sometimes be challenging. Since sexual identity and actual sexual behavior may be discordant, providers should base their risk assessment on a history of specific sexual behaviors, such as anal intercourse, rather than on stated sexual orientation. In the CDC Young Men's Survey, 18% of HIV-positive African-American men reported feelings of isolation and disapproval of their sexual orientation.[17] Coupled with exploration of sexual identity during adolescence, many young men may not consider or may even deny their sexual behavior as being gay. For young women, heterosexual transmission accounts for the majority of HIV infection. Futterman noted that half of the women in a New York City Adolescent AIDS program stated that they had only 1 sexual partner.[18] Teens need to be educated that it is sexual behavior, not sexual identity, that dictates the need for condom use and determines HIV risk.

Regional context may also play a role in youth HIV infection. In a New York City Adolescent AIDS program, 21% of sexually infected youth had an HIV-positive parent.[16] Some providers feel that contemporary youth view HIV/AIDS as a chronic disease rather than a life-threatening problem. Others have raised concern that compared with their older counterparts, teens in the current generation have not had as much exposure to safe-sex messages because of the lack of comprehensive sex education in the United States during the last decade. While national surveys of youth indicate decreasing rates of sexual activity with stable rates of condom use over the last decade,[19] abstinence-only sexual education programs, which proliferated during that same time frame, have been found in scientific reviews to be ineffective in decreasing STI and pregnancy rates.[20]

## Natural History of HIV Infection in Adolescents

In addition to the behavioral risk factors for infection, several biological factors make it more likely for adolescents to become infected with HIV and influence the course of their illness. It is presumed that the inflammation and mucosal breaks from other STIs increase transmission of HIV. Younger women may have an additional biological risk compared with adult women because a larger surface area of their cervical mucosa is made up of a single-layer of columnar cells, making them more susceptible to acquisition of certain STIs.[16] Adolescent males who are not circumcised may have an increased risk of infection since the lining of the foreskin creates a larger mucosal surface that is more susceptible to HIV infection. Circumcision lessens the chances of males acquiring HIV infection. However, although observational studies in Africa suggest that circumcised HIV-infected males have lower HIV transmission rates to female partners, controlled clinical trials have failed to demonstrate this.[21]

Once infected, data suggests that youth ages 13–24 years survive longer with an AIDS diagnosis compared with older adults.[2] Adolescents with HIV may be able to preserve their immune function longer than older patients, perhaps allowing them to remain healthier for a longer period of time. While adolescents have $CD4^+$ cell counts similar to adults, it may be that the adolescent thymus functions differently and slows down the rate of immune system destruction. Younger HIV-infected patients may have a higher thymic volume compared with older adults and have more new thymic emigrants shown by T-cell receptor excision circle (TREC) analysis.[22] Although these differences in the immune system allow individual adolescents to remain asymptomatic for a longer period of time, it may also contribute to further delay in diagnosis, and a longer period of potential HIV transmission before they are aware of their status.

Once infected, most adolescents do not immediately enter care. Luckily, when they are diagnosed and linked to care, they are most often still asymptomatic. In a recent study of newly infected youth at 15 US sites in the Adolescent Trials Network (ATN),[23] 53% of whites were found to be recently infected compared with 28.4% of blacks and 26% of Hispanics. In the subset of young adult MSMs, 48% of black youth were recently infected, compared with 25% of whites and 28% of Hispanics. Overall, 33% of these young people were found to have a recent infection, which is much higher than reports of older adults. In the ATN study, the median CD4 count was 542 in the recently infected patients and 437 in those with established infection.[23] Early diagnosis and entry to care leads to lower patient mortality in adults[24] and has implications in potentially lowering HIV transmission rates. While further data are pending, this study provides encouraging evidence that teens are getting tested and entering into care earlier than their adult counterparts.

### The Other Population of HIV-Infected Teens: Adolescents Infected Perinatally

While much deserved attention has been placed on identifying and treating teens with sexually acquired HIV, there is another growing population of teens with HIV: adolescents who have been infected perinatally. While the landmark 1994 maternal-child HIV transmission trial showed that using AZT (zidovudine) perinatally decreased HIV infection rates in infants from 25% to 6%,[25] thousands of infants had already been infected by their HIV-positive mothers. Fortunately, for those adolescents who survived infancy and childhood, combined highly active antiretroviral treatment (HAART) regimens came into widespread use as early as 1996. The combined medication treatment approach markedly reduced mortality from 5.3% to 0.7% in children with HIV by the year 1999.[26]

Perinatally infected adolescents face some social and medical issues that differ from their uninfected and sexually HIV infected peers. Many of the teens have faced the loss of family members due to HIV, may be subject to placement into the foster care system, and may face long-standing isolation and stigma due to their diagnosis.[27] While increased rates of mental health diagnoses had been previously reported for perinatally infected youth, a recent study found similar rates of mental health diagnoses compared with an uninfected cohort population. However, the perinatally infected youth had higher rates of mental health interventions.[28] Many infected children are closely followed in pediatric HIV treatment programs and may have increased access to health care compared with uninfected peers.

Perinatally HIV-infected teens progress through the same adolescent developmental stages as uninfected teens including exploration of sexuality. While children being treated with HAART have been noted to have fewer infectious medical complications, there have been increasing incident rates of pregnancy and genital dysplasia in perinatally infected adolescents.[29] Although pregnancies occur in perinatally infected teens, the data should be viewed in the context of teen pregnancy rates in the general population. Overall pregnancy rates in one US perinatally infected cohort were substantially lower than uninfected teens.[30] In various reviews of adolescent perinatally infected mothers worldwide, subsequent infant HIV transmission rates have been cited at 0–10%.[31,32]

The often long history of antiretroviral treatment in many perinatally infected teens may lead to other medical complications stemming from treatment toxicities as well as from advancement of the HIV infection. These include conditions such as encephalopathy, pancreatitis, lower bone mineral density, renal disease, dyslipidemia, and cardiac disorders.[29,33] Medication-resistant HIV can also develop due to previous treatment and treatment interruptions. In a sample of 654 perinatally infected patients older than 10 years of age in the United Kingdom, 64% were on antiretrovirals, 18% were off treatment having previously been treated, and 18% were treatment naïve.[34] Of this cohort, 78% of the treated patients had undetectable viral loads with median CD4 count of 554. Only a small number of patients had triple drug class resistance and 12% had CD4 counts <200.

It is encouraging that many perinatally infected teens do not have any mental health or medical complications. In fact, it is not unheard of for many pediatric treatment programs to encounter perinatally infected teens who were not diagnosed until their teen years because they had been previously healthy.[16,35]

## Current Treatment of HIV-Infected Adolescents

*Initial Diagnosis*

Primary care providers are the initial point of contact for many adolescents diagnosed with HIV. For some clinicians, the thought of having to give this type of "bad news" to patients itself becomes a barrier to HIV testing.[36] With the availability of rapid HIV screening, providers are faced with the possibility of providing positive HIV screening results, which will require further confirmatory testing. When a provider discusses a positive screening test result, it is crucial to ensure that there is adequate time to calmly sit with the patient, regardless of their reaction to the news. While many patients will have thought through the possibility of having a positive test result in advance, others may be in shock. The provider will need to evaluate the patient for an acute grief reaction and determine their subsequent safety. Providers should pass on the message of hope in that HIV is not a death sentence and, with good medical care and medication, many people infected with HIV are living relatively normal lives.

The positive screening test must be confirmed by either a Western blot or immunofluorescence assay.[37] The provider must decide whether the confirmatory test will be done in the provider's office or a referral made to an HIV treatment program or local health department program. Specialized HIV treatment programs generally have the advantage of being well equipped to provide mental health support during and after the time of diagnosis, as well as ongoing financial, social work, and case management services. It is often helpful for patients who test preliminarily positive to bring a friend or loved one to help them when they get the confirmatory testing as they may be overwhelmed emotionally with the diagnosis and not able to focus on medical details that are being reviewed. As part of the confirmatory process, the provider should carefully review with the patient the positive and negative potential ramifications of revealing an HIV-positive diagnosis to others in their life. It is common for patients to initially feel that they cannot tell their family or that they will face verbal/physical abuse and/or the loss of home or financial support. For this reason, many patients need some time to reflect and find the right time to disclose to family and friends. Eventually, most teens do disclose to someone and the patient's mother is the most likely person to fulfill this role.[38]

While the overwhelming majority of newly diagnosed patients are asymptomatic, some may present with symptoms of acute HIV infection. According to the U.S. Department of Health and Human Services (DHHS), clinical evidence of acute HIV infection may include fever, lymphadenopathy, skin rash, myalgia/arthralgia, headache, diarrhea, oral ulcers, leukopenia, thrombocytopenia, and/or transaminase elevation. These signs and symptoms usually occur within 2–6 weeks of infection with HIV and may be missed because of overlap with other common infections that occur in young people, including Epstein-Barr virus, cytomegalovirus, influenza, herpes, syphilis, hepatitis, and streptococcal infections. In the scenario of acute infection, HIV antibody testing is usually negative and tests that detect the presence of actual virus as opposed to antibody (eg, p24, DNA polymerase chain reaction, RNA viral load) are far more accurate. While acknowledging that there is not enough research at this time to definitively support immediate drug treatment, the DHHS guidelines state that care providers can consider starting antiretroviral treatment in the setting of acute HIV infection. If treatment is started, it is still recommended that all of the initial laboratory studies listed in Table 1 be sent, including an HIV genotype test, since 6–16% of patients are infected with virus that is resistant to at least one antiretroviral agent.[39]

*Initial Laboratory Evaluation*

It is common for new patients to spend the first visit or two in HIV treatment programs coming to grips with their diagnosis and learning about the biology of HIV and how to take care of their health. This is an important step, and providers should slowly build on the information they provide by frequently asking patients

Table 1
Laboratory tests requested at initial HIV infection evaluation visit

| | |
|---|---|
| Complete blood count | Evaluates for anemia, white blood cell count, blood platelets |
| Blood urea nitrogen, electrolytes, creatine, fasting blood sugar | Evaluates kidney function, blood sugar control |
| Bilirubin, alkaline phosphatase, aspartate aminotransferase | Evaluates liver function |
| Amylase, lipase | Evaluates pancreatic status |
| Serologic tests (syphilis; hepatitis A, B, and C; toxoplasmosis; cytomegalovirus) | Evaluates for prior or latent infections |
| PAP smear | Evaluates for prior human papillomavirus infection |
| PPD skin test | Evaluates for infection with tuberculosis bacteria |
| T-cell subset | (CD4+ count) |
| RNA viral load | Measures amount of free virus (non-cell bound) in the infected host |

From Lyon M, D'Angelo LJ, eds. *Teenagers, HIV, and AIDS*. Westport, CT: Praeger; 2006.

to review the material which was discussed before they leave the office. In a clinically stable patient, discussion about starting medications and potential regimens should be postponed until patient-provider trust is established. A careful and complete medical history and physical examination should be conducted at an early visit, including a genital examination with STI and Pap testing.

In addition to sending the confirmatory HIV testing, providers may send tests to help assess the severity of the infection. (See Table 1) These initial tests include basic baseline serum chemistries, screening titers for baseline of opportunistic or co-infections, and specific testing regarding the severity of HIV disease—the CD4 count and HIV viral load. Genotype testing to detect most drug resistance is also now recommended as a baseline test in newly diagnosed patients. Currently, adolescents and adult testing and treatment guidelines are placed into the same documents by the DHHS. Since the field of HIV care is rapidly evolving, checking the most recent guidelines is helpful (http://www.aidsinfo.nih.gov/ContentFiles/AdultandAdolescentGL.pdf).

*Initial Treatment Considerations*

Guidelines in HIV treatment have swung full circle since the discovery of HAART. When more active antiretrovirals were discovered in the 1980s and 1990s, a philosophy of "hit hard, hit early" emerged. Once drug toxicities and pill burdens were fully realized, however, guidelines were changed to balance the need for treatment with the medical and psychological side effects of the treatment regimens. In the last decade, more antiretrovirals with less frequent dosing requirements and fewer side effects have been discovered. Also, there is mounting evidence in adults that treating HIV at higher CD4 count baselines improves morbidity and mortality from HIV disease.[40,41] In December 2009, the U.S. treatment guidelines were changed to recommend initiation of antiretroviral treatment between CD4 counts of 350 and 500. This was a change from the previous guideline of initiating treatment when the CD4 count had fallen below 350 cells/mm$^3$. Moreover, the advisory panel was split 50/50 over recommending initiating treatment of patients with CD4 >500.

Once the decision to start treatment is made, it is most appropriate for the patient to view this as a lifelong commitment to take medication at the proper time and in correct doses in an attempt to prevent the development of medication resistance. Studies suggest that to prevent the development of resistance, a patient needs to be 95% adherent to therapy.[42] Despite the attractiveness of giving individuals "drug holidays" where they do not take all or some of their medications, scheduled treatment interruption trials have shown that such strategies are harmful to adults.[43] While recent pediatric data shows scheduled treatment interruptions with normal CD4 count percentages may not be as harmful to younger patients, little data exist on scheduled treatment interruptions in adolescents.[44]

The underpinning of all treatment strategies in HIV-infected teens and adults is to use as few pills as possible, as infrequently as possible, preferably with once-a-day dosing. Two of the current recommended preferred initial, or naïve, treatment regimens can be dosed once daily, with one combination packaged as a single pill. All recommended regimens combine three or four medications that span at least two drug classes (Table 2). Even when a medication regimen is reduced to one pill daily, adherence can still be a struggle for many patients. A recent review of adherence in HIV-infected youth across several studies revealed that 40–60% of youth are able to remain adherent 95% of the time. Similar to adherence studies in adults, there are no specific individual demographic factors associated with poor adherence in adolescents.[45] Nonadherence can be associated with housing instability, depression, anxiety, substance use, stigma, and a history of early sexual abuse. Other factors include later stage disease, detectable viral loads, and length of treatment with antiretrovirals. On the other hand, factors associated with adherence include being in school, higher caregiver education level, self-efficacy, a belief that the medications will work, more condom use, fewer drugs in the regimen, and fewer side effects of the medication.[45] To improve ultimate adherence, many providers work to stabilize a patient's mental health and/or social situation before starting antiretrovirals. Besides engaging social work and mental health support services, there is ongoing research to assess modified directly observed therapy programs as a means of improving adherence.[46]

The provider has to consider the developmental context of an infected teen's life, as well as the medical and psychosocial adherence factors applicable to adults, in

Table 2
Antiretroviral regimens recommended for treatment-naïve patients

| Regimen | Comments |
|---|---|
| NNRTI-based regimen | |
| Efavirenz/tenofovir/emtricitabine | Trade name Atripla; 1 pill daily |
| | Efavirenz component not recommended for first trimester of pregnancy |
| PI-based regimens | |
| Atazanavir/ritonavir with tenofovir/ emtricitabine or tenofovir/lamivudine | These can be once-a-day regimens |
| | Tenofovir/emtricitabine is packaged as one pill daily with trade name Truvada |
| Darunavir/ritonavir with tenofovir/emtricitabine or tenofovir/ lamivudine | |
| INSTI-based regimen | |
| Raltegravir with tenofovir/emtricitabine or tenofovir/lamivudine | Twice-a-day dosing regimen only with raltegravir |

NNRTI = nonnucleoside reverse; transciptase inhibitor; PI= Protease, Inhibitor; INSTI = Integrase strand transfer inhibitor. One of the following three types of combination regimens is recommended: Nonnucleoside reverse transcriptase inhibitor + 2 nucleoside reverse transcriptase inhibitors; or Protease inhibitor (preferably boosted with ritonavir) + 2 nucleoside reverse transcriptase inhibitors; or Integrase strand transfer inhibitor + 2 nucleoside reverse transcriptase inhibitors.
Adapted from Panel on Antiretroviral Guidelines for Adults and Adolescents. Guidelines for the use of antiretroviral agents in HIV-1 infected adults and adolescents. Department of Health and Human Services. December 1, 2009; 1–161. Available at http://www.aidsinfo.nih.gov/ContentFiles/AdultandAdolescentGL.pdf. Accessed July 11, 2010, Table 5a.

making decisions about starting antiretroviral therapy. Many adolescents are inexperienced in dealing with the health care system and may have trouble keeping appointments, getting to a pharmacy, or having sufficient "health literacy" to understand information given to them. Adolescents, like some adults, may actually go into denial over their diagnosis ("This can't be happening to me"), have magical thinking about illness ("If I don't have more sex, this will go away"), or be very concrete ("I don't feel sick, so I don't need to take medicine"). Support services that include case management, psychological counseling, social work, and peer advocacy may be helpful in getting patients through these stages.

Besides selecting a regimen for ease of use, providers must be aware of various potential side effects of the medication. Since certain antiretrovirals may affect the kidneys or liver, existing renal or hepatic dysfunction should be considered when choosing a medication regimen. There should be careful attention to patients with active hepatitis B or C since medications used to treat hepatitis might promote drug-resistant HIV. For noncontracepting females, the use of efavirenz, a commonly used nonnucleoside reverse transcriptase inhibitor, should be avoided because the drug is a potent teratogen. Pregnant women need careful evaluation of the side effects of their antiretroviral regimen and should have closer monitoring of their health status, since medication adjustments may be

Table 3
Potential common toxicities of antiretroviral medication

| Antiretroviral | Comments |
|---|---|
| Nonnucleoside Reverse Transcriptase Inhibitors (NNRTIs) | |
| Nevirapine | Hepatotoxicity, especially in patients with CD4 counts over 250, hepatitis coinfection |
| Efavirenz | Neuropsychiatric side effects (eg, vivid dreams, dizziness, headaches, worsened mood symptoms) |
| | Teratogenic |
| Class Effects | Greater risk of developing resistance with treatment interruptions |
| | Skin rash |
| | Transmitted resistance to NNRTI more common than resistance to PIs |
| | Potential CYP450 drug interactions |
| Protease Inhibitors (PIs) | |
| Atazanavir | Indirect hyperbilirubinemia |
| | Nephrolithiasis |
| | Skin rash |
| | Hyperlipidemia |
| | PR interval prolongation |
| | Food requirement |
| | Renal dose adjustments |
| Fosamprenavir | Skin rash |
| | Hyperlipidemia |
| Lopinavir | Higher dose of boosting ritonavir needed may lead to more gastrointestinal upset |
| | Possible risk of myocardial infarction with cumulative use |
| | PR and QT prolongation |
| Darunavir | Skin rash |
| | Food requirement |
| Saquinavir | Highest pill burden of PIs (6 pills a day) |
| | Food requirement |
| Class Effects | Metabolic complications: dyslipidemia, insulin resistance, hepatotoxicity |
| | Gastrointestinal adverse side effects |
| | CYP3A4 drug interactions |
| Nucleoside Reverse Transcriptase Inhibitor (NRTIs) | |
| Abacavir | Hypersensitivity reaction in patients with HLA-B*5701 |
| | Increased cardiovascular events |
| Emtricitabine | Hyperpigmentation of palms and soles of patients with darker skin |
| | Usually well tolerated |
| Lamivudine | Usually well tolerated |
| Tenofovir | Renal impairment |
| | Can decrease bone mineral density |
| Zidovudine | Nausea |
| | Myopathy |
| | Bone marrow suppression |
| Class Effects | Mitochrondrial toxicity- including lipodystrophy, lactic acidosis, hepatic steatosis |
| | Peripheral neuropathy |
| | Renal dose adjustments |

Adapted from Panel on Antiretroviral Guidelines for Adults and Adolescents. Guidelines for the use of antiretroviral agents in HIV-1 infected adults and adolescents. Department of Health and Human Services. December 1, 2009; 1–161. Available at http://www.aidsinfo.nih.gov/ContentFiles/AdultandAdolescentGL.pdf. Accessed July 11, 2010, Table 12.

needed, particularly in the third trimester. There are many other potential side effects of the various antiretrovirals. The more common side effects are listed in Table 3.

In addition to the specific toxicities noted in Table 3, there are numerous drug-drug interactions, both between individual antiretroviral agents and with a variety of commonly used medications. The lists of these are long and complex, but Table 4 shows some of the interactions between the antiretroviral drugs and several other drugs commonly used by adolescents. A good relationship with the patient's pharmacist is advantageous because of the complexity of these inter-

Table 4
Common drug interactions for adolescent HIV-infected patients on antiretrovirals

| Drug or Class | Comments |
|---|---|
| Protease Inhibitors (PIs) | |
| Antacids | Move antacid dosing, can block absorption of PI |
| H2 receptor antagonists | H2 dose limits |
| Proton Pump Inhibitors (PPIs) | PPI dose limits or use not recommended |
| Antifungals | Antifungal dose limits |
| Anticonvulsants | May increase or decrease anticonvulsant levels depending on specific interaction. Monitor anticonvulsant levels and effects carefully |
| Anti-mycobacterials | Prolonged QTc |
| | May decrease antibiotic levels |
| St. John's wort | Do not coadminister with PIs |
| Hormonal contraceptives | Decreased hormone level; consider using 35 $\mu$g or higher estrogen dosing |
| Methadone | Methadone levels may be decreased |
| NNRTI | |
| Antifungals | May need to increase antifungal dose |
| | Hepatotoxicity |
| Anticonvulsants | Monitor clinical and drug levels of anticonvulsants |
| | Some prohibited use combinations |
| Anti-mycobacterials | Decreased NRTI and antibiotic levels |
| | Some prohibited use combinations |
| St Johns Wort | Do not coadminister |
| Hormonal Contraceptive | Increased estrogen levels- clinical significance not known |
| Methadone | Methadone levels may be decreased |
| Nucleoside Reverse Transcriptase Inhibitors (NRTIs) | |
| Antivirals | May increase drug and NRTI levels |
| | May be additive with NRTI toxicities, including bone marrow suppression |
| Methadone | Methadone levels may be decreased |

Adapted from Panel on Antiretroviral Guidelines for Adults and Adolescents. Guidelines for the use of antiretroviral agents in HIV-1 infected adults and adolescents. Department of Health and Human Services. December 1, 2009; 1–161. Available at http://www.aidsinfo.nih.gov/ContentFiles/Adultand-AdolescentGL.pdf. Accessed July 11, 2010, Tables 13 and 14.

actions and the importance of maintaining appropriate antiretroviral drug levels to suppress infection. For some teens, using preloaded pill boxes is helpful. For others, pill counts and using electronic monitoring methods to determine adherence becomes important.

All of these problems may well be of secondary importance when we realize that drug dosing in teens may be different from in adults. This is particularly true in younger teens who have not completed pubertal maturation. Few studies exist on correct antiretroviral drug dosing during puberty. Pediatric weight-based dosing may lead to excessively high dosing, whereas lower adult dosing may lead to suboptimal therapeutic levels of the drug.[47] Currently, DHHS guidelines recommend using pediatric dosing for patients in early puberty, with patients in later puberty (Tanner stages 3–5) using the adolescent and adult treatment guidelines.

After a patient is started on a regimen, close follow-up with phone calls, nurse visits, and provider visits can help support the patient in remaining adherent while monitoring the patient for adverse side effects. Generally an HIV viral load is sent within 2–4 weeks of starting a new medication regimen, and another CD4 count is sent within a month of initiating treatment. After demonstrating that the treatment is working, provider visits that include CD4 counts and viral loads are recommended every 3 months. Again, in the early treatment stages, a provider may want to see an adolescent or young adult more frequently than an older adult to provide additional support.

**The Primary Care of the HIV-Infected Adolescent**

Even when an adolescent or young adult is transferred to a specialized center for HIV treatment, the primary care doctor needs to be aware of their health issues and remain an important part of the treatment team. Adult or pediatric HIV treatment centers may lack familiarity with minor consent processes, adolescent developmental stages, and adolescent sexuality. Depending on the array of services offered in an HIV treatment center, adolescents may still need to rely on a primary care office for contraception, STI screening, immunizations, and treatment of minor illness. Good communication between the primary provider who is well versed in routine adolescent health care and the HIV treatment team will greatly benefit the patient.

*Immunizations*

Currently, for nonpregnant HIV-infected adolescents and young adults, the vaccine schedule is the same as for uninfected adolescents, with the exception that if a patient has a CD4 count <200, measles, mumps, rubella and varicella vaccines are contraindicated. If the CD4 count is over 200, HIV-infected patients should be fully immunized against tetanus, diphtheria, and pertussis (using TdaP), meningococcal disease, human papillomavirus, influenza (using the inactivated vaccine), and hepatitis B, as are other adolescents. Additionally, HIV-infected patients should receive hepatitis A and pneumococcal vaccines. One can view all recommended immunization schedules at http://www.cdc.gov/vaccines/recs/schedules/default.htm.

Catchup vaccinations should be administered for youth who are behind on their immunizations. The provider should also be mindful that HIV-infected youth, especially those with more immune compromise, may have lower antibody response to pneumococcal, hepatitis B, and pertussis vaccinations.[48-50] While there are no guidelines recommending postvaccination antibody titers, a provider may consider sending titers if a patient was vaccinated when they had a lower CD4 count that has now recovered or if a clinical situation warrants proof of coverage (eg, nursing student, community outbreak of disease).

*Pap Smears*

While in 2009, the guidelines from the American College of Obstetricians and Gynecologists changed to recommend the first Pap smear at 21 years old for immunocompetent women, the recommendations for HIV-infected women have not changed. Sexually active immunocompromised women should have a Pap smear at the time of initial diagnosis. The Pap smear should be repeated in 6 months and if both Pap results are normal, then screening can be performed annually. In a study of 638 perinatally infected girls in the United States, 29.7% had an abnormal cytology on their first Pap smear. Despite the lack of differences in HIV disease severity between patients, 32.8% of those with an abnormal Pap progressed to low- or high-grade squamous intraepithelial lesion.[51] Any HIV-infected woman with any abnormal Pap result (including Atypical Squamous Cells of Undetermined Signficance and low-grade lesions) should be referred for colposcopy.[52] Also, since anal cancer is now being identified as one of the most common non-AIDS-defining tumors in HIV-infected persons, many HIV treatment centers are screening for anal dysplasia in both men and women. While the screening technique is similar to female Pap smears, providers should review the appropriate technique and speak with the receiving laboratory to ensure they will accept the sample. Research is ongoing to define anal smear screening guidelines, as well as treatment options for dysplasia and invasive lesions.[53]

*STI Testing*

At the time of diagnosis, all HIV-infected patients should be tested for gonorrhea, chlamydia, Trichomonas, and syphilis. Some providers also consider herpes 1 and 2 serologies for those patients who have undetermined histories for prior herpes infections. For patients who report receptive anal sex, rectal testing for both gonorrhea and chlamydia should be performed. For patients who report receptive oral sex from a male partner, a pharyngeal specimen for gonorrhea testing should be sent. Pharyngeal chlamydia screening is not recommended.

Since Nucleic Acid Amplification Test is not approved by the US Food and Drug Administration for rectal or pharyngeal specimens at this time, providers should use either culture or an approved NAAT test verified by a local laboratory provider. For patients who engage in high-risk sexual behavior, rescreening for STIs should occur every 3–6 months. At a minimum, most HIV providers screen annually for STIs, including syphilis, in all sexually active HIV-infected patients. As the CDC guidelines for STI screening were last updated in 2006, providers should check their website at http://www.cdc.gov/std/treatment/ for future updates.

*Birth Control and Conception Counseling*

Many adolescents and young people are in need of birth control and contraceptive counseling, and HIV-infected teens are no exception. While most providers teach their patients about the role of sexual contact as a mode of transmission of HIV infection, many infected teens remain sexually active. In a longitudinal study of 40 perinatally infected teens with a mean age of 16 years, 28% were sexually active at the beginning of the study and 41% were active 21 months later.[54] In teens infected postnatally through HIV risk behaviors, those numbers are consistently higher, with over 60% remaining sexually active (defined as sex within the past 3 months) after their diagnosis.[55] For all sexually active youth, condom use becomes essential in preventing transmission of their infection to others. However, condoms alone are not a sufficient form of birth control. Other complimentary methods are necessary to effectively prevent pregnancy in HIV infected young women or uninfected young women who are the sexual partners of HIV infected young men.

The immediate question that arises is, "Are these methods safe and effective in HIV-infected patients?" For the most part the answer to this question is, "Yes." Use of progesterone-only based contraceptives have been assessed with HAART and there have not been any clinically significant interactions. Use of the levenonorgestrel-releasing interuterine system has also been found to be an effective birth control option for HIV-infected females, although the World Health Organization does not recommend its placement in women with AIDS due to the suspected risk of pelvic infections.[56] There can be drug interactions between HAART and combined hormonal contraception (methods containing estrogen and progesterone). Protease inhibitors in particular will lower serum levels of steroid contraceptives.[57] However, overall there are limited data about these interactions in the clinical setting. One randomized study of sub-Saharan African women raised concern about the use of hormonal contraception because the data showed more rapid HIV disease progression in untreated HIV-infected women who used either combined hormonal contraceptives or depomedroxyprogesterone acetate when compared with those using a copper intrauterine device.[58] Further research is needed regarding the use of contraception in HIV-infected women, and at this time providers continue to recommend combining condom use with a hormonal contraceptive as the most effective strategy in preventing pregnancy in HIV-infected women.

Although many providers spend their days trying to help adolescents avoid unintended pregnancies, many young patients diagnosed with HIV have real concerns about their future reproductive options, fearing they will not be able to have children or will pass HIV on to a child or their partner. Entering into this discussion is a great method of discussing HIV transmission and the patient's own overall care, emphasizing that the patient should be in the best possible health before conceiving a child. Many young people are relieved to find out that assisted reproductive techniques are available for patients with HIV infection and that good medical care can greatly reduce the possibility of transmission to a child. Providers who work with HIV-infected patients should not avoid the discussion of family planning and should try to provide the most up-to-date information for their patients.[59]

## Treatment of AIDS and "Treatment Failure"

AIDS is defined by the appearance of an opportunistic infection or AIDS-defining illness in a patient who is infected by HIV or by a decline in the infected individual's CD4 lymphocyte count to 200 cells/mm$^3$ or less. Viral load numbers,

Table 5
Staging of HIV infection

| Stage | |
|---|---|
| Stage I | CD4+ lymphocyte count >500 cells/mm |
| | Asymptomatic |
| | Non-AIDS-defining, but serious infections or health conditions[a] |
| | AIDS-defining opportunistic infections or health conditions[b] |
| Stage II | CD4+ lymphocyte count >200 cells/mm, but <500 cells/mm |
| | Asymptomatic |
| | Non-AIDS-defining, but serious infections or health conditions[a] |
| | AIDS-defining opportunistic infections or health conditions[b] |
| Stage III | CD4+ lymphocyte count <200 cells/mm |
| | Asymptomatic |
| | Non-AIDS-defining, but serious infections or health conditions[a] |
| | AIDS-defining opportunistic infections or health conditions[b] |

[a] Conditions include, but are not limited to, bacillary angiomatosis, thrush, persistent vulvovaginitis, cervical dysplasia (moderate or severe), diarrhea >1 month, oral hairy leukoplakia, herpes zoster (second episode or >1 dermatome), idiopathic thrombocytopenia purpura (ITP), listerosis, pelvic inflammation disease (especially with tubo-ovarian abscess), and peripheral neuropathy.
[b] AIDS-defining opportunistic infections or health conditions: *Candida* infection of esophagus, trachea, bronchi, or lungs; cervical cancer; coccidiomycosis (extrapulmonary); cryptococcosis (extrapulmonary); cytomegalovirus infection, herpes simplex >1 month duration; histoplasmosis (extrapulmonary ); dementia; wasting (weight loss >10% of baseline); isoporosis; Kaposi's sarcoma; lymphoma; *Mycobacterium avium*; *Mycobacterium tuberculosis; Pneumocystis carinii* pneumonia; multifocal leukoencephalopathy; *Salmonella* bloodstream infections; toxoplasmosis.
From Lyon M, D'Angelo LJ, eds. *Teenagers, HIV, and AIDS*. Westport, CT: Praeger; 2006.

the quantitative measure of the estimated number of viral particles present in a patient's bloodstream, are not part of the diagnostic criteria for AIDS (Table 5). Between 2003 and 2007, ~70–80 HIV infected patients ages 13–14 years met an AIDS case definition annually, while 300–400 of 15–19 year olds and 1500–1900 of 20–24 year olds met this same diagnostic definition. Since the first cases of AIDS were noted in 1981, over 100 000 of 13–24 year olds have been diagnosed. Although most primary care providers may only encounter HIV-infected patients that are relatively asymptomatic, other youth, particularly those who were perinatally infected, may well have progressed to an AIDS defining point in their illness. Since the defining characteristics of AIDS, with the exception of opportunistic infections, are on a continuum, fitting the criteria for the case definition of AIDS often has little clinical impact on patients. However, these patients are by definition more immunosuppressed and therefore are more likely to develop some of the more severe complications of their infection.

A clinical phenomenon that may occur when initiating or restarting antiretrovirals in patients with low CD4 counts is immune reconstitution inflammatory syndrome (IRIS). IRIS is described as fever with worsened clinical manifestations of an existing opportunistic infection (OI), most likely to be a mycobacterium infection. These signs and symptoms may occur at the site of a previously known OI or from an "unmasked" infection. IRIS is more likely to happen in patients with higher viral loads, lower CD4 counts, and generally occurs within 2–8 weeks of initiation of antiretroviral therapy. The diagnosis of IRIS is only made when progression of the OI alone, a new OI, side effect/allergic reaction to HAART, or unrelated organ dysfunction is ruled out. The only recommended intervention is empiric therapy with anti-inflammatories and steroids, while HAART and the OI treatment are continued. IRIS does not appear to affect clinical outcomes in most patients.[60]

Antiretroviral treatment is recommended in all patients with an AIDS diagnosis. Prophylaxis to prevent opportunistic infections may also be needed. For patients with a CD4 count <200 cells/mm$^3$, prophylaxis with daily double-strength Bactrim is the preferred regimen to prevent *Pneumocystis jirovecii* pneumonia. Bactrim is also used for the prophylaxis of *Toxoplasma gondii* infections, which can appear when the CD4 count falls below 100. Bactrim prophylaxis for both infections can be stopped when a patient's CD4 count remains above 200 for 3 months. When the CD4 count falls below 50, prophylaxis is also started to prevent *Mycobacterium avium* complex disease. The preferred regimens for prophylaxis of mycobacterium avium are azithromycin (1200 mg weekly) or clarithomycin (500 mg twice daily). These medications can also be stopped when the patient's CD4 count is above 100 for 3 months.[52] The 2009 DHHS guidelines includes more detailed information on the treatment of opportunistic infections and alternate regimens for prophylaxis; this topic is outside of the scope of this article.

## Treatment Failure

Although not precisely defined, as described in the DHHS guidelines, a patient is usually considered to be failing a particular treatment regimen when there is a viral load registering >50 copies 48 weeks after treatment initiation or when there is rebound to this level or higher in a patient who has previously had an undetectable serum viral load. Other experts have set a viral load range of 1000–5000 as the definition of failure. Additionally, some providers look for a rising CD4 count after initiating treatment as evidence of successful treatment and consider an increase of <50–100 cells over a year or the lack of return in the CD4 count to over 350 in ~5 years as an "immunologic failure." Since there is less research on treatment changes with isolated immunologic failure, most clinicians use the viral load to guide treatment changes. Even if there is an accepted range of viral load which is used to define treatment failure, it is important to note that isolated "blips" of viral loads in a 51–1000 range have been reported and have not been shown to be associated with long-term progression of HIV. These transient elevations should prompt the provider to closely review adherence and medication tolerability with the patient.

Since many adolescents and young adults struggle to take their antiretroviral medications, treatment failures need to be assessed quickly as poor adherence increases the risk of HIV progression. Most cases of treatment failure can be traced back to patients not taking their medications as prescribed. Poor adherence may come from a patient's lack of understanding about their medications and how to take them, difficulty in remembering to take all doses, difficulty swallowing medications, denial of their illness or the importance of adhering to the prescribed regimen, unpleasant side effects, or some combination of the above. In a small number of cases, pharmacokinetic issues can contribute to medication, and ultimately treatment failure.[61] In some cases, the patient and provider are not able to identify the exact cause of the treatment failure. When an elevated viral load is noted, a repeat genotype should be sent while the patient is taking HAART to determine drug resistance patterns. Interruption of treatment is not recommended while treatment is being switched or reevaluated. When resistance is found, providers should attempt to find as many active drugs as possible while still having the goal of using the most simplified and least toxic regimen. These drug regimens can be called "salvage therapy," especially when few active antiretrovirals are identified for the patient. In this situation, the provider must have a frank discussion with the patient about the timing and potential number of pills and side effects.

It can be challenging to identify the ideal time to make a medication switch, particularly in patients with lower levels of viremia who have not experienced significant illness due to their HIV disease.[39] As children and adolescents face a potentially lifelong need for medication, changing regimens may have significant medical implications. Some providers of pediatric and adolescent patients will admit a patient with treatment failure to the hospital to observe viral loads and CD4 counts for a week and determine if adherence or medication tolerance is a factor.[62] Managing treatment failure is challenging and should be undertaken by experienced clinicians. Again, the reader is referred to the DHHS guidelines for further discussion of this topic.

## Transition Care of Teens with HIV

With the survival of perinatally infected teens and enhanced emphasis on screening and diagnosing teens with HIV, the need to transition the care of HIV-infected adolescents to adult providers in the community has become an important issue. In a qualitative study of perinatally infected patients, their parents, and their providers at an urban, academic medical center, difficulty in adhering to a medication regimen was cited as a barrier to transition. Many adolescents reported that they depended on their parents to remember their medication. Families expressed concern over the potential to experience stigma and discrimination in the adult system. Providers worried that their patients did not have enough autonomy and were also concerned about letting go of their patient relationship and that their patients would not be as comfortable in the adult setting.[63] All of this is understandable when considering the bonds that have been established between providers and patients, particularly in patients who were not expected to survive.

In a study of 65 patients with a mean age of 15 years, participating in an HIV treatment center that closed quickly due to loss of funding, families were initially most concerned about insurance/payment issues, lack of appropriate pediatric providers in their community, and lack of a social worker in their upcoming transition. Once these issues were identified, the program worked to find a primary community physician and social worker and worked with patients to educate them more about their health status, medications, and other issues. With these interventions, there was increased readiness and decreased anxiety in the patients and families at the time of the transition.[64]

As modeled in many other chronic disease treatment programs, the concept of transition needs to be bought up early, usually by at least 14 years of age.[65] Transition to adult services can be achieved in steps, such as starting with adult case management or gynecology services, before leaving the primary pediatric/adolescent team. In many pediatric HIV treatment centers, generalist physicians may have been the main medical providers in a multidisciplinary group where there has been "one-stop shopping," which naturally incorporated primary care with HIV care. In adult centers, physicians tend to be infectious disease specialists who may not be able to provide primary care services. Adult HIV treatment centers are usually larger and may be more intimidating to the teen patient. Inviting the teen and family to tour the prospective adult site before the first visit, taking a trusted pediatric provider to the first visit, or having a member of the adult team come to a pediatric visit may help smooth the transition process. Some centers may have physicians who are dually trained in pediatric and internal medicine or family medicine physicians who can see patients in combined or separate settings. In any transition process, communication between both programs is key. Written documentation may be very important and valuable to the new team especially for the perinatally infected patient who may have an extensive treatment history. Most likely, the transition will take place in steps over time with visits to both systems until a complete and comfortable transfer of care is achieved.

## Prevention of HIV in Youth

The ultimate strategy in combating HIV infection in youth is to reduce the spread of infection. To date, the majority of the trials of HIV preventative vaccines have been mostly discouraging. In one community-based, randomized, double-blind, placebo-controlled trial of a recombinant canarypox vector and glycoprotein 120 subunit vaccine in over 16 000 Thai volunteers over 3 years, vaccine efficacy was 31.2%.[66] This modest result may be one of the first positive steps toward developing an HIV vaccine, but it will be a number of years before such a vaccine is widely available.

Secondary prevention of HIV transmission from those already infected is an important strategy that is currently available. The CDC cites that this strategy is often overlooked in the busy clinical setting. However, pediatric-trained care providers are well poised to take on this work since anticipatory guidance is usually a part of every patient visit. Patients may believe that if their viral load is undetectable they cannot transmit the virus, and may reengage in riskier sexual practices. Providers can point out while it is less likely to transmit HIV if one has an undetectable viral load, transmission is still possible and one can acquire a resistant HIV strain from other HIV-infected partners. Encouraging patients to continue condom use will also reduce other STIs that may act as cofactors in HIV transmission. Treating injection drug use in HIV-infected individuals is another way to promote secondary prevention.

With the onset of the HIV epidemic, a plethora of primary HIV prevention programs were developed. These programs are mostly designed for community settings, outside of the clinical office site. As with sexual health education, HIV prevention programs have undergone science-based program evaluation. The CDC has been instrumental in assisting programs in evaluation and publishes an online compendium of effective HIV prevention programs through the HIV/AIDS Prevention Research Synthesis Project (www.cdc.gov/hiv/topics/research/prs/index.htm). This project has identified 41 programs as best-evidence interventions as of July 2009. Since a "one size fits all" approach may not work in HIV primary prevention, the programs are tailored for various risk groups, such as MSM, drug users, hepatitis-infected individuals, and different ethnic groups and genders. The interventions may be aimed at the group, community, or individual level. In general, programs tend to be more effective for youth when they focus on specific skills needed for reducing HIV risk instead of being packaged or bundled into larger, more global preventative health programs.[67] In a meta-analysis of programs, interventions had higher efficacy if they included condom use skills, partner negotiation/communication skills around condom use, and had condoms available in a community-type setting.[67,68] Condom use skills and needle exchanges have been shown to be cost-effective in terms of the medical costs averted in preventing HIV infections.[69] If a provider is called to help a community or institution pick an HIV prevention program, the CDC also has a program to disseminate materials through local HIV/STD Training and Education Centers. These programs also can be found on the CDC's website.

## CONCLUSIONS

The adolescent provider of the 21st century will encounter HIV-infected teens in their practice. Hopefully, the rates of HIV infection will decrease in the coming years through better treatment and prevention of the disease. However, primary care providers will still play an important role in the health care and transition care of these young people.

## REFERENCES

1. Glynn MK, Lee LM, McKenna MT. The status of national HIV case surveillance, United States 2006. *Public Health Rep.* 2007;122 Suppl 1:63–71
2. Centers for Disease Control and Prevention. *HIV/AIDS Surveillance Report, 2007.* Atlanta: U.S. Department of Health and Human Services, Centers for Disease Control and Prevention; 2009
3. Hall HI, Song R, Rhodes P, et al. Estimation of HIV incidence in the United States. *JAMA.* 2008;300(5):520–529
4. Rangel MC, Gavin L, Reed C, Fowler MG, Lee LM. Epidemiology of HIV and AIDS among adolescents and young adults in the United States. *J Adolesc Health.* 2006;39(2):156–163
5. Branson BM, Handsfield HH, Lampe MA, et al. Revised recommendations for HIV testing of adults, adolescents, and pregnant women in health-care settings. *MMWR Recomm Rep.* 2006; 55(RR-14):1–17
6. Campsmith ML, Rhodes PH, Hall HI, Green TA. Undiagnosed HIV prevalence among adults and adolescents in the United States at the end of 2006. *J Acquir Immune Defic Syndr.* 2010;53(5): 619–624
7. Qaseem A, Snow V, Shekelle P, Hopkins R Jr, Owens DK. Screening for HIV in health care settings: a guidance statement from the American College of Physicians and HIV Medicine Association. *Ann Intern Med.* 2009;150(2):125–131
8. Mahajan AP, Stemple L, Shapiro MF, King JB, Cunningham WE. Consistency of state statutes with the Centers for Disease Control and Prevention HIV testing recommendations for health care settings. *Ann Intern Med.* 2009;150(4):263–269
9. Guttmacher Institute. State policies in brief: Minors' access to STD services. Available at: http://www.guttmacher.org/statecenter.spibs/spib_MASS.pdf, accessed July 11, 2010.
10. Minniear TD, Gilmore B, Arnold SR, Flynn PM, Knapp KM, Gaur AH. Implementation of and barriers to routine HIV screening for adolescents. *Pediatrics.* 2009;124(4):1076–1084
11. Peralta L, Deeds BG, Hipszer S, Ghalib K. Barriers and facilitators to adolescent HIV testing. *AIDS Patient Care STDS.* 2007;21(6):400–408
12. Moyer M, Silvestre A, Lombardi E, Taylor C. High-risk behaviors among youth and their reasons for not getting tested for HIV. *J HIV AIDS Prev Child Youth.* 2007;8(1):59–73

13. Kowalcyzk Mullins T, Braverman P, Dorn L, Kollar L, Kahn J. Adolescents preferences for human immunodeficiency virus testing methods and impact of rapid tests on receipt of results. *J Adolesc Health.* 2010;46(2):162–168
14. Grant AM, Jamieson DJ, Elam-Evans LD, Beck-Sague C, Duerr A, Henderson SL. Reasons for testing and clinical and demographic profile of adolescents with non-perinatally acquired HIV infection. *Pediatrics.* 2006;117(3):e468–475
15. Tanney M, Naar-King S, Murphy DA, Parsons J, Janisse H. Multiple risk behaviors among youth living with human immunodeficiency virus in five U.S. cities. *J Adolesc Health.* 2010;46:11–16
16. Futterman DC. HIV and AIDS in adolescents. *Adolesc Med Clin.* 2004;15(2):369–391
17. Centers for Disease Control and Prevention. HIV/STD risks in young men who have sex with men who do not disclose their sexual orientation–six U.S. cities, 1994–2000. *MMWR Morb Mortal Wkly Rep.* 2003;52(5):81–86
18. Futterman DC. HIV in adolescents and young adults: half of all new infections in the United States. *Top HIV Med.* 2005;13(3):101–105
19. Eaton DK, Kann L, Kinchen S, et al. Youth risk behavior surveillance–United States, 2007. *MMWR Surveill Summ.* 2008;57(4):1–131
20. Ott MA, Santelli JS. Approaches to adolescent sexuality education. *Adolesc Med State Art Rev.* 2007;18(3):558–570
21. Wawer MJ, Makumbi F, Kigozi G, et al. Circumcision in HIV-infected men and its effect on HIV transmission to female partners in Rakai, Uganda: a randomised controlled trial. *Lancet.* 2009; 374(9685):229–237
22. Lee JC, Boechat MI, Belzer M, et al. Thymic volume, T-cell populations, and parameters of thymopoiesis in adolescent and adult survivors of HIV infection acquired in infancy. *AIDS.* 2006;20(5):667–674
23. Sill A, Constantine N, Wilson C, Peralta L. Demographic profiles of newly acquired HIV infections among adolescents and young adults in the U.S. *J Adolesc Health.* 2010;46:93–96
24. Battegay M, Wirz M, Steuerwald MH, Egger M. Early participation in an HIV cohort study slows disease progression and improves survival. The Swiss HIV Cohort Study. *J Intern Med.* 1998;244(6):479–487
25. Connor EM, Sperling RS, Gelber R, et al. Reduction of maternal-infant transmission of human immunodeficiency virus type 1 with zidovudine treatment. Pediatric AIDS Clinical Trials Group Protocol 076 Study Group. *N Engl J Med.* 1994;331(18):1173–1180
26. Gortmaker SL, Hughes M, Cervia J, et al. Effect of combination therapy including protease inhibitors on mortality among children and adolescents infected with HIV-1. *N Engl J Med.* 2001;345(21):1522–1528
27. Levenson R Jr, Mellins C. Pediatric HIV disease: What psychologists need to know. *Prof Psychol Res Pr.* 1992;23(5):410–415
28. Chernoff M, Nachman S, Williams P, et al. Mental health treatment patterns in perinatally HIV-infected youth and controls. *Pediatrics.* 2009;124(2):627–636
29. Nachman SA, Chernoff M, Gona P, et al. Incidence of noninfectious conditions in perinatally HIV-infected children and adolescents in the HAART era. *Arch Pediatr Adolesc Med.* 2009; 163(2):164–171
30. Brogly SB, Watts DH, Ylitalo N, et al. Reproductive health of adolescent girls perinatally infected with HIV. *Am J Public Health.* 2007;97(6):1047–1052
31. Vogler MA. Pregnancy in a perinatally infected woman: preventing second-generation mother-to-child transmission of HIV. *AIDS Read.* 2007;17(11):536–540
32. Williams SF, Keane-Tarchichi MH, Bettica L, Dieudonne A, Bardeguez AD. Pregnancy outcomes in young women with perinatally acquired human immunodeficiency virus-1. *Am J Obstet Gynecol.* 2009;200(2):149 e141–145
33. Hazra R, Siberry GK, Mofenson LM. Growing up with HIV: children, adolescents, and young adults with perinatally acquired HIV infection. *Annu Rev Med.* 2010;61:169–185
34. Foster C, Judd A, Tookey P, et al. Young people in the United Kingdom and Ireland with perinatally acquired HIV: the pediatric legacy for adult services. *AIDS Patient Care STDS.* 2009;23(3);159–166

35. Lyon M, D'Angelo LJ, eds. *Teenagers, HIV, and AIDS*. Westport, CT: Praeger; 2006
36. Jain CL, Wyatt CM, Burke R, Sepkowitz K, Begier EM. Knowledge of the Centers for Disease Control and Prevention's 2006 routine HIV testing recommendations among New York City internal medicine residents. *AIDS Patient Care STDS*. 2009;23(3);167–176
37. Greenwald JL, Burstein GR, Pincus J, Branson B. A rapid review of rapid HIV antibody tests. *Curr Infect Dis Rep*. 2006;8(2):125–131
38. D'Angelo LJ, Abdalian SE, Sarr M, Hoffman N, Belzer M. Disclosure of serostatus by HIV infected youth: the experience of the REACH study. Reaching for Excellence in Adolescent Care and Health. *J Adolesc Health*. 2001;29(3 Suppl):72–79
39. Panel on Antiretroviral Guidelines for Adults and Adolescents. Guidelines for the use of antiretroviral agents in HIV-1-infected adults and adolescents. Available at: http://www.aidsinfo.nih.gov/contentfiles/adultandadolescentgl.pdf. Accessed June 27, 2010
40. Kitahata MM, Gange SJ, Abraham AG, et al. Effect of early versus deferred antiretroviral therapy for HIV on survival. *N Engl J Med*. 2009;360(18):1815–1826
41. Sterne JA, May M, Costagliola D, et al. Timing of initiation of antiretroviral therapy in AIDS-free HIV-1-infected patients: a collaborative analysis of 18 HIV cohort studies. *Lancet*. 2009;373(9672):1352–1363
42. Garcia de Olalla P, Knobel H, Carmona A, Guelar A, Lopez-Colomes JL, Cayla JA. Impact of adherence and highly active antiretroviral therapy on survival in HIV-infected patients. *J Acquir Immune Defic Syndr*. 2002;30(1):105–110
43. El-Sadr WM, Lundgren JD, Neaton JD, et al. CD4+ count-guided interruption of antiretroviral treatment. *N Engl J Med*. 2006;355(22):2283–2296
44. Paediatric European Network for Treatment of AIDS (PENTA). Response to planned treatment interruptions in HIV infection varies across childhood. *AIDS*. 2010;24(2):231–241
45. Reisner SL, Mimiaga MJ, Skeer M, Perkovich B, Johnson CV, Safren SA. A review of HIV antiretroviral adherence and intervention studies among HIV-infected youth. *Top HIV Med*. 2009;17(1):14–25
46. Garvie PA, Lawford J, Flynn PM, et al. Development of a directly observed therapy adherence intervention for adolescents with human immunodeficiency virus-1: application of focus group methodology to inform design, feasibility, and acceptability. *J Adolesc Health*. 2009;44(2):124–132
47. Rakhmanina NY, Capparelli EV, van den Anker JN. Personalized therapeutics: HIV treatment in adolescents. *Clin Pharmacol Ther*. 2008;84(6):734–740
48. Kamchaisatian W, Wanwatsuntikul W, Sleasman JW, Tangsinmankong N. Validation of current joint American Academy of Allergy, Asthma & Immunology and American College of Allergy, Asthma and Immunology guidelines for antibody response to the 23-valent pneumococcal vaccine using a population of HIV-infected children. *J Allergy Clin Immunol*. 2006;118(6):1336–1341
49. Abzug MJ, Warshaw M, Rosenblatt HM, et al. Immunogenicity and immunologic memory after hepatitis B virus booster vaccination in HIV-infected children receiving highly active antiretroviral therapy. *J Infect Dis*. 2009;200(6):935–946
50. Abzug MJ, Song LY, Fenton T, et al. Pertussis booster vaccination in HIV-infected children receiving highly active antiretroviral therapy. *Pediatrics*. 2007;120(5):e1190–1202
51. Brogly S, Williams P, Seage GR 3rd, Oleske JM, Van Dyke R, McIntosh K. Antiretroviral treatment in pediatric HIV infection in the United States: from clinical trials to clinical practice. *JAMA*. 2005;293(18):2213–2220
52. Kaplan JE, Benson C, Holmes KH, Brooks JT, Pau A, Masur H. Guidelines for prevention and treatment of opportunistic infections in HIV-infected adults and adolescents: recommendations from CDC, the National Institutes of Health, and the HIV Medicine Association of the Infectious Diseases Society of America. *MMWR Recomm Rep*. 2009;58(RR-4):1–207
53. Siekas LL, Aboulafia DM. Establishing an anal dysplasia clinic for HIV-infected men: initial experience. *AIDS Read*. 2009;19(5):178–186

54. Wiener LS, Battles HB, Wood LV. A longitudinal study of adolescents with perinatally or transfusion acquired HIV infection: sexual knowledge, risk reduction self-efficacy and sexual behavior. *AIDS Behav.* 2007;11(3):471–478
55. Rogers AS, Futterman DK, Moscicki AB, Wilson CM, Ellenberg J, Vermund SH. The REACH Project of the Adolescent Medicine HIV/AIDS Research Network: design, methods, and selected characteristics of participants. *J Adolesc Health.* 1998;22(4):300–311
56. Heikinheimo O, Lahteenmaki P. Contraception and HIV infection in women. *Hum Reprod Update.* 2009;15(2):165–176
57. El-Ibiary SY, Cocohoba JM. Effects of HIV antiretrovirals on the pharmacokinetics of hormonal contraceptives. *Eur J Contracept Reprod Health Care.* 2008;13(2):123–132
58. Stringer EM, Levy J, Sinkala M, et al. HIV disease progression by hormonal contraceptive method: secondary analysis of a randomized trial. *AIDS.* 2009;23(11):1377–1382
59. Barreiro P, Duerr A, Beckerman K, Soriano V. Reproductive options for HIV-serodiscordant couples. *AIDS Rev.* 2006;8(3):158–170
60. Kelley CF, Armstrong WS. Update on immune reconstitution inflammatory syndrome: progress and unanswered questions. *Curr Infect Dis Rep.* 2009;11(6):486–493
61. Ding H, Wilson CM, Modjarrad K, McGwin G Jr, Tang J, Vermund SH. Predictors of suboptimal virologic response to highly active antiretroviral therapy among human immunodeficiency virus-infected adolescents: analyses of the reaching for excellence in adolescent care and health (REACH) project. *Arch Pediatr Adolesc Med.* 2009;163(12):1100–1105
62. Glikman D, Walsh L, Valkenburg J, Mangat PD, Marcinak JF. Hospital-based directly observed therapy for HIV-infected children and adolescents to assess adherence to antiretroviral medications. *Pediatrics.* 2007;119(5):e1142–1148
63. Vijayan T, Benin AL, Wagner K, Romano S, Andiman WA. We never thought this would happen: transitioning care of adolescents with perinatally acquired HIV infection from pediatrics to internal medicine. *AIDS Care.* 2009;21(10):1222–1229
64. Wiener LS, Zobel M, Battles H, Ryder C. Transition from a pediatric HIV intramural clinical research program to adolescent and adult community-based care services:assessing transition readiness. *Soc Work Health Care.* 2007;46(1);1–19
65. Rosen DS, Blum RW, Britto M, Sawyer SM, Siegel DM. Transition to adult health care for adolescents and young adults with chronic conditions: position paper of the Society for Adolescent Medicine. *J Adolesc Health.* 2003;33(4):309–311
66. Rerks-Ngarm S, Pitisuttithum P, Nitayaphan S, et al. Vaccination with ALVAC and AIDSVAX to prevent HIV-1 infection in Thailand. *N Engl J Med.* 2009;361(23):2209–2220
67. Johnson BT, Carey MP, Marsh KL, Levin KD, Scott-Sheldon LA. Interventions to reduce sexual risk for the human immunodeficiency virus in adolescents, 1985–2000: a research synthesis. *Arch Pediatr Adolesc Med.* 2003;157(4):381–388
68. Sales JM, Milhausen RR, Diclemente RJ. A decade in review: building on the experiences of past adolescent STI/HIV interventions to optimise future prevention efforts. *Sex Transm Infect.* 2006;82(6):431–436
69. Holtgrave DR, Curran JW. What works, and what remains to be done, in HIV prevention in the United States. *Annu Rev Public Health.* 2006;27:261–275

*Note:* Page numbers of articles are in **boldface** type. Page references followed by "*f*" and "*t*" denote figures and tables, respectively.

## A

AAP. *See* American Academy of Pediatrics (AAP)
Assortive mating, 337
Abnormal transillumination, for sinusitis, 191
Abscess
  epidural, 198
  in incision and drainage, 323
  intracerebral, 198
  orbital, 195
  subdural, 198
Acellular pertussis (ap) vaccines
  filamentous hemagglutinin, 224
  fimbriae, 224
  pertactin, 224
  pertussis toxin, 224
Acetaminophen, 257
ACIP. *See* Advisory Committee on Immunization Practices (ACIP)
ACOG. *See* American Congress of Obstetricians and Gynecologists (ACOG)
Acquired immune deficiency syndrome (AIDS), treatment, 379–380
  failure, 380–381
Acute disseminated encephalomyelitis (ADEM), 288
Acute respiratory distress syndrome (ARDS), 321
Acute sinusitis, **187–201**
Acyclovir, 257, 311
Adacel, 175, 231
Adefovir, 275
ADEM. *See* Acute disseminated encephalomyelitis (ADEM)
Adolescents
  MCV4 vaccine, 182
  quadrivalent HPV vaccine, 182
  supine position, 182
  Tdap vaccine, 182
Adolescent pneumonia, **202–219**
Adolescent Trials Network (ATN), 368
Adult respiratory distress syndrome, 240

Advisory Committee on Immunization Practices (ACIP), 173, 231, 243, 266, 269, 310, 342, 356
African-American, HIV incidence, 364–365
AIDS. *See* Acquired immune deficiency syndrome (AIDS)
Airway obstruction, 255–256
Alan Guttmacher Institute, 366
"Alice in Wonderland" syndrome, 256
All-inactivated polio vaccine, 180
Amantadine, 243
*Amblyomma americanum* (the lone star tick), 293
American Academy of Family Physicians, 173
American Academy of Pediatrics (AAP), 173, 231, 243, 266, 269, 302, 325
American Congress of Obstetricians and Gynecologists (ACOG), 178, 342, 352
American Medical Association, 173
American Society for Colposcopy and Cervical Pathology, 351
Amoxicillin, 256
  for acute uncomplicated sinusitis, 192
Ampicillin, 256
  for pyogenic bacterial pneumonia, 208
Amsel criteria, 340
Anal cancer
  associated with HPV, 356
  screening, 358
Anaphylactic reaction
  for diphtheria, 176
  for pertussis, 176
  for tetanus, 176
*Anaplasma phagocytophilum*, 293, 303
Anerobes, 189
Annual routine vaccination, 177
Antibiotics, 257, 311
  for sinusitis in primary level, 191

Anticoagulation, for venous sinus thrombosis, 199
Anticonvulsants, for subdural abscess, 198
Anti-early antigen (EA) antibodies, 348
Antigenpresenting cells (APCs), 348
Anti-HAV, 267t
Anti-HBc, 267t, 272
Anti-HBs, 267t, 272
Anti-HCV, 267t
Antimicrobial medication, 210
  for pleural effusions, 211
Anti-NMDAR antibody, 297
Antiretroviral therapy, 246, 369, 373–374, 379
  adverse effects, 379t
  drug interactions, 374t
  for influenza, 241
Antiviral therapy, for influenza, 242t
APCs. See Antigenpresenting cells (APCs)
ARDS. See Acute respiratory distress syndrome (ARDS)
Arthropod vectors
  mosquitoes, 293
  ticks, 293
Arthus reaction, 175
Aseptic meningitis, 302
Aspirin, 256
Association of Public Health Laboratories, 339
Asthma, 240
ATN. See Adolescent Trials Network (ATN)
Auscultation, 205
Azithromycin
  for pertussis, 230
  for pneumonia in adolescents, 208
AZT (zidovudine), 368

**B**

Bacteremia, 320
Bacterial (septic) meningitis, 287
Bacterial culture, for pertussis, 227, 227f
Bacterial Meningitis Score, 302
Bacterial pneumonia, diagnosis of, 207
Bacterial sinusitis, major and minor clinical criteria of, 190t
Bacterial vaginosis (BV), 340
*Bacteroides* spp., 340
Bactrim, 380
Baker's yeast, 179
Bayview Networks Study, 338
BDProbeTec ET assay, 338, 339
β-hemolytic streptococci (GAS), 256
Bilirubin, 255

Birth control and conception counseling, 378–379
Bivalent vaccine, 174
Bleach baths, 327
Blood ammonia level, 241
Blood cultures, to determine the bacterial etiology, 207
Booster vaccine, 175
  for diphtheria, 175
  for pertussis, 175
  for tetanus, 175
Boostrix, 175, 231
Bordetella pertussis
  causative agent of whooping cough, 220
  clinical illness of, 224
  catarrhal, 224
  convalescent, 224
  paroxysmal, 224
*Borrelia borgdorferi*, 293
*Borrelia burgdorferi* infection, 309
British Thoracic Society, 210
Broad-spectrum antibiotics
  for epidural abscess, 198
  for intracerebral abscess, 198
  for subdural abscess, 198
  for venous sinus thrombosis, 199
Brudzinski's sign, 298
Burkitt's lymphoma, 257
BV. See Bacterial vaginosis (BV)
BVBlue Test, 340

**C**

California Encephalitis Project, 292
CA-MRSA. See Community acquired methicillin-resistant *S. aureus* (CA-MRSA)
Cardinal symptoms of acute sinusitis, 191
Catch up schedule, 175
Catchup vaccination, 356, 377
Cavernous sinus thrombosis, 199
CD4 count, 372, 376, 381
CDC. See Centers for Disease Control and Prevention (CDC)
Cefadroxil, 192
Cefdinir, 192
Cefepime, 306
Cefpodoxime, 192
Cefprozil, 192
Ceftobripole, 326
Cefuroxime, 192
Centers for Disease Control and Prevention (CDC), 173, 191, 214, 222, 289, 333, 341, 351–352, 364, 383
  recommendations for HIV screening, 365–366
  Young Men's Survey, 366

Centers for Medicare and Medicaid
  Services (CMS), 339
Central nervous system (CNS)
  complications, 240
  infections, 287
Cephalexin, 192
Cephalosporins, 192, 311
  for pneumonia in hospitalized
    patients, 212
Cerebrospinal fluid (CSF)
  for children and adults, 300*t*
  glucose concentration, 301
  Gram stain of, 300
  WBC count range in, 301
Cervarix, 174
Cervarix, 174, 342
  vaccine efficacy of, 354*t*
Cervical cancer
  rates, 350
  screening, 350, 351–352
  vaccine efficacy against, 353–354, 353*t*
Cervical intraepithelial neoplasia
  (CIN), 348, 351, 352
CFS. *See* Chronic fatigue syndrome
  (CFS)
Chemoprophylaxis, 246, 246*t*, 309
  for household contacts, 230
  *N. meningitidis,* 309
  rifampin, 309
  and vaccination, 311
Chest radiographs, 205*f*, 325
  for pleural effusion, 210
Chlamydia, 334
  screening, 341
Chlamydia Rapid Test, 340
*Chlamydia trachomatis*, 333
*Chlamydia trachomatis,* 348
Chlamydophila pneumoniae, 212–213
Chlorhexidine bath, 327
Chronic fatigue syndrome (CFS), 257
Chronic pelvic pain, 333
CIN. *See* Cervical intraepithelial
  neoplasia (CIN)
Cirrhosis, Hepatitis C progression to, 278
Clarithromycin
  for pertussis, 230
CLIA. *See* Clinical Laboratory
  Improvement Amendments
  (CLIA)
Clindamycin, 208, 324, 326
Clinical Laboratory Improvement
  Amendments (CLIA)
  compliance, 339
CMS. *See* Centers for Medicare and
  Medicaid Services (CMS)
CNS. *See* Central nervous system
  (CNS)
Color vision testing, for subperiosteal
  abscess, 197
Columnar epithelium, 350
Community acquired methicillin-
  resistant *S. aureus* (CA-MRSA),
  214, 318
  transmission of, 319
Composite reference standard (CRS), 340
Computed tomography (CT), 195, 325
  for Periorbital cellulites, 196
  for pot's puffy tumor, 196
  for subperiosteal abscess, 197
Comvax, 275, 276*t*
Condom use, 336–337
Condyloma, 356
Contraception, in HIV-infected
  individuals, 378–379
Corticosteroids, 256, 257
Council of State and Territorial
  Epidemiologists, 226
C-reactive protein (CRP), 207, 302
CRP. *See* C-reactive protein (CRP)
CRS. *See* Composite reference
  standard (CRS)
*Cryptococcus gatti*, 293
CSF. *See* Cerebrospinal fluid (CSF)
CT. *See* Computed tomography (CT)
Cystic fibrosis, 188, 240
Cytomegalovirus infections, 251, 258–259
  clinical manifestations, 259
  complications and prevention, 259–260
  epidemiology, 258–259
  reactivation, 258, 259
  transmission, 258–259
  virology, 258

# D

Daptomycin, 324, 326
Dendritic cells, 348
*Dermacentor andersoni* (Rocky
  Mountain wood tick), 293
*Dermacentor variabilis* (the American
  dog tick), 293
Dermoid cysts, 294
Dexamethasone, 307
DFA. *See* Direct fluorescent antibody
  (DFA)
Direct fluorescent antibody (DFA), 228
Directly observed therapy (DOT), 215
Dissortive mating, 337
Doppler ultrasound, 325
DOT. *See* Directly observed therapy
  (DOT)

Doxycycline, 324
　for pertussis, 230
　for tick-borne meningoencephalitis, 302
D-test, 324, 324f

## E

EBNA. *See* Epstein-Barr nuclear antigen (EBNA)
EBV. *See* Epstein-Barr virus (EBV) infections
Ectopic pregnancy, 333
EEG. *See* Electroencephalogram (EEG)
*Ehrlichia chaffensis,* 293, 303
*Ehrlichia ewingii,* 293, 303
EIA. *See* Enzyme immunoassay (EIA)
Electroencephalogram (EEG), 292
Empyema, 240
Encephalitis, 240, 256, 302
　definition of, 287
　causes of, 287
Encephalitis
　adjunctive measures, 307–308
　antimicrobial therapy, 304–307
　clinical manifestations, 295–298, 290–292*t*
　diagnosis, 299–304, 290–292*t*
　identification of pathogens, 302–304
　interpretation of CSF findings, 299–302
　epidemiology, 289–294, 290–292*t*
　lumbar puncture and initial management, 298–299
　management algorithm for, 299f
　pathophysiology, 294–295
　prevention, 309–311
　chemoprophylaxis, 309
　immunoprophylaxis, 309–311
　prognosis, 308–3090
Encephalopathy, 240, 287
Endocarditis, 321
Engerix-B, 275, 276*t*
　for Hepatitis B virus, 179
Entecavir, 275
Enterovirus 71 (EV-71), 293
Enzyme immunoassay (EIA), 241, 340
Epidermoid cysts, 294
Epidural abscess, 198
Epstein-Barr nuclear antigen (EBNA), 254
Epstein-Barr virus, cytomegalovirus, and infectious mononucleosis, **251–264**
Epstein-Barr virus (EBV) infections, 252–258, 260
　acute complications, 255–256
　neurologic, 256
　antibody tests, 253–254, 254*t*
　chronic and latent infection, 257–258
　clinical syndrome, 253
　differential diagnosis, 253
　epidemiology, 252–253
　laboratory evaluation, 253–255
　management, 256–257
　virology, 252
Erythrocyte sedimentation rate (ESR), 207
Erythromycin, 230
ESR. *See* Erythrocyte sedimentation rate (ESR)
Ethmoid paranasal sinuses, 187
EV-71. *See* Enterovirus 71 (EV-71)
Extension from the orbit, 198
Extragenital screening, with NAAT, 339

## F

FDA. *See* U.S. Food and Drug Administration (FDA)
Flaccid paralysis, 295
Fluoroquinolones, for pertussis, 230
Focal neurologic abnormalities, 297
Foscarnet, 260
Frontal paranasal sinuses, 187

## G

Ganciclovir, 260
Gardasil, 174, 342
　vaccine efficacy of, 353*t*
*Gardnerella vaginalis,* 340
GAS. *See* β-hemolytic streptococci (GAS)
GBS. *See* Guillain-Barre' syndrome (GBS)
Genital warts, 174
Genitourinary (GU) tract infections, 333
Gen-Probe APTIMA Combo 2 assay, 339
Gentamicin, for *S. aureus* infections, 325
German measles. *See* Rubella
"Glandular fever," 251
Glycerol monolaurate, for tampons, 320
Gonococcal Isolate Surveillance Program, 334
Gonorrhea, 334, 335–336
Gram-stainnegative bacterial meningitis, 302
Group A streptococci, 240
Group B meningococcus, 310

Guillain-Barre' syndrome (GBS), 175, 232, 240, 310

# H

H1N1 vaccine, 177–178
HAART. See Highly active antiretroviral therapy (HAART)
*Haemophilus influenzae*, 189, 308
  type B (Hib), 289
HA-MRSA. See Hospital acquired methicillin-resistant *S. aureus* (HA-MRSA)
Havrix, 179, 269*t*
HBcAg, 267*t*
HBeAg, 267*t*, 270, 272, 273
HBIG. See Hepatitis B immunoglobulin (HBIG)
HBsAg, 267*t*, 270, 271–272, 273, 275
HCV RT-PCR, 267*t*
Health maintenance organization (HMO), 341
Health plan employer data, 183
Healthy People 2010, 273
Hematogenous osteomyelitis, 320
Hemophagocytic syndrome, 258
*Hepadnaviridae*, 270
Hepatitis A virus infections, 265–269
  clinical manifestations, 266–267
  diagnosis, 267–268
  epidemiology, 265–266
  prevention, 268–269
  postexposure prophylaxis, 269
  preexposure prophylaxis, 268–269
  transmission, 265–266
  treatment, 268
  vaccine, 179, 268–269
  recommended doses for, 269*t*
Hepatitis B immunoglobulin (HBIG), 276–277
Hepatitis B virus infections, 270–277
  acute, 271, 272*f*, 273*f*
  chronic, 178, 271, 272–273, 273*f*
  clinical manifestations, 271
  diagnosis, 271–273
  epidemiology, 270
  prevention, 275–277
  postexposure prophylaxis, 276–277
  preexposure prophylaxis, 275–276
  serologic tests for, 274*t*
  transmission, 270–271
  treatment, 273–275
  vaccines, 178–179, 275
  recommended doses for, 276*t*
Hepatitis C virus infections, 277–280
  antibody, 278, 279*f*
  clinical manifestations, 278
  diagnosis, 278
  epidemiology, 277–278
  prevention, 280
  transmission, 277
  treatment, 278–280
Herpes simplex virus 1 (HSV-1), 293
Herpes simplex virus 2 (HSV-2), 334
Heterophile antibody test, 251, 253–254
Heteroresistant vancomycin intermediate *Staphylococcus aureus* (hVISA), 326
Higher-grade squamous intraepithelial lesions (HSIL), 348, 349, 352
Highly active antiretroviral therapy (HAART), 259, 368, 369, 371
Hispanics, HIV incidence, 365
HIV. See Human immunodeficiency virus (HIV)
HME. See Human monocytic ehrlichiosis (HME)
HMO. See Health maintenance organization (HMO)
Hospital acquired methicillin-resistant *S. aureus* (HA-MRSA), 318
HPV. See Human papillomavirus (HPV)
HSIL. See Higher-grade squamous intraepithelial lesions (HSIL)
HSV-1. See Herpes simplex virus 1 (HSV-1)
HSV-2. See Herpes simplex virus 2 (HSV-2)
Human immunodeficiency virus (HIV) infection, 364
  adherence and nonadherence factors, 372
  in adolescents, **364–387**
  adolescents infected perinatally, 368–369
  age group, 364
  antiretroviral regimens, 373*t*
  behavioral risk factors, 367
  biological factors, 367–368
  circumcision, 367
  current treatment
    initial diagnosis, 369–370
    initial laboratory evaluation, 370–371
    initial treatment considerations, 371–375
  and higher risk sexual behavior, 366
  immune function period, 367–368
  incidence of, 364
  men who have sex with men (MSM), 364
  natural history of, 367–368
  primary care
    birth control and conception counseling, 378–379

immunizations, 376–377
Pap smears, 377
STI testing, 377–378
and problem-level substance use, 366
regional context, 367
signs and symptoms, 370
staging, 379t
prevention in youth, 383–384
teens, with HIV
diagnoses, 364–367
transition care of, 382–383
testing in, 365–367
barriers to, 366
trichomoniasis and, 334
in young women, 365
Human monocytic ehrlichiosis (HME), 293
Human papillomavirus disease and vaccines in adolescents, **347–363**
Human papillomavirus (HPV), 334
anal cancer associated with, 354
screening, 358
anogenital HPV in males
epidemiology, 357–358
natural history of, 357–358
biological vulnerabilities to, 349–350
biology of, 347–348
cervical cancer
rates, 350
screening, 350, 351–352
vaccine efficacy against, 353–354, 353t
cervical intraepithelial neoplasia, 348, 351, 352
epidemiology, 348–349
higher-grade squamous intraepithelial lesions, 348, 349, 352
low-grade squamous intraepithelial lesion, 348, 349, 352
management of, 352
natural history of, 348–349
oropharyngeal cancer associated with, 357
penile cancer associated with, 357
screening, 358
prevention of, 352–353
advances in, 342
risk factors, 351
screening, advances in, 342
vaccines, 174, 352, 353
efficacy, 353–356
indications for noncervical genital disease in females, 356
in males, 358
hVISA. See Heteroresistant vancomycin intermediate *Staphylococcus aureus* (hVISA)
Hygiene, and *S. aureus* infections, 327
Hypoxemia, 209

**I**

ICP. See Increased intracranial pressure (ICP)
IDSA. See Infectious Diseases Society of America (IDSA)
Ig. See Immunoglobulin (Ig)
IM. See Infectious mononucleosis (IM)
Immune function, and EBV infection, 260
Immune reconstitution inflammatory syndrome (IRIS), 380
Immunizations, 173–184, 376–377
hepatitis A vaccine, 179
hepatitis B vaccine, 178–179
human papillomavirus vaccines, 179
influenza and h1n1 vaccines, 176–178
meningococcal vaccine, 175–176
MMR and varicella vaccines, 179–180
pertussis vaccine (tdap), 175
pneumococcal vaccine, 181
polio vaccine, 180–181
vaccination efforts, 182–183
vaccine safety, 181–182
Immunizations in adolescents, **173–186**
Immunofluorescence assay, 370
Immunoglobulin (Ig), 204, 268
Immunoglobulin G (IgG) antibody, 154
anti-HBc, 272
Immunoglobulin M (IgM) antibody, 253, 254, 303
anti-HAV, 267t
anti-HBc, 267t
Immunoprophylaxis, 309–311
Inactivated virus vaccine, for H1N1, 178, 245
Incision and drainage, for SSTI, 323
Increased intracranial pressure (ICP), 294
Infants, Hepatitis B transmission in, 270–271
Infectious Diseases Society of America (IDSA), 298
Infectious mononucleosis (IM), 251
cytomegalovirus, 251, 258–260
Epstein-Barr virus, 251, 258–260
Infertility, 333
Inflammatory edema. See Periorbital cellulitis
Influenza, 173, **236–250**, 321

diagnosis, 241–242
epidemiology, 237–238
h1n1 vaccines, 176–178
increased risk of complications from, 244t
infection control, 246
management, 242–243
manifestations, 239–241
central nervous system complications, 240
myositis, 240
pulmonary complications, 240
reye syndrome, 241
uncomplicated influenza, 239
pathogenesis and host immune response, 238–239
in pregnancy, 178
-positive illness, 245
prevention, 243–246
chemoprophylaxis, 246
vaccines, 243–246
symptoms and signs, 239, 239t
vaccines, 243–244
for asthma, 177
comparison of, 245t
for diabetes, 177
for human immunodeficiency virus, 177
for sickle cell anemia, 177
virology, 236–237
Influenza A virus, 237
Influenza viruses
influenza A virus, 236–237
hemagglutinin, 236
neuraminidase, 236
influenza B virus, 236
influenza C virus, 236
Influx of leukocytes, 294
Initial diagnosis, 369–370
Initial laboratory evaluation, 370–371
Initial treatment considerations, 371–376
Institute of Medicine, 260
Interferon alfa-2b, 275
Interferon-$\alpha$, 279
Intracerebral abscess, 198
Intraepithelial lesions, 357
Intraepithelial neoplastic (IN) lesions, 358
Intravenous acyclovir, for encephalitis, 306
IRIS. See Immune reconstitution inflammatory syndrome (IRIS)
Ixodes black-legged ticks (deer ticks), 293

## J

Japanese encephalitis virus, 293
Joint task force on Practice Parameters for Sinusitis, 193

## K

Kernig's sign, to screen for meningitis, 368
Kids' inpatient database, 209
"Kissing disease," 252

## L

La Crosse virus
arthropodborne viruses, 293
mosquito-borne arboviruses, 293
LAIV. See Live attenuated influenza vaccine (LAIV)
Lamivudine, 275
Langerhans, 348
Leukocytosis, 228–229
Levenonorgestrel-releasing interuterine system, 378
Levofloxacin, 208
Lidocaine, 323
Linezolid, 324, 326
antibiotic for pneumococcus, 306
for methicillin-resistant Staphylococcus aureus, 208
Live attenuated influenza vaccine (LAIV), 244, 255
for seasonal influenza, 177
for H1N1, 178
Local insult factors, 188
Long-term prognosis, for subdural abscess, 198
Low-grade squamous intraepithelial lesion (LSIL), 348, 349, 352
LSIL. See Low-grade squamous intraepithelial lesion (LSIL)
lukFPV, 319
lukSPV, 319
Lumbar puncture, 198
adjunctive therapy for, 298
antimicrobial therapy for, 298
in children, 301
and initial management, 298–299
Lungs, and CA-MRSA infection, 321
Lyme meningitis
ceftriaxone for, 307
intravenous penicillin for, 306, 307
Lymphocytic meningitis, 297
Lymphocytosis, 228–229
and heterophile antibody test, 254

## M

Macrolide, for community-acquired pneumonia, 208
Magnetic resonance imaging (MRI), 195, 325
gadolinium-enhanced, 195
for pot's puffy tumor, 196
Massachusetts Department of Public Health, 228

Maternal-child HIV transmission, 196
Maxillary aspiration
Maxillary paranasal sinuses, 187
MCV4. See Meningococcal conjugate vaccine (MCV4)
Measles, 179
Measles, Mumps, and Rubella (MMR) vaccine, 173
 and varicella vaccines, 179–180
Mechanical obstruction factors, 188
Medication-resistant HIV, 369
MenACWY-CRM, 310
Meningitis, 288f
 adjunctive measures, 307–308
 antimicrobial therapy, 304–307
 clinical manifestations, 295–298, 290–292t
 complications, 198–199
 venous sinus thrombosis, 199
 diagnosis, 299–304, 290–292t
 identification of pathogens, 302–304
 interpretation of CSF findings, 299–302
 epidemiology, 289–294, 290–292t
 lumbar puncture and initial management, 298–299
 management algorithm for, 299f
 pathophysiology, 294–295
 prevention, 309–311
 chemoprophylaxis, 309
 immunoprophylaxis, 309–311
 prognosis, 308–309
 definition of, 287
 symptoms of, 287
 classified into, 287
 etiology of, 292
 caused by N. meningitidis, 296
 due to spirochetes, 297
 penicillin G for, 304
Meningitis and encephalitis in adolescents, **287–317**
Meningococcal conjugate vaccine (MCV4), 176
Meningococcal polysaccharide vaccine (MPSV4), 176
Meningococcal strains, 289
Meningococcal vaccine, 175–176
Meningoencephalitis, 302
Menomune, 176
Men who have sex with men (MSM), 339, 357, 364, 368
Meropenem, 306
Metaplastic epithelium, 350
Methicillin-resistant *staphylococcus aureus* (MRSA), 213–214, 318
Methicillin-susceptible *Staphylococcus aureus* (MSSA), 315

MIC. See Minimum inhibitory concentration (MIC)
Minimum inhibitory concentration (MIC), 326
MLI. See Mononucleosis-like illnesses (MLI)
MMR. See Measles, Mumps, and Rubella (MMR) vaccine
Mononucleosis-like illnesses (MLI), 252
"Monospot" test, 251
Moraxella catarrhalis, 189
Morbidity and Mortality Weekly Report, 215
Moxifloxacin, 208
MPSV4. See Meningococcal polysaccharide vaccine (MPSV4)
MRI. See Magnetic resonance imaging (MRI)
MRSA. See Methicillin-resistant *staphylococcus aureus* (MRSA)
MSM. See Men who have sex with men (MSM)
MSSA. See Methicillin-susceptible *Staphylococcus aureus* (MSSA)
Mucoceles, 193–195
 primary, 193
 secondary, 193–194
Mucosal antibody responses, 238
Multidrug resistant (MDR) tuberculosis, 214
Multifocal osteomyelitis, 320
Mupirocin, 327
Musculoskeletal Infections, 320
*Mycobacterium avium*, 380
Mycobacterium tuberculosis (TB), 214, 293
*Mycoplasma pneumoniae*, 212–213
Myositis, 240, 320, 3221f

# N

NAAT. See Nucleic acid amplification tests (NAAT)
Nafcillin, 325
Nasal HA-specific immunoglobulin (Ig), 238
Nasal saline, for acute sinusitis, 192
Nasotracheal intubation, 190
National Health and Nutrition Examination Survey (NHANES), 223, 334, 200
National Health Interview Survey, 336
National Immunization Survey–Teens, 232
National Longitudinal Study of Adolescent Health (Add Health), 334, 335–336

National Survey of Family Growth (NSFG), 336
National Vaccines for Children program, 182–183
Necrotizing pneumonia, 321
Necrotizing pneumonitis, 240
Negative predictive value, 242
*Neisseria gonorrhea*, 333–334
*Neisseria meningitides*, 289
  bacterial meningitis due to, 289
  meningococcal conjugate vaccine, 176
  meningococcal polysaccharide vaccine, 176
Neuraminidase inhibitors, antiviral medications, 243
Newborn. *See* Infants
New York City Adolescent AIDS program, 367
NHANES. *See* National Health and Nutrition Examination Survey (NHANES)
N-methyl-D-aspartate receptor, 289
N-N-diethyl-*m*-toluamide, 309
Nonbacterial (aseptic) meningitis
  in adults, 293
  definition of, 288
  in immunocompetent adolescents, 293
  infectious etiologies of, 288
  rare causes of, 293
NSFG. *See* National Survey of Family Growth (NSFG)
Nucleic acid amplification tests (NAAT), 338, 377–378
  extragenital screening with, 339
Nugent criteria, 340

**O**

Obesity, 238
Ophthalmologic consultation, for orbital cellulitis, 196
Oral polio vaccine, 180
Orbital abscess, 197
Orbital cellulitis, 196–197
Oropharyngeal cancer, associated with HPV, 357
Orthomyxoviridae, 236
Oseltamivir, 243
OSOM Trichomonas Rapid Test, 340
Osteomyelitis, 320, 321*f*

**P**

Pandemic influenza, 238
Panton-Valentine Leukocidin (PVL), 319
Pap smear, 182, 277
Paranasal sinuses
  ethmoid, 187
  frontal, 187
  maxillary, 187
  sphenoid, 187
Pathogens, identification of, 302
  aseptic Meningitis, 302
  encephalitis, 302
  meningoencephalitis, 302
  septic meningitis, 302
Pathogen-specific antimicrobial therapy, recommendations for, 305–306*t*
PCR. *See* Polymerase chain reaction (PCR)
PCV7. *See* Pneumococcal conjugate vaccine
Pediatric health information system, 211
Pediatrix, 275, 276*t*
Peginterferon alfa-2a, 275
Pelvic inflammatory disease (PID), 333
Penicillin, 256
  for pneumonia in hospitalized patients, 212
Penile cancer, associated with HPV, 357
  screening, 358
Perichondritis, 320
Periorbital cellulitis, 196
Per Protocol studies, 353
Pertussis, 173, 175, 120–233
  in age groups, 223*f*
  antibiotic therapy, 229–230
  complications of, 224, 226
  contraindications, precautions, and deferral of, 232–233
  diagnosis, 226–229
  clinical case definition, 226
  differential, 229
  laboratory criteria for, 226
  epidemiology, 220–223
  presentation, 224–225
  etiology, 224
  symptoms, 224–225
  prevention, 230–233
  active immunization, 230–232
  antibiotic prophylaxis, 230
  stages and communicability of, 225*f*
  symptoms in, 225–226
  treatment, 229
  vaccines, 221–222
Pertussis in adolescents and prevention using Tdap, **392–407**
Pertussis vaccine (tdap), 347
Pharyngeal chlamydia screening, 377
PID. *See* Pelvic inflammatory disease (PID)

Plan-Do-Study-Act rapid cycle, 341
Pleural effusions, 209–211
 antimicrobial therapy for, 211
 definition of, 209
 etiology of, 209
 laboratory evaluation of, 210
  biochemical methods, 210
  culture, 210
  hematologic methods, 210
  special pathologic staining techniques, 210
 management of, 210
  algorithm for, 206f
  radiography of, 209–210
  video-assisted thoracoscopic surgery for, 210–211
Pleural fluid sample, 210
Pneumococcal conjugate vaccine (PCV7), 289
 purified capsular polysaccharide, 181
Pneumococcal disease, 289
Pneumococcal vaccine, 181
*Pneumocystis jirovecii*, 380
Pneumonia, 202–216
 causes of, 203t, 211–216
  bacterial, 211–215
  prevention, 216
  viral, 215–216
 complications, 209
 definition of, 202
 diagnosis of, 203t, 207
 epidemiology, 202–203
 etiology, 204–205
 general principles, 202–204
 hospitalization, 209
 laboratory evaluation, 207–208
 management, 208
 manifestations, 205–207
 microbiologic diagnosis, 204
 outpatient and inpatient treatment of, 204f
 pathogenesis, 203–204
 pleural effusions, 209–211
 radiography, 207
Polio vaccine, 180–181
Polymerase chain reaction (PCR), 226, 228, 287, 334
Positive IgG immunoblot, 304
Positive predictive value, 242
Postexposure prophylaxis
 hepatitis A infections, 269
 hepatitis B infections, 276–277
Pott's puffy tumor, 195–196
 common pathogens for, 196
PPSV23, 181
Preexposure prophylaxis
 hepatitis A infections, 268–269
 hepatitis B infections, 275–276

Pregnancy, 369
 and cytomegalovirus infection, 260
Preseptal cellulites. *See* Periorbital cellulitis
*Prevotella* spp, 340
Primary care
 birth control and conception counseling, 378–379
 immunizations, 376–377
 Pap smears, 377
 STI testing, 377–378
ProQuad, combination MMR/varicella vaccine, 180
Protease inhibitors, 378
Pulmonary defense system, 204
Pulmonary disease, 321
PVL. *See* Panton-Valentine Leukocidin (PVL)
Pyomyositis, 320

## Q

Quadrivalent vaccine, 174
 gardasil, 174
QuantiFERON-TB, for diagnosing M. tuberculosis infection, 315
Quinupristin/dalfopristin, 326

## R

Rapid antigen tests, 212
Rapid diagnostic tests, 339–341
Rapid immunochromatographic test, 212
RBCs. *See* Red blood cells (RBCs)
Recombivax HB, 179, 275, 276t
Red blood cells (RBCs), 199
Respiratory viruses, 295
Reverse-transcriptase polymerase chain reaction (RT-PCR)
 for influenza, 242
Reye Syndrome, 241, 292
Rhinosinusitis. *See* Sinusitis
Rhinovirus, 189
RIBA, 267t
Ribavirin, 279–280
*Rickettsia rickettsii,* 293, 303
Rifampin, 325
 for latent tuberculosis, 215
Rimantadine, 243
RT-PCR. *See* Reverse-transcriptase polymerase chain reaction (RT-PCR)
Rubella, 180

## S

Salicylates, 242
Salivary gland virus, 258
Salvage therapy, 381
Sanofi Pasteur, 176

SCC. *See* Staphylococcal chromosomal cassette (SCC)
Seasonal influenza, 238, 321
Secondary bacterial pneumonias, 240
Separate monovalent vaccine, 245
Septic arthritis, 320
Septic meningitis, 172
Serology, 228
Serum creatine kinase, 240
7-valent pneumococcal vaccine (PCV7), for pneumonia, 211
Severe sepsis syndrome, 320, 321–322
  diagnosis and treatment, 324–325
Sexual behavior, 366
Sexual education programs, 366
Sexual identity, 366
Sexually transmitted disease (STD), and Hepatitis C vaccine, 276
Sexually transmitted infection, 348, 367
  age factor, 336–337
  condom use, 336–337
  diagnosis, advances in
  extragenital screening with NAAT, 339
  rapid diagnostic tests, 339–341
  vaginal swab specimens, 338–339
  epidemiology, advances in, 332–335
  *Chlamydia trachomatis*, 333
  *Neisseria gonorrhea*, 333–334
  *Trichomonas vaginalis*, 334–335
  female military recruits, 335
  National Job Training Program (Job Corps), 335
  prevalence, 35
  screening, advances in, 341–342
  testing, 365–366, 377–378
  understanding racial/ethnic disparities, advances in
  behavioral risk factors, 336
  contextual risk factors, 337–338
  individual risk factors, 335–337
Sexually transmitted infections in adolescents: advances in epidemiology, screening, and diagnosis, **332–346**
Sinusitis, acute, 187–200
  acute, 187
  anatomy, 187–188
  causative agents of sinusitis
  *Candida* species, 189
  *Escherichia coli*, 189
  *Proteus mirabilis*, 189
  *Pseudomonas* species, 189
  *Streptococcus aureus*, 189
  *Streptococcus viridans*, 189
  chronic, 187
  complications, 193–199, 194f
  intracranial, 197–198
  local, 193–196
  meningitis, 198–199
  orbital, 196–197
  diagnosis, 190–191
  definition of, 187
  microbiology, 189–190
  predisposing factors, 188
  local insult, 188
  mechanical obstruction, 188
  systemic, 188
  prevention, 199
  recurrent, 187
  referral indications, 193
  subacute, 187
  treatment, 191–192
Sinus ostia, 187
Sinus with nasal and pharyngeal symptoms, 194f
Skin and soft tissue infections (SSTIs), 318, 320
  diagnosis and treatment, 323–324
Society for Adolescent Medicine, 182
Sphenoid paranasal sinuses, 187–188
Spider bites, and SSTI, 320
Splenic rupture, 255
SSTIs. *See* Skin and soft tissue infections (SSTIs)
Staphylococcal chromosomal cassette (SCC), 214, 319
*Staphylococcus aureus* infections, 188, 240, 318
  clinical presentation
  endocarditis, 321
  musculoskeletal Infections, 320
  pulmonary disease, 321
  severe sepsis syndrome, 321–322
  skin and soft tissue infections, 320
  toxic shock syndrome, 322–323
  diagnosis and treatment
  invasive infections, 324–327
  skin and soft tissue infections, 323–324
  epidemiology, 318–320
  prevention, 327
  risk factors, 319–320
*Staphylococcus aureus* infections in adolescents, **318–331**
STD. *See* Sexually transmitted disease (STD)
Steven Johnson syndrome, 324
*Streptococcus pneumoniae*, 181, 188, 240
  bacterial meningitis due to, 289
  for pleural effusion, 209
Subdural abscess, 198
Subperiosteal abscess, 197

Superior sagittal sinus. *See* Cavernous sinus thrombosis
Surgical drainage
  for epidural abscess, 198
  for intracerebral abscess, 198
  for subdural abscess, 198
  for venous sinus thrombosis, 199
Surveillance Epidemiology and End Results statistics, 350
Sustained virologic response (SVR), 118
SVR. *See* Sustained virologic response (SVR)
Symptomatic neuroinvasive disease, 297
Symptomatic treatment
  acetaminophen, 242
  ibuprofen, 242
Syncope, after vaccination, 182
Systemic antibody responses, 238

## T

Tachypnea, 205
Tampons use, 320
Tattooing, and CA-MRSA infection, 319–320, 319*f*
TB. *See* Mycobacterium tuberculosis (TB)
T-cell receptor excision circle (TREC) analysis, 367
Tdap. *See* Tetanus, diphtheria, and pertussis vaccine (Tdap)
Teens, with HIV
  diagnoses, 364–367
  transition care of, 382–383
Telbivudine, 275
Telvavancin, 326
Tenofovir, 275
Tetanus, diphtheria, and pertussis vaccine (Tdap), 173, 175, 231, 232
  for adults, 232
  contraindications, precautions, and deferral of, 232–233
  for diphtheria, 175
  objective of, 231
  for pertussis, 175
  for tetanus, 175
Thimerosal, 182
Thoracocentesis, 207
Thymic volume, 367
Tigecycline, 324, 326
TIV. *See* Trivalent inactivated influenza vaccine (TIV)
TLRs. *See* Toll-like receptors (TLRs)
TMP-SMX. *See* Trimethoprim-sulfamethoxazole (TMP-SMX)
TNF. *See* Tumor necrosis factor (TNF)
Toll-like receptors (TLRs), 348
Toxic shock syndrome (TSS), 320, 322–323
Toxic shock toxin-1 (TSST-1), 320
*Toxoplasma gondii*, 380
Transition care of teens with HIV, 382–383
Transverse myelitis, 240
Treatment, of HIV
  initial diagnosis, 369–370
  initial laboratory evaluation, 370–371
  initial treatment considerations, 371–376
*Trichomonas vaginalis*, 334–335
*Trichomonas vaginalis*, 340
Tricyclic amines, antiviral medications, 243
Trimethoprim-sulfamethoxazole (TMP-SMX), 324
Trivalent inactivated influenza vaccine (TIV), 244, 245
  for seasonal influenza, 177
TSS. *See* Toxic shock syndrome (TSS)
TSST-1. *See* Toxic shock toxin-1 (TSST-1)
Tuberculin skin testing, 180
Tuberculosis, 214
Tumor necrosis factor (TNF), 294
Twinrix, 179, 269*t*, 275, 276*t*

## U

Ultrasound, 323
Uncomplicated influenza, 239
USA300, 319
U.S. Department of Health and Human Services (DHHS) guidelines, 370, 376
U.S. Food and Drug Administration (FDA), 243, 310, 326
U.S. Preventative Services Task Force, 365

## V

Vaccination
  efficacy against cervical cancer, 353–356, 353*t*
  for human papillomavirus, 352
Vaccination efforts, 182–183
Vaccine Adverse Event Reporting System (VAERS), 177, 181
Vaccines
  hepatitis A, 179
  hepatitis B, 178–179
  human papillomavirus, 174
  influenza and h1n1, 176–178
  meningococcal, 175–176

MMR and varicella, 179–180
pertussis, 175
pneumococcal, 181
polio, 180–181
Vaccine safety, 181–182
data link, 177
VAERS. See Vaccine Adverse Event Reporting System (VAERS)
Vaginal intraepithelial neoplastic (VAIN) lesions, 356
Vaginal swab specimens, 338–339
Vancomycin, 311, 324, 325–326
for methicillin-resistant Staphylococcus aureus, 208
Vaqta, 179, 269$t$
Varicella zoster virus (VZV), 179, 293
Varivax, 180
VATS. See Video-assisted thoracoscopic surgery (VATS)
VCA. See Viral capsid antigen (VCA)
Venous sinus thrombosis, 199
Video-assisted thoracoscopic surgery (VATS), for pleural effusions, 210–211
Viral capsid antigen (VCA), 254
Viral hepatitis infections, 265, 280
hepatitis A, 265–269
hepatitis B, 270–277
hepatitis C, 277–280
markers, 267$t$
symptoms of, 266$t$
Viral hepatitis A, B, and C: grown-up issues 265–286
Viral infections, 301
Viral isolation, 242
Viral-like particles (VLP), 352–353
Viral load numbers, 379
Viral meningitis, 296

nonspecific symptoms, 296
Viral pneumonia, diagnosis of, 216
VLP. See Viral-like particles (VLP)
Vulvar intraepithelial neoplastic (VIN) lesions, 356
VZV. See Varicella zoster virus (VZV)

# W

WBCs. See White blood cells (WBCs)
Western blot, 370
West Nile virus (WNV)
arthropodborne viruses, 293
mosquito-borne arboviruses, 293
Wheezing, 206
White blood cells (WBCs), 189
WHO. See World Health Organization (WHO)
Whole-cell pertussis (wp) vaccines, 222
WNV. See West Nile virus (WNV)
World Health Organization (WHO), 205

# X

Xenostrip-Tv, 340
X-linked lymphoproliferative syndrome, 257–258

# Y

Young women
biological risk, 367
heterosexual transmission, 366–367
Youth Risk Behavior Survey (YRBS), 336
YRBS. See Youth Risk Behavior Survey *(YRBS)*